D0871643

Alternative Medicine Guide

Heart Disease, Stroke & High Blood Pressure

BURTON GOLDBERG

and the Editors of

ALTERNATIVE MEDICINE DIGEST

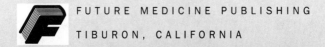

FUTURE MEDICINE PUBLISHING

TIBURON, CALIFORNIA

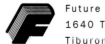 Future Medicine Publishing, Inc.
1640 Tiburon Blvd., Suite 2
Tiburon, CA 94920

Copyright © 1998 by Future Medicine Publishing, Inc.
All rights reserved.
No part of this book may be reproduced in any form
without the expressed written consent of the publisher,
except by a reviewer, who may quote brief passages in
connection with a review.

Editor: Richard Leviton
Senior Editor: Stephanie Marohn
Assistant Editor: Nina Giglio
Research Editor: John Anderson
Art Director: Janine White
Cover and book design: Amparo Del Rio Design
Indicated images: LifeART Images Copyright©1989-1997
by TechPool Studios, Inc. USA

Manufactured in the United States of America.

10 9 8 7 6 5 4 3 2 1

ISBN 1-887299-27-0 (hard cover)

Portions of this book were previously published,
in a different form, in *Alternative Medicine: The
Definitive Guide* and *Alternative Medicine Digest*.

Important Information

BURTON GOLDBERG and the editors of *Alternative Medicine Digest* are proud of the public and professional praise accorded Future Medicine Publishing's series of books. This latest book continues the groundbreaking tradition of its predecessors.

The health of you and your loved ones is important. Treat this book as an educational tool that will enable you to better understand, assess, and choose the best course of treatment when heart disease strikes, and how to prevent heart disease from striking in the first place. It could save your life.

Remember that this book on heart disease is different. It is not another catalog of mainstream medicine's conventional treatments and drugs used to treat heart disease. This book is about *alternative* approaches to heart disease–approaches generally not understood and, at this time, not endorsed by the medical establishment. We urge you to discuss the treatments described in this book with your doctor. If your doctor is open-minded, you may actually educate him or her. We have been gratified to learn that many of our readers have found their physicians to be open to new ideas.

Use this book wisely. Because many of the treatments described in this book are, by definition, alternative, they have not been investigated, approved or endorsed by any government or regulatory agency. National, state, and local laws may vary regarding the use and application of many of the treatments that are discussed. Accordingly, this book should not be substituted for the advice and care of a physician or other licensed health care professional. Pregnant women, in particular, are especially urged to consult with a physician before commencing any therapy. Ultimately, you, the reader, must take responsibility for your health and how you use the information in this book.

Future Medicine Publishing and the authors have no financial interest in any of the products or services discussed in this book, other than the citations to Future Medicine's other publications. All of the factual information in this book has been drawn from the scientific literature.

Contents

PART ONE— Heart Disease

PART TWO— High Blood Pressure

PART THREE— Stroke

PART FOUR— Alternative
Practitioner Listings

You Don't Have to Die of Heart Disease

HEART DISEASE is a disease of the 20th century. Atherosclerosis, the hardening, thickening, and clogging of the arteries, was virtually unknown in 1900. Today, it is a major killer of Americans. This book will show you why heart disease is rampant, how to reverse it using natural, alternative modalities, and how to prevent it from returning or occuring in the first place. This book will explain—and give you the proof—why heart disease is a function of nutrient deficiency and toxicity, and how you can avoid bypass, angioplasty, heart transplants, and other highly invasive cardiac procedures.

Today, an estimated 57.4 million Americans have one or more types of heart disease. Heart disease is responsible for half of all deaths in the United States. In addition to the huge cost in human suffering, the medical costs of treating this epidemic are astronomical. As you will learn in this book, conventional medicine is making little progress in stemming the tide of this epidemic. This is because, for the most part, it only offers assistance when an individual's heart disease has become a serious problem. And that assistance fails as a solution because it does not address the underlying causes of heart disease.

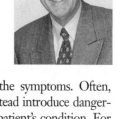

Cholesterol-lowering drugs, high blood pressure medication, angioplasty to clean out the arteries, and coronary artery bypass surgery—the most common "solutions"—may temporarily relieve the symptoms. Often, however, they don't even accomplish that, but instead introduce dangerous side effects and further complications in the patient's condition. For example, cholesterol-lowering drugs have been found to actually increase your risk of heart attack and stroke. Channel blockers, the drug of choice for high blood pressure, increase your risk of developing cancer.

As you will learn in this book, invasive medical procedures such as angioplasty and coronary artery bypass surgery are frequently unnecessary and produce no benefit to the patient at all. Some people endure multiple operations (one patient whose case is discussed in this book underwent 14 angioplasties) without result or their condition returns later. In addition, bypass surgery is dangerous, many people suffering strokes or other damage to their brain as a result of the operation.

Much of this is needless suffering because heart disease is one of the most preventable chronic degenerative diseases. This is both the good news and the bad news; bad news because many of the nearly one million annual deaths from heart disease didn't need to happen, but good news because the epidemic can be brought to a halt. Alternative medicine has practical solutions for reversing and preventing heart disease. The message is: you don't have to die from or even be sick with heart disease.

The doctors in this book have years of experience treating heart disease and will show you how you can keep your heart healthy and, if you already have heart disease, how you can reverse it. They don't use just one therapy, but draw on a range of alternative medicine approaches. As heart disease is not caused by one factor alone, the best treatment will involve multiple methods to remove each contributing cause. The doctors in this book know that in order to permanently reverse any health condition, you must find and remove the multiple factors that created it. This is a basic principle of alternative medicine and the reason why it succeeds where conventional medicine often fails in the treatment of chronic disease.

The first place many alternative physicians begin is with diet, exercise, and lifestyle habits. Sometimes, reversing heart disease is as simple as making changes in these areas. In other cases, supplements are needed to address specific nutritional deficiencies which have contributed to the patient's condition. Therapies which have proven

Much of this is needless suffering because heart disease is one of the most preventable chronic degenerative diseases. This is both the good news and the bad news; bad news because many of the nearly one million annual deaths from heart disease didn't need to happen, but good news because the epidemic can be brought to a halt.

particularly invaluable in the treatment of heart disease include chelation and hyperbaric oxygen. Chelation therapy is a highly effective and noninvasive method of clearing the arteries and reversing atherosclerosis (clogging of the arteries due to plaque, or buildup, on the arterial walls), the main cause of heart disease. Hyperbaric oxygen therapy has been remarkably successful in reversing the damage caused by stroke, even years afterward, by getting oxygen to oxygen-deprived brain tissues.

You may well ask—Why haven't I heard about these treatments? The answer is: politics and greed. The U.S. medical monopoly, comprised of the major pharmaceutical companies, physicians' trade groups, insurance companies, and government bodies such as the National Institutes of Health and the Food and Drug Administration, have a literal investment in keeping nonpatentable and inexpensive treatments from the public. Widespread use of chelation and hyperbaric oxygen therapies would cut deeply into the conventional medical profit pie—because these therapies work and by using them people can avoid very costly (and highly profitable) medical procedures such as coronary artery bypass surgery and angioplasty, not to mention years of taking expensive heart medications.

You don't need to take my word for it. In this book, you will learn how some of the best treatments have been suppressed. Consider the case of David A. Steenblock, D.O., a specialist in hyperbaric oxygen therapy, who was driven into bankruptcy by state medical authorities to the detriment of his many patients (see Chapter 16, pp. 244-249). Or look at what happened to heart researcher Kilmer S. McCully, M.D., when he published an article in a prestigious scientific journal on his discovery that it was homocysteine, not high cholesterol, that was really behind atherosclerosis. If this idea were to gain widespread acceptance, where would that leave the huge industry devoted to lowering cholesterol? Dr. McCully was fired from his job at Harvard University after the article was published (see Chapter 1, pp. 33-37).

It is important for you, the reader, to understand what is going on in the U.S. regarding health care because you are being denied access to medical treatment that can save your life. You have the right to these treatments and I am doing everything possible to see that you get them. One way I can do that is by publishing this book. The more information you have about your options, the more you can make informed choices and then demand the medical care you deserve, because you don't have to live with heart disease—and you certainly don't have to die from it. God bless.

—Burton Goldberg

You may well ask—Why haven't I
heard about these treatments? The
answer is: politics and greed. Widespread
use of chelation and hyperbaric
oxygen therapies would cut deeply into the
conventional medical profit pie—because
these therapies work and
by using them people can avoid very
costly (and highly profitable) medical
procedures such as coronary artery bypass
surgery and angioplasty, not
to mention years of taking expensive
heart medications.

User's Guide

One of the features of this book is that it is interactive, thanks to the following 11 icons:

Here we refer you to our book, *An Alternative Medicine Definitive Guide to Cancer*, for more information on a particular topic.

This means you can turn to the listed pages elsewhere in this book for more information on the topic. For example, if you are reading about toxicity as a contributing cause for cancer in Chapter 25, this icon directs you to Chapter 33 for practical information on detoxification protocols; it also guides you to those cancer doctors in Part One who have detailed programs for detoxification.

This tells you where to contact a physician, group, or publication, or how to obtain substances mentioned in the text. This is an editorial service to our readers. Most importantly, the use of this icon empowers you right now, by giving you a source to acquire something vital to your health, quickly and easily. Whenever possible, we give you complete contact information for all substances mentioned in the text. All items are based on recommendations from the clinical practice of physicians in this book. The publisher has no financial interest in any clinic, physician, or product discussed in this book.

Many times the text mentions a medical term that requires explanation. We don't want to interrupt the text, so instead we put the explanation in the margins under this icon. This gives you the option of proceeding with the text or taking a moment to learn more about an important term. You will find some of the key definitions repeated at different places in the book so you don't have to search for the definition.

This sign tells you there may be some risks, uncertainties, side effects, or special contraindications regarding a procedure or substance. **Pay close attention to these icons.**

Here we refer you to our best-selling book, *Alternative Medicine: The Definitive Guide*, for more information on a particular topic.

This icon will alert you to an article published in our bimonthly magazine, *Alternative Medicine Digest*, that is relevant to the topic under discussion.

This icon asks you to give a particular point special attention in your thinking. It is important to the overall discussion at hand.

This icon highlights a particularly noteworthy point and bids you to remember it.

In many cases, alternative medicine is far less expensive than conventional treatments. This icon means that the widespread acceptance of the therapy or substance under discussion could save considerable health-care money.

More research on this topic would be valuable and should be encouraged to further substantiate or clinically prove a promising possibility of benefit to many.

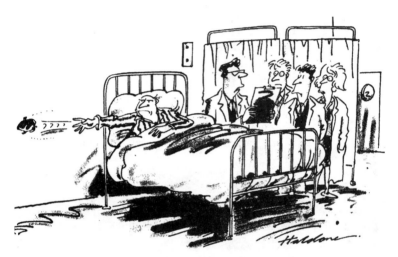

"It looks as though Mr. Markham has rejected his new heart."

Reprinted from *Stitches* by Dr. John Cocker with permission from Stoddart Publishing Co. Limited, 1993

PART ONE

Heart
Disease

What Causes Heart Disease?

THE UNITED STATES leads the world in death rates from cardiovascular disease (pertaining to the heart and blood vessels). More loosely called heart disease, it is the leading killer of Americans, now causing half of all U.S. deaths.[1]

Among the conditions included in the category of cardiovascular disease (CVD) are coronary heart disease (decreased blood flow to the heart usually caused by atherosclerosis), congestive heart failure (cardiomyopathy), heart attack (myocardial infarction), stroke, chest pain (angina pectoris), high blood pressure (hypertension), arrhythmia (irregular heartbeat), rheumatic heart disease, and hardening of the arteries (arteriosclerosis, of which atherosclerosis, involving fatty arterial wall deposits, is the most common).

There are an estimated 1,500,000 new and recurrent cases of heart attack every year. The majority occur with no warning. This makes it vital to practice good heart health.

According to the American Heart Association (AHA), every 33 seconds an American dies of CVD—that's about 954,000 deaths annually or about 42% of all mortalities. Every 20 seconds, an American suffers a heart attack, and every 60 seconds, somebody dies from one, reports AHA. Among deaths attributed to CVD, 52.3% are women and 47.7% are men. African Americans suffer CVD at much higher rates than whites: the rate of death from CVD among black males is 47.4% higher and among black females it's 69.1% higher.

Before we look more specifically at heart disease and what causes it, here's a preview of the alternative medicine techniques we cover in this book to help you on your way to a healthy heart. In the following section, **James R. Privitera, M.D.**, of Covina, California, explains a revolutionary technology to detect a heart attack in the making and outlines a program to reduce your risk.

Preventing a Heart Attack

Heart attacks are a particularly lethal outcome of cardiovascular disease. In 1994 alone, 487,490 people died from heart attacks and there are an estimated 1,500,000 new and recurrent cases every year.[2] The majority of heart attacks occur with no warning, making it vital to practice good heart health.

If you think you're prone to a heart attack or have health factors suggesting the possibility of one, there is a simple, inexpensive way to "ask" your body if conditions exist to make a heart attack possible. Even better, once you know your level of risk, it's easy to take preventive steps, using nutrition, to keep it from ever happening.

This simple, inexpensive technique is called darkfield live blood microscopy. We draw a drop of your blood from your fingertip and place it on a microscope slide. Then a special lens inside the microscope projects an intimate view of your living blood onto a television or computer screen by way of a video camera. A Polaroid camera is hooked up to the device enabling us to take photographs of a patient's blood condition before and after treatment. The result is a *living* picture of the cellular you.

What Silent Clots Can Do Without Warning

The advantage of using a darkfield microscope instead of the more conventional brightfield is that we can see much more detail, such as the contours and shapes of red blood cells and platelets. In a cubic centimeter of blood from a

QUICK DEFINITION

A **red blood cell**, or erythrocyte, contains the pigment hemoglobin which carries oxygen to the body's tissues. The erythrocyte is the main component in blood; 1 cubic millimeter of blood contains between 4 and 4.5 million (in women) and 4.5 to 5 million (in men) red blood cells. The red blood cell is a biconcave disc that is highly flexible in shape, allowing it to squeeze through capillaries, which are narrower than blood vessels. Healthy red blood cells are like sacks that can be endlessly reshaped without damage.

Darkfield microscopy is a way of studying *living* whole blood cells under a specially adapted microscope that projects the dynamic image, magnified 1400 times, onto a video screen. With a darkfield light condenser, images of high contrast are projected, so that the object appears bright against a dark background. The skilled physician can detect early signs of illness in the form of microorganisms in the blood known to produce disease. The amount of time the blood cell stays viable and alive indicates the overall health of the individual. Specifically, darkfield microscopy reveals distortions of red blood cells (which in turn indicate nutritional status), possible undesirable bacterial or fungal life forms, and blood ecology patterns indicative of health or illness.

15

A "silent" heart attack can be prevented through a darkfield examination of your blood, followed by a precise nutritional prescription to reduce platelet clustering.

healthy individual, there are usually close to 300,000 platelets, which are disc-shaped elements essential for blood clotting.

In most cases, clotting is good because it stops uncontrolled bleeding; but if excess clotting happens in a blood vessel, it can cause a heart attack. When platelets start clustering (aggregating) and sticking together in the blood, they form a clot, which can block the flow of blood through that vessel. Then, if the platelet aggregation is three to four times larger than a red blood cell (which is often the case), it will block the movement of the red blood cells through a capillary (a tiny tributary blood vessel) and stop them from releasing oxygen to the tissues, producing a lower oxygen concentration. This clinical condition, characterized by a shortage of blood flow to the heart, is called ischemia (iss-KEY-mee-uh).

The biggest problem about blood clotting inside your blood vessels is that you probably will have no idea it's happening. When patients come to the office with chest pains (a strong indication of risk), I immediately have a look at their blood. But about 80% of heart attacks are painless, which means the ischemia due to blood clotting

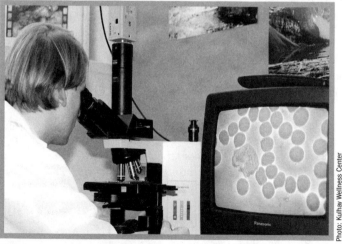

Photo: Kulhay Wellness Center

Darkfield microscopy reveals distortions of red blood cells (which in turn indicate nutritional status), possible undesirable bacterial or fungal life forms, and blood ecology patterns indicative of health or illness.

Dr. Privitera's Program
to Reduce the Risk of Heart Attack

- Kyolic EPA: EPA (eicosapentaenoic acid, a fatty acid) with garlic and fish oil; 280 mg, 5 times daily
- Karuna GLA-240: GLA (gamma-linolenic acid, a fatty acid), containing 1,000 mg of pure borage seed oil and 10 IU of vitamin E; 250 mg, once daily
- Kyolic Garlic: 6 capsules daily; 240 mg each
- CardioSpare: magnesium and potassium aspartate; 500 mg, 2 capsules after each meal, providing 49 mg of elemental potassium and 33 mg of elemental magnesium
- Thyroid Chew: porcine thyroid glandular extract; ¼ g daily
- Natur Practic Super Enzyme: containing pancrelipase, pancreatin, pepsin, betaine HCL, papain, amylase, ox bile extract, and others; 2 after each meal
- Vitamin E: 1,000 IU daily
- L-carnitine: 250 mg, 2 before each meal
- Raw Heart: glandular extract from cattle heart, plus added magnesium, manganese, and potassium; 3 times daily
- Vitamin C: 5,000 mg daily, divided into 2 doses
- PhytoPharmica: aqueous liver glandular extract, containing 100 mcg vitamin B12 and 550 mg liquid liver fractions; 2 times daily
- Selenium: 200 mcg, once daily
- Karuna Maxxum-4: multivitamin and antioxidant; 2 after each meal

For more information about **Karuna GLA-240** and **Maxxum-4**, contact: Karuna, 42 Digital Drive, Suite 7, Novato, CA 94949; tel: 800-826-7225 or 415-382-0147; fax: 415-382-0142. For **Kyolic EPA** and **Kyolic® Aged Garlic Extract™**, contact: Wakunaga of America Co., Ltd., 23501 Madero, Mission Viejo, CA 92691; tel: 714-855-2776; fax: 714-458-2764. For **CardioSpare**, contact: G, Y, and N Industries, 2407 Grandad Way, Carlsbad, CA 92008; tel: 800-526-3030 or 619-434-6360; fax: 619-434-0816. For Thyroid Chew, contact: Merit Pharmaceuticals, 2611 San Fernando Road, Los Angeles, CA 90065; tel: 800-696-3748 or 213-227-4831; fax: 213-227-4833. For Natur Practic Super Enzyme, contact: Randal Products, P.O. Box 7328, Santa Rosa, CA 95407; tel: 707-528-1800; fax: 707-528-0924. For L-carnitine, contact: DaVinci Laboratories, 20 New England Drive, Essex Junction, VT 05453; tel: 800-325-1776 or 802-878-5508; fax: 802-878-0549. For **Raw Heart**, contact: Licata Enterprises, 5242 Bolsa Avenue, Suite 3, Huntington Beach, CA 92649; tel: 800-926-7455 or 714-893-0017; fax: 714-897-5677. For **PhytoPharmica aqueous liver glandular extract**, contact: PhytoPharmica, P.O. Box 1745, Green Bay, WI 54305; tel: 800-376-4418 (consumer information), 800-553-2370 (licensed healthcare practitioners) or 414-469-9099; fax: 414-469-4418.

produces no pain or gasping and therefore gives you no warning.

You may be driving the car and suddenly slump over the wheel with a silent heart attack. This frightening event may be prevented through a darkfield examination of your blood, followed by a precise nutritional prescription to reduce platelet aggregation. In the darkfield blood pictures (see p. 18), the platelet cluster looks like a blob of oatmeal poured onto a black surface. This is what blood clotting looks like, and it's also the face of a condition that could produce a heart attack.

How Carlon Avoided a Triple-Bypass Surgery

Carlon, 62, came to me with high blood pressure (170/70), chest pains, and a five-year history of serious heart problems, including a moderate heart attack. He had undergone numerous mainstream treatments, which hadn't helped him, and now his conventional physician was urging him to have triple-bypass surgery.

"A total of 14 doctors of the highest degree told me I couldn't live without this surgery, that it was imperative," Carlon reported. "They all agreed that this was the 'only' way they had to keep me alive." They told him if he did not have the surgery in two weeks or less, he would probably die.

Carlon didn't buy this pessimistic forecast and refused the surgery. He came to me for help. "I believe God built a cage over my heart for a reason. It doesn't need to be messed up with a knife," said Carlon.

I performed a comprehensive mineral analysis from a sample of Carlon's hair and a darkfield examination of his blood. He was seriously low in selenium, magnesium, zinc, chromium, and manganese, and he had some large clots which, incidentally, are asso-

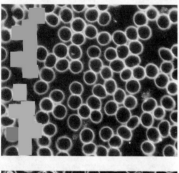

In this initial picture of Carlon's blood, there are signs of severe clotting indicated by the gray mass.

After taking supplements, Carlon's blood is free of clots, and healthy red blood cells prevail.

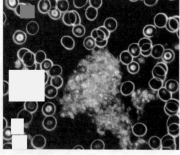

When Carlon temporarily discontinued supplements for 2 weeks, some clotting returned.

Photo: James M. Privatera, M.D.

"A total of 14 doctors of the highest degree told me I couldn't live without [bypass] surgery," Carlon reported. It took only three months of chelation and supplementation for his chest pains to disappear. That was five years ago. He bypassed the bypass and is doing well.

ciated with a magnesium deficiency. My treatment program for Carlon had two major aspects: chelation therapy and a nutritional prescription.

First, Carlon started having intravenous chelation twice weekly to improve his circulation and remove heavy metals from his system. Chelation therapy is a clinically proven method of binding up ("chelating") and draining toxins and metabolic wastes from the body while at the same time increasing blood flow and removing arterial plaque. In chelation, a nontoxic substance called EDTA is intravenously infused over a $1\frac{1}{2}$- to $3\frac{1}{2}$-hour period; usually 20-30 treatments are recommended at the rate of one to three sessions per week.

Second, I developed a nutritional supplementation formula for Carlon to help thin his blood and dissolve the clots. Although the nutrients and dosages must be adjusted to the conditions of individual patients, the list (see p. 17) will give the reader a practical idea of how a nutrient program can help prevent heart attacks.

It took Carlon three months of chelation and supplementation for his chest pains to disappear. Even better, at that point he was able to ride his bicycle 25 miles a day with no discomfort. That was five years ago. He bypassed the bypass and is doing well. Carlon follows a reduced dosage maintenance plan for supplements and has chelation about once monthly. "I have skipped the scalpel five times in my life," Carlon told me recently. "I thank God I was stubborn enough to choose my own doctors." ∎

To contact the author: NutriScreen, Inc., **James R. Privitera, M.D.**, director, 105 North Grandview, Covina, CA 91723; tel: 818-966-1618; fax: 818-966-7226. Dr. Privitera provides detailed instruction manuals in darkfield microscopic interpretation and nutritional prescribing to licensed healthcare professionals. Dr. Privitera is the author (with Alan Stang, M.A.) of *Silent Clots: Life's Biggest Killers* (1996), The Catacombs Press™ (same address as NutriScreen, Inc.).

For more about **chelation**, see Chapter 3: Scrubbing the Arteries Naturally, pp. 70-92.

The Heart Disease Epidemic

Conventional medicine believes that the answer to fighting heart disease lies in treating certain symptoms such as high blood pressure or in lowering cholesterol with medication. Americans make about 147 million office visits to doctors every year for hypertension and heart

How Your Heart Pumps Blood

The heart is a hollow muscular organ in the chest that contracts rhythmically to circulate blood through the body. The heart sends blood rich with oxygen and nutrients out to the body's tissues and also pumps blood from the rest of the body to the lungs to be re-oxygenated.

The average heart measures 3½" x 4¾" and weighs between 8 and 14 ounces. At rest, the heart normally beats 60 to 80 times per minute (100,000 times per day) and during exercise or stress may beat up to 200 times per minute. The average amount of blood pumped per beat of the heart (at rest) is 2.5 ounces (1,980 gallons per day).

The heart is really two pumps side by side. Each pump consists of two chambers, the *atrium* above and the *ventricle* below. There are left and right atria, and left and right ventricles. These chambers are connected by valves which allow blood flow in one direction only. The rhythm of each heartbeat is regulated by a part of the heart muscle that is connected to the central nervous system; this rhythmic action serves as a natural pace-maker.

Blood flows through the heart on the following course: Blood that has been oxygenated in the lungs flows into the left atrium, then is pumped through the left ventricle out through the aorta to replenish the whole body. Oxygen-depleted blood returns from all parts of the body to the

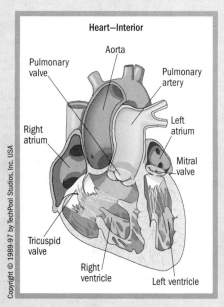

Heart—Interior

Aorta

Pulmonary valve

Pulmonary artery

Right atrium

Left atrium

Mitral valve

Tricuspid valve

Right ventricle

Left ventricle

Copyright © 1989-97 by TechPool Studios, Inc. USA

disease, according to a report in *American Health*. Expensive coronary artery bypass surgeries and angioplasties are performed with increasing regularity, while cholesterol-lowering drugs further fuel the skyrocketing costs associated with heart disease. Coronary artery bypass surgery is called an "overprescribed and unnecessary surgery" by many leading authorities.[3] Complications from such treatments are common and the expense to the health care system is extraordinarily high.

In 1994, an estimated 501,000 bypass surgeries at $44,000 each were performed on Americans, and 47% of these were done on men right atrium, where it is pumped through the right ventricle via the pulmonary artery to the lungs.

Each heartbeat has two phases, diastole (the resting phase) and systole (the contraction). During the diastolic or resting phase, the left atrium fills with oxygenated blood from the lungs and the right atrium fills with oxygen-depleted blood from the body. The contraction begins from the top of the heart as both atria squeeze the blood into the ventricles: the right atrium through the tricuspid valve into the right ventricle, the left atrium through the mitral valve into the left ventricle.

The contraction then continues from the bottom of the heart, squeezing both ventricles upward. The right ventricle moves blood through the pulmonary valve and into the pulmonary artery, then to the lungs. Blood from the left ventricle is pumped through the aortic valve and into the aorta, then out to all parts of the body. The diastolic or resting phase starts again as all valves close and the atria begin to refill.

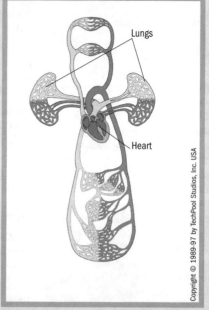

Lungs

Heart

Copyright © 1989-97 by TechPool Studios, Inc. USA

Blood flow through the body. **The heart pumps blood rich with oxygen (the darker shade) to the tissues of the body through the arteries; blood from the body (the lighter shade) moves through the veins back to the heart and on to the lungs to be re-oxygenated.**

and women under age 65. In the same year, 404,000 angioplasties at $21,000 each were performed (65% on men, 53% on people under age 65). Total costs of cardiovascular disease for 1994, both direct (hospitalization, procedures, and drugs) and indirect (lost working time), were an estimated $259 billion.

Some physicians choose to reduce a patient's risk factors for heart disease by considering preventive measures such as stress reduction, exercise, dietary improvement, weight control, and the elimination of smoking. "Although these methods have resulted in some leveling off

Heart Catheterization Increases Risk of Death

According to a study published in the *Journal of the American Medical Association (JAMA)*, the conventional medical procedure called "right heart catheterization" may increase a patient's risk of death. Performed for information-gathering purposes, the test involves inserting a catheter (tube) through the neck to measure blood pressure inside the heart.

The method has never undergone strict scientific trials and should therefore be considered experimental. However, it is widely used as a diagnostic tool in conventional cardiac treatment. Over 500,000 people are estimated to receive this test every year in the U.S.

Reviewing over 5,000 critically ill heart patients, the *JAMA* study concluded that those who have right heart catheterization may be more likely to die. "If you had 1,000 patients, you would have ended up in our population with about 50 more deaths," states researcher Dr. Joanne Lynn of George Washington University. "That's a substantial number, and we should be very concerned about it." Apply these numbers to the total who have the test and the result is 30,000 more deaths every year. The researchers state that, as people don't die during the test, but later, the cause of the increased risk is unknown at this time and will require further study.[5]

of the rate of heart disease," says Garry F. Gordon, M.D., D.O., (H) M.D., of Payson, Arizona, co-founder of the American College of Advancement in Medicine, "the 'epidemic' of heart disease continues and conventional medicine continues to use drugs and surgery as the primary treatments." Equipped to treat heart disease only when it has reached its most serious and life-threatening stages, conventional medicine is largely failing in its battle against the epidemic.

90% of Patients Receive No Benefit from Bypass Surgery

When it comes to thinking about modern medicine, outrage is a useful attitude, says Lynne McTaggart, editor of the popular and outspoken British medical newsletter *What Doctors Don't Tell You*.

The content of her daily mail frequently makes McTaggart "livid" because her readers tell her about the latest way in which they have been damaged by conventional medicine and the inexcusable failure on the part of physicians to tell their patients the dangers inherent in a drug or procedure. These letters prompted McTaggart to write a book (also entitled *What Doctors Don't Tell You*).[4] She wrote it because, as she states it, "I don't want you to be another statistic."

McTaggart warns the reader that her book is likely to be unsettling, especially in the revelation

The "miracle cure" of beta blockers to lower high blood pressure also evaporates when you look at the outcomes, McTaggart says. A British study of 2,000 patients with high blood pressure showed that in barely 50% of the cases blood pressure dropped to a moderately healthy level as a result of taking hypertension drugs.

that "much of what your doctor tells you isn't true." Her goal is usefully subversive, too: she wants every reader to become an informed medical consumer, able to distinguish between when a doctor is needed and when their advice is best ignored.

To facilitate this radicalization of the medical consumer, McTaggart exposes the "diagnostic excesses" of X rays, MRIs, lab tests, and ultrasounds; she analyzes the shortcomings of medicine's "miracle cures" (antibiotics, steroids, antidepressants, and chemotherapy); and she critiques the routine use of surgery for breast and prostate cancer, hernias, and heart disease, among other topics.

For example, bypass surgery for heart disease, at an average cost of $44,000 per operation, is "one of the most unnecessary operations of all," says McTaggart. Heart surgeons have known since the 1970s that bypass does not improve survival except for patients with severe left ventricle coronary disease, while U.S. government statistics state that about 90% of patients receive no benefit. The "miracle cure" of beta blockers to lower high blood pressure (hypertension) also evaporates when you look at the outcomes, McTaggart says. A British study of 2,000 patients with high blood pressure showed that in barely 50% of the cases blood pressure dropped to a moderately healthy level as a result of taking hypertension drugs.

Study Finds 50% of Bypass Operations Unnecessary

Researchers at the Maine Medical Center found that the number of bypass surgeries and angioplasties performed in a region of the U.S. depends en-tirely upon the amount of diagnostic testing of patients, but not necessarily upon actual medical need, according to the *Journal of the American Medical Association*. The researchers estimated that 80% of all heart testing procedures are inappropriate and that 50% of all bypass operations in the U.S. are unnecessary. The total 1993 cost of Medicare billings of diagnosis and treatment of heart disease was $1 billion.

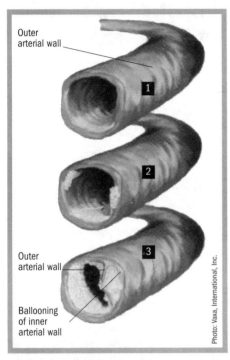

Photo: Vaxa, International, Inc.

How Arteries Thicken
1. A normal, healthy artery with open and clear passages.
2. The beginning of cholesterol plaque buildup within the artery. The inner artery wall is also beginning to weaken and bulge with cholesterol and toxic deposits.
3. Severely restricted artery with cholesterol plaque filling the majority of the passage. Note further breakdown and ballooning of inner artery wall.

In a similar European study of 12,000 patients, only 30% reached their target blood pressure levels with drugs; and in 1993, an American study stated that only 20% of patients on blood pressure drugs experienced the intended results. Further, for hypertension drugs are the major cause of hip fractures among the elderly, while they are linked with an elevenfold increase in diabetes cases, reports McTaggart.

"Our faith in medical science is so ingrained that it has become woven into the warp and woof of our daily routine," says McTaggart. But we may be deeply imperiling our health by putting our faith in a medical approach based on "unscience," she argues. Outcome statistics suggest that in many cases "Western medicine not only won't cure you but may leave you worse off than you were before."

Many treatments we take for granted—for heart disease, breast cancer, and asthma, for example—have been adopted without a single valid scientific study demonstrating their safety or efficacy, says McTaggart. In fact, *New Scientist* estimated that 80% of today's medical procedures have never been properly tested. McTaggart comments: "For all the attempts to cloak medicine in the weighty mantle of science—a good deal of what we regard as standard medical practice today amounts to little more than 20th-century voodoo."

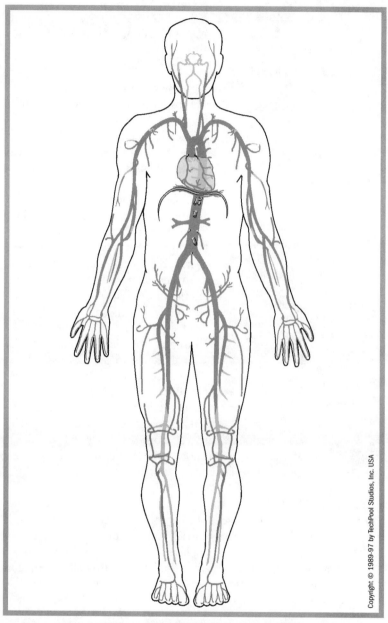

The circulatory system. A network of arteries (shown here) carries oxygenated blood from the heart to all parts of the body. A system of veins carries blood back to the heart.

Copyright © 1989-97 by TechPool Studios, Inc. USA

Drugs Associated With a Higher Incidence of Congestive Heart Failure

According to the *Physicians' Desk Reference*, the following drugs are associated with congestive heart failure. (Statistics refer to the percentage of individuals affected.)[7]

Emcyt Capsules (3%)

Ethmozine Tablets (1%-5%)

Lupron Depot 3.75 mg (among most frequent) Injection (5% or more)

Novantrone for Injection Concentrate (up to 5%)

Rythmol tablets (0.8%-3.7%)

Tambocor Tablets (approximately 5%)

Tonocard Tablets (4%)

Zoladex (5%)

How Atherosclerosis Leads to Cardiovascular Disease

A common precursor of heart disease is atherosclerosis (thickening of the arterial walls, the most common form of arteriosclerosis). In atherosclerosis, the inner arterial walls harden and thicken due to deposits of fatty substances. These substances form a plaque that, with buildup, causes a narrowing of the arteries.[6] Over time, plaque can block the arteries and interrupt blood flow to the organs they supply, including the heart and brain (see illustration, p. 24).

Atherosclerosis of the coronary arteries (the arteries supplying the muscle of the heart), known as coronary heart disease, is one of the most common forms of heart disease in the United States today. Coronary heart disease can lead to heart attack, coronary occlusion, and angina, while atherosclerosis of the cerebral arteries (the arteries that supply blood to the brain) can precipitate strokes. Coronary occlusion and heart attacks can in turn lead to another heart condition, congestive heart failure.

See Chapter 14: What Causes Stroke?, pp. 230-236.

Heart Attack

When atherosclerosis occurs in the coronary arteries, it can deprive the heart of oxygen-rich blood until the affected area of the heart literally dies, causing a heart attack (myocardial infarction), sometimes leading to cardiac arrest (heartbeat stops) that can result in death. Often, a diminished blood supply to the heart exhibits few symptoms until the blockage is so great that a heart attack results. However, while a heart attack may appear to come on suddenly, it often begins with years of physical neglect, such as a poor diet and lack of exercise. Genetic predisposition can also be a crucial factor.

Coronary Occlusion

In coronary occlusion (blockage of the heart arteries), arteries that course over the surface of and penetrate into the heart muscle become narrowed so that blood flow through them is restricted. The heart muscle stops receiving adequate amounts of oxygen and nutrients and the person develops angina. This means the heart muscle's pumping capacity has been exceeded. Coronary occlusion is commonly caused by atherosclerosis, the buildup of plaque and clogging in the arteries that can lead to heart attacks.

Angina

Angina (discomfort, heaviness, pain, or pressure in the chest or throat) can result when there are lesions in the coronary arteries or in the walls or valves of the heart. These lesions diminish the supply of oxygenated blood to the heart muscle, causing discomfort to radiate from the throat or chest to the shoulder and, in some cases, down the left arm. Angina is a warning sign that there are problems with the heart, but it is not necessarily a precursor of a heart attack if appropriate treatment is initiated.

There is also "silent angina," which means a person may have shortness of breath, numbness in the arm, dizziness, or other vague symptoms that appear when they overexert or become emotionally stressed. About one-half of all people with coronary clogging develop this silent angina form of coronary occlusion. Unfortunately, often the first time they know they have heart disease is when they have a sudden heart attack. That's why coronary disease is such a common killer, because half the people die before they ever reach the hospital.

Congestive Heart Failure

Congestive heart failure (cardiomyopathy) means failure of the heart muscle. The heart becomes literally congested with blood and dangerously weakened. The most common cause of this is coronary occlusion and heart attacks. After you "kill" a large section of your heart muscle through repeated heart attacks, there is not enough heart muscle left to pump blood out of the heart. The pressure and volume of blood inside the heart's pumping chamber build up, putting additional pressure on arteries and veins in the lungs; fluid leaks into the lungs, and the congestive heart failure process begins. A typical sign of congestive heart failure is shortness of breath either with minimal exertion or when lying down at night.

How Plaque Forms in Arteries

Atherosclerosis may be well underway even at birth. In investigating the deaths of newborn babies in Scandinavia from a variety of causes, it was found that nearly 97% had some degree of arterial thickening, the first step in heart disease.[8] Plaque formation in arteries usually follows prior damage to the inner lining of the arteries.

According to William Lee Cowden, M.D., an internist and cardiologist based in Richardson, Texas, deficiencies of nutrients such as vitamin C, vitamin E, and magnesium make this inner lining more susceptible to damage and plaque formation. "Small tears can occur in the lining of the arteries after a sudden very high blood pressure episode brought on by stress," explains Dr. Cowden, who adds that "the vessels cannot always dilate rapidly enough to accommodate the sudden increase in pressure, and tearing occurs."

Dr. Cowden explains how collagen (a protein of the connective tissue), clotting proteins, and other chemical substances are released into the bloodstream to repair the tear. These substances adhere at the site and attract platelets, special blood cells responsible for clotting. "Other cells are attracted to the repair site, including white blood cells laden with oxidized cholesterol which is deposited at the site and initiates soft plaque formation," says Dr. Cowden. "Calcium is then drawn to the site and solid plaques, which are more difficult to remove, are formed."

Matthias Rath, M.D., author of *Eradicating Heart Disease*,[9] calls atherosclerotic desposits the body's "blood vessel repair mechanism" and traces its development back to the Ice Age. According to Dr. Rath, animals don't have heart attacks or strokes because they can manufacture vitamin C and therefore maintain high body levels of this important antioxidant. The human body, on the other hand, lost the ability to manufacture vitamin C thousands of generations ago through what Dr. Rath terms a "genetic accident," the enzymes needed to produce vitamin C becoming defective.

Humans became dependent on diet to supply sufficient vitamin C until the Ice Age when plants were destroyed and people could not get any fruits or vegetables. An epidemic of scurvy (caused by severe vitamin C deficiency) followed. In scurvy, blood vessel walls grow weak and become leaky. A compensation mechanism, atherosclerotic deposits, evolved in the human body, says Dr. Rath. Today, our diet is generally not deficient enough in vitamin C to produce scurvy, but our vitamin C intake is low enough to produce heart disease.

That vitamin C plays a vital role in heart health is supported by a

Despite the evidence to the contrary, dietary cholesterol is regarded by many as the single most important factor in heart disease. This view persists even though a significant percentage of coronary heart disease occurs in people with normal or low cholesterol.

study of more than 11,000 Americans tracked for an average of ten years.[10] Dr. James Enstrom (of the University of California at Los Angeles, School of Public Health) and his colleagues compared the heart disease rate of those eating an average diet (which in our modern world is low in vitamin C) and those supplementing their diet with an average

See **Vitamin C**, Chapter 5: Nutritional Supplements, pp. 109-111.

of 300 mg of vitamin C daily. Among men, the supplementation cut their heart disease rate in half. Among women, it was reduced by one-third. Dr. Enstrom's study is one of the largest, and a significant body of research lends weight to the importance of vitamin C in reversing heart disease and maintaining cardiovascular health.

Cholesterol is Not All Bad

Cholesterol, which has long been cast as the villain in heart disease, is a waxy, oily compound vital to the body's health and functioning. Contrary to popular belief, the body, in fact, needs cholesterol. It is an essential component in cell membranes. Your body also needs it to make bile salts which help absorb the fat-soluble vitamins (A, D, E, K) and essential fatty acids from your small intestine. Cholesterol, a steroid, is also involved at the beginning of the pathway that manufactures key male and female sex hormones and steroidal hormones, including pregnenolone, testosterone, estradiol, estrone, progesterone, and cortisol. These are critical for the health of the immune system, the mineral-regulating functions of the kidneys, and the smooth running of the hormonal systems in men and women.

Cholesterol is not only obtained through the diet, but produced by the liver. According to Dr. Cowden, the human liver synthesizes about 3,000 mg of new cholesterol in any 24-hour period, a quantity equivalent to the amount contained in ten eggs. "This new cholesterol is used to repair cells," he says. "In fact, in most people less than 5% of the cholesterol in the bloodstream gets there through diet." Dr. Cowden adds that "when cholesterol levels get too low, depression, lung disease, and even cancer can be the result."

Cholesterol levels in the body are determined by measuring the

Cholesterol's contribution to heart disease appears to depend on the presence of oxidized cholesterol in the bloodstream. LDL cholesterol becomes harmful only after it has been oxidized (the process of a substance combining with oxygen).

Lipoproteins are in two principal forms. Low-density lipoproteins (LDLs) are combination molecules of proteins and fats, particularly cholesterol. LDLs circulate in the blood and act as the primary carriers of cholesterol to the cells of the body. An elevated level of LDLs, the so-called bad cholesterol, is a contributing factor in causing atherosclerosis (plaque deposits on the inner walls of the arteries). A diet high in saturated fats can lead to an increase in the level of LDLs in the blood. High-density lipoproteins (HDLs) are also fat-protein molecules in the blood, but contain a larger amount of protein and less fat than LDLs.

HDLs are able to absorb cholesterol and related compounds in the blood and transport them to the liver for elimination. HDL, the so-called good cholesterol, may also be able to take cholesterol from plaque deposits on the artery walls, thus helping to reverse the process of atherosclerosis. A higher ratio of HDL to LDL cholesterol in the blood is associated with a reduced risk of cardiovascular disease.

levels of lipoproteins in the blood (proteins that carry fats in the bloodstream). These include high-density lipoproteins (HDLs) and low-density lipoproteins (LDLs). Testing cholesterol levels allows physicians to determine how effectively the body is metabolizing cholesterol and how much remains in the bloodstream. LDL cholesterol is often referred to as "bad" cholesterol because it appears to deposit fats on arterial walls and causes the most arterial damage.[11] HDLs are often called "good" cholesterol because high levels are associated with a reduced risk of heart disease. HDLs may contribute to the removal of "bad" cholesterol from the body.[12]

The Cholesterol Myth

Despite the evidence to the contrary, dietary cholesterol is regarded by many as the single most important factor in heart disease.[13] This mistaken view persists even though a significant percentage of coronary heart disease occurs in people with normal or low cholesterol. It should also be noted that in the first decade of this century consumption of animal fat and cholesterol in the United States was close to mid-century levels. Yet the epidemic spread of atherosclerosis and cornonary heart disease did not appear until the middle of the century. In addition, after coronary heart disease peaked in the 1950s, it slowly declined between 1960 and 1980 even though dietary cholesterol levels rose slightly during those years.

The so-called French paradox further refutes the cholesterol myth. Despite a high intake of total fat, the French have a low incidence of coronary heart disease. It has been suggested that this may be due to the limited presence of hydrogenated fats (damaging trans-fatty acids) in the French diet. Similar "paradoxes" are found in other populations. Eskimos consume huge amounts of dietary cholesterol, have high blood cholesterol and yet low rates of mortality due to coronary heart disease. Northern

Asiatic Indians eat a high percentage of their calories as fat, mostly from butter, yet have an exceptionally low incidence of cardiovascular disease.[14]

Dr. Cowden cites one of many medical examples which refute the notion that all cholesterol is bad and high levels will lead to heart disease. "I have a man in my practice who had a cholesterol count of 300 to 400 for many years," reports Dr. Cowden. "But because he's taking high levels of antioxidant nutrients and avoiding processed foods high in oxidized cholesterol, he's had no plaque formation and has even had plaque regression." Clearly, you would be well advised to consider these facts before turning to a cholesterol-lowering drug as the solution to your heart condition.

Do Cholesterol-Lowering Drugs Even Work?—Since many people with heart disease also have elevated blood cholesterol levels, physicians have traditionally prescribed cholesterol-lowering drugs as part of their treatment program, although new research suggests that it is not the levels of cholesterol but the levels of *oxidized* cholesterol which represent high risk for heart disease.

There is also new information concerning the safety, side effects, and efficacy of cholesterol-lowering drugs. It has been found, for instance, that the drugs used to lower LDL (low-density lipoprotein) cholesterol actually raise it in people who already have the highest levels.[15] In addition, these medications can lead to serious complications. A study conducted in Finland reported that deaths from heart attacks and strokes were 46% higher in those taking cholesterol-lowering drugs.[16]

Newer drugs being touted as safer also have harmful side effects. Studies have shown that Mevacor (lovastatin) lowers the levels of coenzyme Q10, an antioxidant that helps the body resist heart damage, in the bloodstream.[17] A coQ10 deficiency can accelerate congestive heart failure, according to Dr. Cowden. "Studies show that most people with congestive heart failure have a deficiency of coQ10 in their heart muscle," he says. "The lower the levels, the worse the congestive heart failure. But studies also show that patients who were supposed to die 15 years ago from congestive heart failure are still alive, primarily because of taking coenzyme Q10 daily." This may be why many people in Japan use coenzyme Q10 in the place of cardiac drugs.

Trans-fatty acids are found in margarine and other oils which have been hydrogenated (combined with hydrogen) to lengthen shelf-life. Ingredient lists on food labels often designate these oils as "partially hydrogenated," but the partial is a misnomer as far as the body is concerned. When vegetable or animal oils are highly processed and hydrogenated, they are partially converted into an abnormal form called trans. These trans-fatty acids can block the normal digestion pathways of fatty acids. This, in turn, can contribute to the development of heart disease and cancer and interfere with the immune system.

For more about **coenzyme Q10**, see Chapter 5: Nutritional Supplements, pp. 115-119.

Oxysterols can also be generated internally through exposure to environmental pollutants and pesticides such as DDT. Chemicals that oxidize cholesterol include chlorine and fluoride, both of which are ingested from tap water.

Widely used cholesterol-lowering drugs such as Mevacor and gemfibrozil (Lopid) can cause cancer in mice and rats and possibly humans, state researchers at the University of California at San Francisco. Rodent exposure that was carcinogenic was at the same order of magnitude as the maximum dose typically given to humans, reports *Science News*. The researchers noted major discrepancies for carcinogenicity in the listings for these drugs in the 1994 versus 1992 editions of the *Physicians' Desk Reference*, supposedly the standard for accurate drug information.

Sidney M. Wolfe, M.D., advises that drugs should not be the first choice for lowering cholesterol unless other circumstances exist. "A change from animal to vegetable proteins often corrects high cholesterol," says Dr. Wolfe. "Supplementation [of fiber] can significantly lower total cholesterol and LDL cholesterol by absorbing water and softening the stools in your intestine."[18]

The Real Problem is *Oxidized* Cholesterol

Cholesterol's contribution to heart disease appears to depend on the presence of oxidized cholesterol in the bloodstream. LDL cholesterol becomes harmful only after it has been oxidized (the process of a substance combining with oxygen), according to Dr. Cowden. Once oxidized, LDL cholesterol can initiate plaque formation on arterial walls which in turn can lead to atherosclerosis and ultimately to heart attacks and strokes.[19]

Overwhelming evidence shows that the risk of heart attacks and strokes can be greatly decreased through dietary changes, exercise, stress reduction, and nutritional supplementation to help prevent excessive oxidation of cholesterol in the blood. "We've been living on cholesterol phobia for 20 years," says Richard Passwater, Ph.D., of Berlin, Maryland, "but nothing matters unless you prevent the oxidation of cholesterol."

One way oxidized cholesterols (known as oxysterols) enter the bloodstream is from processed foods.[20] According to medical researcher Joseph Hattersley, M.A., of Olympia, Washington, many oxysterols reach people through the air-dried powdered milk and eggs used in processed foods, as well as in fast food products.[21] Lard, kept hot and used repeatedly to cook French fries and potato chips, is loaded with oxysterols, as are gelatin preparations, says Hattersley. "Scrambled eggs and hamburgers are big culprits in the production of oxysterols," states Dr. Privitera. "Oxygen and intense heat from cooking quickly oxidizes unsaturated fats."

Oxysterols can also be generated internally through exposure to environmental pollutants and pesticides such as DDT.[22] Chemicals that oxidize cholesterol include chlorine and fluoride, both of which are ingested from tap water.[23] Chlorine has been shown to have an effect on the arteries, and fluoride lowers thyroid function which in turn allows levels of cholesterol and homocysteine (see the following section) to rise.[24] Chlorine in drinking water also forms trihalomethanes (THMs, carcinogens formed when chlorine interacts with organic chemicals in water) which, according to Hattersley, create oxysterols.[25]

> **A German study (1991) looked at the coronary arteries of 163 males with chest pain and concluded that the arterial narrowing was due more to blood levels of homocysteine than of cholesterol.**

Electromagnetic stress (overexposure to electromagnetic fields emitted by power lines, household appliances, and computers, among other electical devices) is another source of oxysterols. Various stressors such as infections, traumas, and emotional stress can also raise oxysterol levels.[26]

The Homocysteine Connection

There is a significant and growing body of evidence that the biggest culprit responsible for oxidizing cholesterol and producing atherosclerosis, and, therefore, heart disease, is homocysteine, a substance naturally found in the body. In 1969, heart researcher Kilmer S. McCully, M.D., published an unorthodox conclusion in the *American Journal of Pathology* regarding this new possible cause of heart disease. The move soon cost him his job at Harvard University.

Dr. McCully proposed that homocysteine could, when allowed to accumulate to toxic levels, degenerate arteries and produce heart disease. Homocysteine, an amino acid, is a normal by-product of protein metabolism; specifically, of the amino acid methionine,

QUICK DEFINITION

Oxidation-reduction refers to a basic chemical mechanism in the cell by which energy is produced from foods. Electrons (negatively charged particles in an atom) are removed from one atom, resulting in "oxidation" of this first atom, and then are added to or transferred to another atom, resulting in "reduction" of this second atom. This continual process of energy metabolism is actually a flow of electrons, or a minute electrical current within the cell.

Elevated homocysteine has the potential of displacing high cholesterol levels as the major dietary factor in heart disease. Dr. Cowden notes that this problem is overlooked, in his view, largely because there is no pharmaceutical drug to "fix" elevated homocysteine levels. "If there was, homocysteine would become just as big a problem as cholesterol."

QUICK DEFINITION

A **free radical** is an unstable molecule with an unpaired electron that steals an electron from another molecule and produces harmful effects. Free radicals are formed when molecules within cells react with oxygen (oxidize) as part of normal metabolic processes. Free radicals then begin to break down cells, especially if there are not enough free-radical quenching nutrients, such as vitamins C and E, in the cell. While free radicals are normal products of metabolism, uncontrolled free-radical production plays a major role in the development of degenerative disease, including cancer and heart disease. Free radicals harmfully alter important molecules, such as proteins, enzymes, fats, even DNA. Other sources of free radicals include pesticides, industrial pollutants, smoking, alcohol, viruses, most infections, allergies, stress, even certain foods and excessive exercise.

which is found in red meat, milk, and milk products and which does not create a problem when present in *small* amounts. Methionine is converted in the body to homocysteine, which is normally then converted to cystathionine, a harmless amino acid. But in individuals deficient in the enzyme necessary to convert homocysteine to cystathionine, homocysteine will be abnormally high. Excess homocysteine may generate free radicals which are capable of producing oxysterols.

The conversion in the body of homocysteine to cystathionine requires sufficient levels of vitamin B6, folic acid, and vitamin B12.[27] Also, if sufficient antioxidants are present in the bloodstream (vitamins C and E, and beta-carotene, for example), oxysterols can be neutralized and prevented from damaging the vessel walls. But stress depletes the body of vitamin B6 and vitamin C, and this depletion can lead to a further buildup of homocysteine, which can in turn cause the generation of oxysterols.

Dr. McCully observed that children with elevated levels of homocysteine showed signs of blood vessel degeneration similar to that observed in middle-aged adults with heart disease. He next demonstrated that when rabbits were injected with homocysteine, they developed arterial plaque within three to eight weeks. Homocysteine apparently curtails the ability of blood vessels to expand, keeping them restricted and narrow. It produces this effect by increasing connective tissue growth and by degenerating the elastic tissue in the arterial walls, says Dr. McCully.

Dr. McCully argues that high-protein diets, more than fats and cholesterol, seem to be a prime cause of heart disease. In "honor" of his novel theory, subsequently backed by considerable clinical support, Harvard denied him tenure and effectively fired him.

The Hypothyroidism Connection

An underactive thyroid gland can contribute to heart disease and the propensity to sustain a heart attack, according to Broda O. Barnes, M.D., a Connecticut physician who specialized in identifying and treating the many unsuspected connections between low thyroid activity and numerous health problems. "I am convinced that we are seeing today many more people with low thyroid function than ever before," explained Dr. Barnes in 1976, "and that the rising incidence of heart attacks is related to the rising incidence of hypothyroidism."

Dr. Barnes demonstrated the correlation of low thyroid function and heart disease in a study of 1,569 patients in his practice, grouped according to six categories of age or heart status. As a frame of reference, Dr. Barnes used the statistics reported by the now classic Framingham Heart Study (begun in 1949) which tracked the health status of many thousands of men and women over several decades. Dr. Barnes found that among women 30-59 years old, while there were 7.6 expected coronary cases according to the Framingham results (where no thyroid treatment was given), among his thyroid-treated patients, there were no cases.

Similarly, for those women with high risk (high cholesterol or high blood pressure), Framingham results predicted 7.3 cases, but there were none among Dr. Barnes' patients. For women over 60, Framingham predicted 7.8 cases to zero observed in Dr. Barnes' group; for men 30-59 years old, the ratio was 12.8 (Framingham) to 1 (Barnes); for high-risk males, it was 18.5 to 2; and for men 60 and over, it was 18 to 1. In summary, out of an equivalent patient population, Framingham results expected 72 coronary cases; among Dr. Barnes' thyroid-treated patients, there were only four cases.[28]

The evidence continues to mount in support of Dr. McCully's homocysteine theory. It has been found that men with high homocysteine levels have three times more heart attacks than men with low levels.[29] In 1992, researchers at Harvard University School of Public Health showed that men with homocysteine levels only 12% higher than average had a 3.4 times greater risk of heart attack than those with normal levels. Also that year, a study in the *European Journal of Clinical Investigation* showed that 40% of stroke victims had elevated homocysteine levels compared to only 6% of the controls.

The *Journal of the American Medical Association* (1995) reviewed 209 studies linking homocysteine with heart disease and concluded that the evidence demonstrates that homocysteine represents a strong independent risk

To reach **Kilmer S. McCully, M.D.**, contact: Veterans' Affairs Medical Center, 830 Chalkstone Avenue, PL & M (113), Providence, RI 02908; fax: 401-457-3069.

For more about the **thyroid**, see "The Reason Behind Weight Gain, Fatigue, Muscle Pain, Depression, Food Allergies, Infections...." *Digest* #16, pp. 52-56.

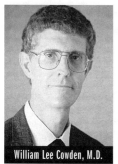

William Lee Cowden, M.D.

A possible dental involvement is another factor to consider. A large percentage of people who have heart disease have some type of abnormal dental process (such as a root canal tooth or previous tooth extraction site) in the mouth.

factor. In 1996, *The Lancet* stated that homocysteine was to be considered an independent risk factor for stroke even after adjustment for other risk factors.

Put simply, the homocysteine theory suggests that heart disease is attributed to "abnormal processing of protein in the body because of deficiencies of B vitamins in the diet," says Dr. McCully. In short, "protein intoxication" starts damaging the cells and tissues of arteries, "setting in motion the many processes that lead to loss of elasticity, hardening and calcification, narrowing of the lumen and formation of blood clots within arteries."

See **Essential Fatty Acids**, Chapter 5: Nutritional Supplements, p. 119-120.

Elevated homocysteine has the potential of displacing high cholesterol levels as the major dietary factor in heart disease. A German study (1991) looked at the coronary arteries of 163 males with chest pain and concluded that the arterial narrowing was due more to blood levels of homocysteine than of cholesterol. Recently, Dr. McCully declared: "Elevated blood homocysteine is estimated to account for at least 10% of the risk of coronary heart disease in the U.S. population." Dr. Cowden notes that this problem is overlooked, in his view, largely because there is no pharmaceutical drug to "fix" elevated homocysteine levels. "If there was, homocysteine would become just as big a problem as cholesterol."

An effective way to lower homocysteine is through vitamin B6, often combined with folic acid and vitamin B12, Dr. McCully further discovered. Excess levels of homocysteine are correlated with deficiencies in these nutrients which, as mentioned, are required for the conversion of homocysteine into a nontoxic form. Dr. McCully recommends 350-400 mcg daily of folic acid, 3-3.5 mg of vitamin B6, and at least 3 mcg daily of vitamin B12.[30] Dr. Cowden additionally recommends taking betaine hydrochloride (the stomach's principal digestive acid) and vitamin C to lower homocysteine levels in the blood.

According to Mark Nehler, M.D., and colleagues at Oregon

Health Sciences University in Portland, at least 50,000 annual deaths from coronary disease could be prevented by supplementation with oral folate (folic acid), based on their analysis of patient outcomes (and mortalities) of other published studies.[31]

Before we go on to talk about all the ways you can prevent and treat heart disease, here is a look at another doctor's heart treatment protocol to illustrate the *multimodal* approach most alternative physicians use. In the following section, **William Lee Cowden, M.D.**, discusses his comprehensive program to promote heart health.

The Healthy Heart

All the causes of heart failure are reversible, to some degree, using a multifactorial process. There are many people whose heart problems get steadily worse until the only thing conventional medicine can offer is a heart transplant. Yet several patients in my practice who were told this was their last option have never had to have a transplant. Instead, they used natural techniques to improve their heart muscle function to the point where they became active people again. Here's what you need to do.

Your diet needs to move away from standard American fare toward one more plentiful in uncooked vegetables, fruits, and raw grains, seeds, and nuts, but no peanuts. Reduce your intake of dairy products, most animal meats, and refined white flour and sugar. Increase your intake of cold-water fish oil (such as sardine, herring, or mackerel), which is high in an omega-3 fatty acid called EPA (eicosapentaenoic acid). EPA prevents the formation of a clot-forming substance involved in heart disease. Flaxseed contains another omega-3 fatty acid called alpha linolenic acid (ALA) which is normally converted by the body into eicosapentaenoic acid, but stress and nutrient deficiencies block this conversion. For this reason, I recommend that most people living in a city (or an equivalently stressful environment) should take EPA supplements.

Completely avoid all fried foods and hydrogenated vegetable oils because their trans-fatty acids increase atherosclerosis, probably more so than butter. Another nutrient important for reversing heart disease is magnesium, to pre-

QUICK DEFINITION

Omega-3 and **omega-6 oils** are the two principal types of essential fatty acids, which are unsaturated fats required in the diet. The digits "3" and "6" refer to differences in the oil's chemical structure with respect to its chain of carbon atoms and where they are bonded. A balance of these oils in the diet is required for good health. The primary omega-3 oil is called alpha-linolenic acid (ALA) and is found in flaxseed (58%), canola, pumpkin and walnut, and soybeans. Fish oils, such as salmon, cod, and mackerel, contain the other important omega-3 oils, DHA (docosahexaenoic acid) and EPA (eicosapentaenoic acid). Omega-3 oils help reduce the risk of heart disease. Linoleic acid or cis-linoleic acid is the main omega-6 oil and is found in most plant and vegetable oils, including safflower (73%), corn, peanut, and sesame. The most therapeutic form of omega-6 oil is gamma-linolenic acid (GLA), found in evening primrose, black currant, and borage oils. Once in the body, omega-6 is converted to prostaglandins, hormone-like substances that regulate many metabolic functions, particularly inflammatory processes.

The Thyroid Gland

The **thyroid gland**, one of the body's seven endocrine glands, is located just below the larynx in the throat with interconnecting lobes on either side of the trachea. The thyroid is the body's metabolic thermostat, controlling body temperature, energy use, and, for children, the body's growth rate. The thyroid controls the *rate* at which organs function and the *speed* with which the body uses food; it affects the operation of all body processes and organs. Of the hormones synthesized in and released by the thyroid, T3 (triiodothyronine) represents 7%, and T4 (thyroxine) accounts for almost 93% of the thyroid's hormones active in all of the body's processes. Iodine is essential for forming normal amounts of thyroxine. The secretion of both these hormones is regulated by thyroid-stimulating hormone, or TSH, secreted by the pituitary gland in the brain. The thyroid also secretes calcitonin, a hormone required for calcium metabolism.

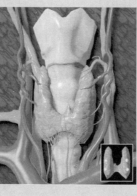

Hypothyroidism is a condition of low or underactive thyroid gland function that can produce numerous symptoms. Among the 47 clinically recognized symptoms are: fatigue, depression, lethargy, weakness, weight gain, low body temperature, chills, cold extremities, general inappropriate sensation of cold, infertility, rheumatic pain, menstrual disorders (excessive flow or cramps), repeated infections, colds, upper respiratory infections, skin problems (itching, eczema, psoriasis, acne, dry, coarse, and scaly skin, skin pallor), memory disturbances, concentration difficulties, paranoia, migraines, oversleep, "laziness," muscle aches and weakness, hearing disturbances, burning/prickling sensations, anemia, slow reaction time and mental sluggishness, swelling of the eyelids, constipation, labored and difficult breathing, hoarseness, brittle nails, and poor vision. A resting body temperature (measured in the armpit) *below* 97.8°F indicates hypothyroidism; menstruating women should take the underarm temperature only on the second and third days of menstruation.

Copyright © 1989-97 by TechPool Studios, Inc. USA

vent the coronary arteries from going into spasm, which can produce a heart attack. Magnesium deficiency is common in the U.S. because magnesium is lost from the kidneys whenever a person is under stress. There is also a relationship between magnesium and EPA levels. If you are deficient in EPA fish oil, you will become deficient in magnesium: this is guaranteed. You can never catch up on a magnesium deficiency

There is also a relationship between magnesium and EPA levels, says Dr. Cowden. If you are deficient in EPA fish oil, you will become deficient in magnesium: this is guaranteed. You can never catch up on a magnesium deficiency if you are EPA-deficient, so make sure you take EPA and magnesium together.

if you are EPA-deficient, so make sure you take EPA and magnesium together.

Selenium deficiency is another common cause for atherosclerotic disease. For heart health, you need about 200 mcg of elemental selenium a day. Other heart-healing nutrients include the antioxidant vitamins E and C, beta carotene, vitamins B3 and B6, bioflavonoids, and sulfur-containing amino acids such as L-taurine, N-acetyl cysteine, or glutathione. Particularly helpful in reversing plaque formation in the arteries are the amino acids L-lysine and L-proline and the antioxidant pycnogenol, from grape seeds or maritime pine bark. The amino acid L-carnitine, which helps to transport other amino acids and fatty acids into the cells, is also useful. People who have congestive heart failure are often deficient in L-carnitine. Keep in mind that all these nutrients work in concert with one another and it's important to develop a total supplement program.

In addition to diet and nutritional supplementation, the alternative medicine techniques of chelation and hyperbaric oxygen therapy can both prevent and treat heart disease by painlessly and noninvasively clearing the arteries.

A possible dental involvement is another factor to consider. A large percentage of people who have heart disease have some type of abnormal dental process (such as a root canal tooth or previous tooth extraction site) in the mouth. Most commonly this is an infection of the jawbone, usually located at the third molar, or wisdom tooth site, in any of the four jaw locations. These infections usually cause an inflammatory response that speeds up the process of artery hardening. Typically, the teeth on the left side of the mouth affect the left side of the heart; those on the right side affect the right side of the heart. If doctors would recognize and treat this, and work with biological dentists, many people who have heart attacks, arrhythmia, or congestive heart failure could see improvement in their conditions.

Often in a case of coronary disease, I recommend that patients have all the mercury amalgams removed from their teeth. Aside from the documented effect that mercury can leach from dental fillings and

QUICK DEFINITION

An **antioxidant** (meaning "against oxidation") is a natural biochemical substance that protects living cells against damage from harmful free radicals. Antioxidants work against the process of oxidation — the robbing of electrons from substances. If unblocked or left uncontrolled, oxidation can lead to cellular aging, degeneration, arthritis, heart disease, cancer, and other illnesses. Antioxidants in the body react readily with oxygen breakdown products and free radicals, and neutralize them before they can damage the body. Antioxidant nutrients include vitamins A, C, and E, beta carotene, selenium, coenzyme Q10, L-glutathione, superoxide dismutase, catalase, and bioflavonoids such as grape seed extract and pine bark extract (pycnogenol). Plant antioxidants include *Ginkgo biloba* and garlic. When antioxidants are taken in combination, the effect is stronger than when they are used individually.

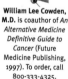

William Lee Cowden, M.D. is coauthor of *An Alternative Medicine Definitive Guide to Cancer* (Future Medicine Publishing, 1997). To order, call 800-333-4325. To contact Dr. Cowden: Conservative Medicine Institute, P.O. Box 832087, Richardson, TX 75083-2087; fax: 214-238-0327.

be distributed throughout the body, it can also leak into specific nerve ganglia (stelate, vagus, or cardiac) which regulate heart function, as I've observed in some of my heart patients. Mercury in these ganglia can cause autonomic nervous system (ANS) imbalance and therefore affect heart function. Spasms can occur in blood vessels or the heart itself as a result of an ANS imbalance. As mentioned earlier, this type of spasm can cause a heart attack.

In these patients, the mercury was poisoning those ganglia, which led to heart problems such as impaired blood supply or disturbed heart rhythm. When we got the mercury out of their teeth, then used chelating (binding-up) agents such as DMPS to get the mercury out of their body tissues, the heart problems cleared up and they were able to discontinue using their various heart medications for arrhythmia and angina. Some people who are helped by EDTA chelation (an effective alternative to angioplasty for atherosclerosis) may be benefiting because it pulls heavy metals from the nerve ganglia serving the heart.

One of my patients with a heart rhythm disturbance had considerable mercury distributed in his body, but it was especially concentrated in the submandibular nerve ganglion (below the jaw). In addition, an infection in the third molar socket of the patient's jaw at the site of a previous wisdom tooth extraction was also contributing to the heart problem.

Through the energy lines called meridians in acupuncture, this site was energetically linked with his heart and the jaw infection was harming that organ. When the infection and mercury leakage and poisoning were corrected (including mercury amalgam removal), his heart arrhythmia resolved. ■

The Mercury Hazard for the Heart

Health researcher H. L. Queen cautions that "the possibilities for involvement of mercury in cardiovascular ailments are so broad" that doctors, from family practitioners to cardiologists, are advised to "routinely address the issue of chronic mercury toxicity (and other heavy metal toxicities) early in the patient's treatment program."

Queen cites Russian research, first reported in 1974, showing that when electrocardiograms were prepared from rabbits exposed to mercury vapor, abnormal changes were apparent in the readings, probably due to an inactivation by mercury of certain heart enzymes necessary for heart muscle contraction. Other research has identified mercury as a contributing factor in arterial disease as well as other problems affecting the heart and arteries; mercury appears to interfere with the normal processing of nutrients that supply arterial smooth muscle, leading to their becoming rigid, Queen says.

QUICK DEFINITION

DMPS (2,3-dimercapto-propane-1-sulfonate) is the chelating (binding-up) agent of choice for the removal of elemental mercury from the human body. It can be given orally, intravenously, or intramuscularly and is useful for people who have been exposed to mercury amalgam through their dental fillings or for those who show evidence or suspicion of heavy metal toxicity from other sources.

Mercury toxicity may also interfere with the processing of cholesterol from arterial cell walls (called Type II hyperlipoproteinemia) and in depositing cholesterol in the liver for removal from the body, says Queen. Further, because it interferes with certain fat-removing enzymes, "mercury may be contributing to the high total serum cholesterol" characteristic of those people vulnerable to arterial disease. In fact, Queen advises that any time there is an unexplained elevated cholesterol level that a physician check for mercury toxicity.

Queen also warns that it can be highly dangerous to suddenly lower a patient's cholesterol (such as with conventional cholesterol-lowering drugs) if they have a preexist-

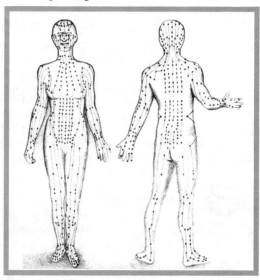

Acupuncture meridians are specific pathways in the human body for the flow of life force or subtle energy, known as *qi* (pronounced CHEE). In most cases, these energy pathways run up and down both sides of the body, and correspond to individual organs or organ systems, designated as Lung, Small Intestine, Heart, and others. There are 12 principal meridians and eight secondary channels. Numerous points of heightened energy, or *qi*, exist on the body's surface along the meridians and are called acupoints. There are more than 1,000 acupoints, each of which is potentially a place for acupuncture treatment.

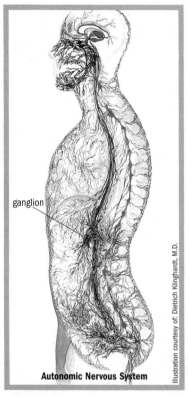

ganglion

Autonomic Nervous System

Illustration courtesy of: Dietrich Klinghardt, M.D.

A *ganglion* is a bundle, knot, or plexus of nerve cell bodies with many interconnections that acts like a sorting and relay station for nerve impulses. There are several dozen ganglia throughout the body. The *autonomic nervous system (ANS)* involves elements of both the central nervous system (CNS) and peripheral nervous system (PNS), is controlled by the brain's hypothalamus gland, and pertains to the automatic regulation of all body processes such as breathing, digestion, and heart rate. It can be likened to the body's automatic pilot, keeping you alive without your being aware of it or participating in its activities. Neural therapy focuses its injections of anesthetics into body structures whose nerve supply is linked with the autonomic nervous system.

Within the ANS, there are two branches—the parasympathetic and sympathetic branches, which are believed to counterbalance each other. The parasympathetic nervous system slows heart rate, inhibits activity, conserves energy, and calms the body, but stimulates gastric secretion and intestinal activity.

See Chapter 3: Scrubbing the Arteries Naturally; Chapter 4: The Dental Connection; Chapter 5: Nutritional Supplements; and Chapter 7: Other Alternatives for Heart Health.

ing but untreated mercury toxicity. "Because mercury has an affinity for lipoproteins and lipoidal tissues, any sudden lowering of cholesterol without a reduction in the body burden of mercury would encourage a transfer of previously circulating mercury to the lipoidal tissues of nerve and brain cells." This in turn could produce behavioral problems including, potentially, violent or impulsive behavior, or other symptoms of chronic mercury toxicity, Queen comments.[32]

An underactive thyroid gland can contribute to heart disease and the propensity to sustain a heart attack, according to Broda O. Barnes, M.D., a Connecticut physician who specialized in identifying and treating the many unsuspected connections between low thyroid activity and numerous health problems. "I am convinced that we are seeing today many more people with low thyroid function than ever before," explained Dr. Barnes, "and that the rising incidence of heart attacks is related to the rising incidence of hypothyroidism."

Caring for Yourself

USE DIET, EXERCISE, AND LIFESTYLE CHANGES TO IMPROVE YOUR HEART

ANY DISCUSSION OF HEART health needs to address diet, exercise, and lifestyle issues such as stress level and emotional well-being. Research has demonstrated the relationship between heart disease prevention and healthy practices in these three areas. For example, eating a vegetarian diet lowers your risk of death from heart disease; exercising just ten minutes daily can significantly reduce the likelihood of heart disease; but anxiety and stress increase the risk of having heart problems.

"The average American lifestyle, combining too little exercise, too much stress, and a diet of highly processed foods often deficient in essential nutrients, has rendered this nation's population especially vulnerable to the ravages of heart ailments," says William Lee Cowden, M.D.

During the teenage and young adult years when bad dietary and exercise habits can most easily be altered, much can be done to protect the body against heart disease. Although initial damage done to the arteries can cause the buildup of plaque, it can be corrected through modifying your diet, building an exercise program into your life, and attending to emotional and psychological concerns.

The Modern Diet and a New Understanding of Nutrition

"Nutrient density is the hallmark of good food," says Paul McTaggart, a nutrition researcher from Ventura, California. Defined

Although initial damage done to the arteries can cause the buildup of plaque, it can be corrected through modifying your diet, building an exercise program into your life, and attending to emotional and psychological concerns.

as the relative ratio of nutrients to calories, foods low in nutrient density are often termed "empty-calorie" or "junk" foods.

The leading nutritional problem in the United States today is "overconsumptive undernutrition," or the eating of too many empty-calorie foods, says Jeffrey Bland, Ph.D., a biochemist and nutrition expert from Gig Harbor, Washington. Although people in the United States consume plenty of food, it is not the right kind of food. Studies have concluded that almost two-thirds of an average American's diet is made up of fats and refined sugars having low to no nutrient density. Consequently, the remaining one-third of the average diet is counted on for the essential nutrients needed to maintain health, which may or may not be from high-nutrient-density food. The result is often nutrient deficiencies which can rob the body of its natural resistance to disease, lead to premature aging, and weaken overall physiological and psychological performance.

The American diet is full of trans-fatty acids which numerous studies have linked to heart-disease risk. These harmful fats are oils which have been hydrogenated to lengthen shelf-life. This altered form is foreign to human metabolism and can block the normal digestion pathways of essential fatty acids, necessary for numerous metabolic functions. Trans-fatty acids are found in margarine and processed, packaged foods such as cakes, cookies, crackers, cereals, donuts, and potato chips, among many other products. Margarine, long promoted as a heart-friendly substitute for butter, has now been proven to be just the opposite. Intake of margarine is significantly associated with risk of heart disease.[1] *Science* reports that hydrogenated fats increase the risk of coronary heart disease.[2]

QUICK
DEFINITION

Trans-fatty acids are found in margarine and other oils which have been hydrogenated (combined with hydrogen) to lengthen shelf-life. Ingredient lists on food labels often designate these oils as "partially hydrogenated," but the partial is a misnomer in terms of the effect on the body. When vegetable or animal oils are highly processed and hydrogenated, they are partially converted into an abnormal form called *trans*. These trans-fatty acids can block the normal digestion pathways of fatty acids. This, in turn, can contribute to the development of heart disease and cancer and interfere with the immune system.

Lipoproteins are in two principal forms. *Low-density lipoproteins (LDLs)* are combination molecules of proteins and fats, particularly cholesterol. LDLs circulate in the blood and act as the primary carriers of cholesterol to the cells of the body. An elevated level of LDLs, the so-called bad cholesterol, is a contributing factor in causing atherosclerosis (plaque deposits on the inner walls of the arteries). A diet high in saturated fats can lead to an increase the level of LDLs in the blood. *High-density lipoproteins (HDLs)* are also fat-protein molecules in the blood, but contain a larger amount of protein and less fat than LDLs. HDLs are able to absorb cholesterol and related compounds in the blood and transport them to the liver for elimination. HDL, the so-called good cholesterol, may also be able to take cholesterol from plaque deposits on the artery walls, thus helping to reverse the process of atherosclerosis. A higher ratio of HDL to LDL cholesterol in the blood is associated with a reduced risk of cardiovascular disease.

Studies have found that total fat intake, independent of type, is not strongly associated with coronary heart disease. However, trans-fatty acids raise LDL (low-density lipoprotein) cholesterol and result in reductions of HDL (high-density lipoprotein) cholesterol. In other words, the *type* of fat, not the total fat, is the significant factor.[3]

Dietary management can be highly effective in reversing heart disease. "Ninety percent of heart attacks are caused by blood clots at the site of an atherosclerotic lesion, and 90% of strokes are caused by platelet aggregation [blood clotting]," says James R. Privitera, M.D., noting that dietary changes and nutritional supplements can be used to correct these problems. Dr. Privitera suggests eating foods low in saturated fats (fats from animal products such as butter, milk, and meat) and high in complex carbohydrates, and taking vitamins C, B6, and E, garlic, and the essential fatty acids EPA and DHA.

Soy products can significantly lower cholesterol. Although cholesterol itself may not be the cause of heart disease, the more LDL cholesterol you have in your blood, the more there is available for oxidation, which is where heart problems can begin. By eating three servings a day of any soy product, you can lower your cholesterol level by nine points, according to a report of 38 studies published in the *New England Journal of Medicine*. As a reference point, a tofu burger and a glass of soy milk provide one serving each and one soy protein drink is equal to three servings. The report further stated that the more soy people ate, the more their cholesterol level went down.[4]

Simply eating a lot of fruit and vegetables can help prevent heart problems, according to researchers at the University of Otago in Dunedin, Scotland. "At least ten prospective studies have shown that high intakes of fruits and vegetables confer protection against cancer, cardiovascular disease, and stroke."[5]

Dean Ornish, M.D., assistant clinical professor of medicine at the University of California at San Francisco, used a vegetarian diet, exercise, and stress-reduction techniques to reverse arterial buildup of plaque.[6] His "reversal diet" is almost entirely free of cholesterol, animal fats, and oils. Dr. Ornish found that the condition of those patients who followed the diet improved, while the condition of those who continued eating a diet high in fat got worse.[7]

According to Dr. Cowden, however, the success of Dr. Ornish's

QUICK DEFINITION

DHA (docosahexaenoic acid), is the primary structural fatty acid in the retina of the eye and the most abundant fat in the gray matter of the brain. (DHA, which is an omega-3 long-chain fatty acid, is unrelated to DHEA, which is a hormone.) Adequate levels of DHA are required for proper brain and eye development and function. DHA is important for signal transmission in the brain, eye, and nervous system. Research has shown that DHA has benefits for patients with depression, Alzheimer's, or attention deficit disorder, and for pregnant and lactating women. Initially, DHA is obtained fetally through the placenta; after birth, DHA comes from breast milk; then later from dietary sources such as fish (tuna, salmon, and sardines, or fish oils), red meats, animal organs, and eggs. DHA is also available in capsule form from a single nutrient source: microalgae, the fish's original source.

diet is due not primarily to low levels of cholesterol and fats but to both low levels of methionine (an amino acid found in red meat, milk, and milk products, and a precursor to homocysteine, a free-radical generator capable of oxidizing cholesterol) and a high intake of vegetables and grains. These foods are rich in the vitamins (B6, C, E, and beta carotene) necessary to act as co-factors for antioxidants and antiatherogenics (substances preventing atherosclerosis).

Dr. Cowden offers the following dietary guidelines to help prevent heart disease:

■ Eat minimally-processed foods (avoid additives and preservatives and foods containing powdered eggs or powdered milk).

■ Buy organic foods (free of pesticides, herbicides, steroids, and antibiotics) whenever possible.

■ Avoid irradiated foods whenever possible.

■ Increase fiber from sources like green leafy vegetables, fresh raw fruits, bran, whole grains, and psyllium.

■ Reduce fat intake, especially fried foods, animal fats, and partially hydrogenated oils. Increase complex carbohydrates such as whole grains, beans, seeds, and potatoes.

■ Use monounsaturated oils (such as cold-pressed olive oil and canola oil), omega-3 oils (from flaxseed or deep ocean fish), and omega-6 oils (from borage, black currant, or evening primrose). Oils must be fresh and cold-pressed—rancid oils can be harmful.

■ Reduce meat, sugar, tobacco, and alcohol consumption—all are sources of free radicals. For example, sugar can cause damage to gallbladder and bowel functions, which can in turn lead to reduced absorption of fat-soluble antioxidant nutrients like vitamin E and

Good News for Chocolate Lovers?

The results of a recent study are a chocolate lover's dream come true. Researchers at the University of California at Davis found that chocolate has high amounts of phenol, a chemical that helps reduce heart disease risk by preventing cholesterol in the bloodstream from oxidizing. It is oxidized cholesterol that clogs the arteries. The phenol in 1.5 ounces of milk chocolate is equal to that in five ounces of red wine, known for its beneficial effects on heart health (to the delight of wine lovers). The study further discovered that chocolate contains a significant amount of antioxidants which also help prevent oxidation.[8]

Unfortunately, chocolate is high in calories and saturated fat along with the heart-enhancing phenol. Since obesity and a diet high in saturated fat increase your chances of heart disease, eating more candy bars as part of your total heart-health program is probably not a good idea.

Margarine, long promoted as a heart-friendly substitute for butter, has now been proven to be just the opposite. Intake of margarine is significantly associated with risk of heart disease.

the increased absorption of free radicals produced by bacterial action in the stagnant colon.

Dr. Cowden also puts many of his heart patients through a detoxification regimen consisting of a vegetarian diet, vegetable juices mixed with garlic, and, in some cases, cayenne, as well as low-temperature saunas. Detoxification in this context means cleansing the internal organs, especially the liver, gall bladder, and intestines, of accumulated toxins. This program helps to cleanse the body of toxins which may be contributing to free radical damage to the artery walls and the buildup of arterial plaque. He also often uses homeopathic remedies to aid in the detoxification.

Weight and Longevity

Leaner men live longer, says a Harvard School of Public Health poll of 19,000 men. Those men with the lowest mortality rate had weights 20% below the average for their age while men whose weights were 20% above the ideal body weight had a 2.5 times higher risk for cardiovascular disease.

To reduce the level of oxidized cholesterol in the bloodstream, noted health educator Richard Passwater, Ph.D., suggests combining a dietary regimen (under 30% of daily calories from fat so as not to raise LDL cholesterol levels) with a personalized nutritional supplementation program. "What needs to be done is to first control the LDL cholesterol through diet, then raise the antioxidant level to prevent oxidized cholesterol from doing damage," says Dr. Passwater. Clearly, a healthy diet that limits sources of homocysteine-generating fat, such as red meat and fried food, can keep the body's systems operating more smoothly.

Eating onions and apples and drinking black tea can also contribute to heart health. These items contain high concentrations of quercetin, a bioflavonoid, and are inversely associated with coronary heart disease mortality rates. In other words, the more onions, apples, and black tea you consume, the lower your risk of dying from heart disease. A bioflavonoid is a pigment within plants and fruits that acts as an antioxidant to protect against damage from free radicals and excess oxygen. In the body, bioflavonoids enhance the beneficial activities of vitamin C and therefore help keep the immune system strong.[9]

A recent study found that men in the highest third of dietary quercetin levels had a 53% lower risk of coronary heart disease than those in the lowest third.[10]

Grapeseed Oil is Good for the Heart

Although there are a number of products that lower total cholesterol, there are few that operate selectively, raising HDL (the "good" cholesterol) while lowering LDL (the "bad" cholesterol that deposits fats on arterial walls). According to both the Helsinki and Framingham Heart Studies performed on thousands of patients over several years, each percentage increase in HDL is correlated with a significant decrease in the incidence of cardiac events.

Grapeseed oil has a high concentration of vitamin E (60-120 mg/100 g), making it a significant source for this nutrient. Grapeseed oil is 76% linoleic acid, an essential fatty acid also known as omega-6, and as the body doesn't produce linoleic acid, it must be acquired through the diet. Linoleic acid is important for producing prostaglandins, hormone-like substances in the body involved in reducing platelet aggregation (blood clotting) and inflammation.

Reducing your intake of saturated fats can help lower your risk of developing heart and circulatory problems. Substituting grapeseed oils for your usual cooking or salad oil can contribute to this healthful goal. Among cooking oils, grapeseed oil has one of the lowest levels of saturated fats at only 9%.

Grapeseed oil is one of the few foods that can simultaneously reduce LDL and increase HDL cholesterol levels; both of these change are beneficial to heart health. In a study published in *Arteriosclerosis* in 1990, researchers at the State University of New York Health Science Center at Syracuse studied the effects of grapeseed oil on 33 men and women with initially low HDL levels. They were tested for cholesterol and triglyceride levels, then instructed to use one ounce of grapeseed oil daily for four weeks. In just this short period, blood tests of the subjects showed a 17.2% reduction in triglycerides and a 10.4% increase in the level of HDL cholesterol.

QUICK DEFINITION

Omega-3 and **omega-6 oils** are the two principal types of essential fatty acids, which are unsaturated fats required in the diet. The digits "3" and "6" refer to differences in the oil's chemical structure with respect to its chain of carbon atoms and where they are bonded. A balance of these oils in the diet is required for good health. The primary omega-3 oil is called alpha-linolenic acid (ALA) and is found in flaxseed (58%), canola, pumpkin and walnut, and soybeans. Fish oils, such as salmon, cod, and mackerel, contain the other important omega-3 oils, DHA (docosahexaenoic acid) and EPA (eicosapentaenoic acid). Omega-3 oils help reduce the risk of heart disease. Linoleic acid or cis-linoleic acid is the main omega-6 oil and is found in most plant and vegetable oils, including safflower (73%), corn, peanut, and sesame. The most therapeutic form of omega-6 oil is gamma-linolenic acid (GLA), found in evening primrose, black currant, and borage oils. Once in the body, omega-6 is converted to prostaglandins, hormone-like substances that regulate many metabolic functions, particularly inflammatory processes.

Detoxification involves a variety of techniques to rid the body of poisons accumulated as a result of a polluted environment (air, water, and food), exposure to toxic chemicals and pesticides, accumulated stress, faulty dietary practices, and chronic constipation or poor elimination, among other factors. Detoxification methods include fasting, intestinal cleansing, enemas and colonics, lymph drainage procedures, chelation, biological dentistry, water and heat therapies, therapeutic massage, and bodywork techniques.

Grapeseed oil is one of the few foods that can simultaneously reduce LDL and increase HDL cholesterol levels; both of these changes are beneficial to heart health.

For a source of **grapeseed oil**, contact: Salute Santé! Grapeseed Oil, Food & Vine, Inc., 301 Poplar Avenue, Suite 6, Mill Valley, CA 94941; tel: 415-388-7792; fax: 415-388-9933. Napa Valley Grapeseed Oil Co., P.O. Box 561, Rutherford, CA 94573; tel: 707-963-0544; fax: 707-963-3150.

Another study by the same team again showed the beneficial effect of grapeseed oil on cholesterol levels. This study (*Journal of the American College of Cardiology*, 1993) involved 56 men and women with initially low HDL levels. The subjects were instructed to substitute in their daily diet up to 45 ml of grapeseed oil for the oil they normally used for cooking and salads. Blood tests were taken at the beginning of the study and after three weeks. At the end of the test period, the subjects showed no significant changes in total cholesterol levels or weight. However, there was a 7% reduction in the level of LDL ("bad") cholesterol and a 13% increase in HDL (the "good" cholesterol) levels. "The use of grapeseed oil in a daily diet appears to improve both HDL and LDL levels in weight-stable subjects with initially low HDL levels," concluded David T. Nash, M.D., lead researcher on the study.

Raising the amount of HDL in your blood is important because there seems to be a strong correlation between HDL level and the risk of both heart disease and impotence. The effect on cardiovascular health was shown in a long-term study of heart disease called the Helsinki Heart Study. This study called thousands of volunteers to assess their risk of heart disease based on cholesterol levels. The study followed 4,081 men, 40 to 55 years old, over a five-year period. Cholesterol levels were artificially altered (LDL level lowered, HDL level raised) using a drug called gemfibrozil. Every three months, the subjects were examined and tested for signs of heart disease.

The results showed that LDL/HDL levels in the blood are an important indicator of health. Over the five-year period of the study, there were 34% fewer incidents of heart disease in the treated group compared to the placebo group and also fewer deaths (14 vs. 19). During the fifth year of the study, the treated group had 65% fewer heart attacks than the placebo group.

A low level of HDL (and corresponding higher level of LDL) is a major danger sign for the development of heart problems, according to the study, more so than overall cholesterol level. "The increase in the concentration of serum HDL cholesterol and the fall in that of LDL cholesterol were both associated with reduced risk, whereas the changes in the amounts of total cholesterol and triglycerides in the serum were not," stated the researchers. "The risk of coronary heart disease increased with decreasing concentration of HDL."

The study showed that raising your HDL level can have a significant impact on lowering your chances of developing heart disease: for each single percentage point increase in the level of HDL there was a corresponding 3% to 4% decrease in the incidence of heart disease. These same results can be provided by a dietary source like grapeseed oil, which, by increasing your level of HDL by 10% to 13%, as demonstrated in Dr. Nash's studies, can reduce your risk for cardiovascular problems by 30% to 52%.

Low HDL level is also a risk factor for impotence. A 1994 study published in the *Journal of Urology* assessed the risk factors for developing impotence. Based on questionnaires from 1,290 men, 40 to 70 years old, living in Massachusetts, the study found several factors that contributed to a higher probability for impotence. Age was the predominant factor, as the prevalence of complete impotence tripled from 5% to 15% between ages 40 and 70 years. After adjusting for age, the other main factors were heart disease, hypertension, diabetes, and personality type.

Research found that one ounce daily of grapeseed oil raises HDL and lowers LDL and each percentage increase in HDL is correlated with a significant decrease in the incidence of cardiac events.

The researchers also found that the HDL level in the blood was inversely related to the probability of impotence. For the younger men in the study (40 to 55 years old), the likelihood of developing moderate impotence quadrupled from 6.7% to 25% as their HDL level decreased from 90 mg to 30 mg (per deciliter of blood). For the older men in the study (56 to 70 years old), the probability of complete impotence increased from near zero to 16% as their HDL level correspondingly decreased. "The probability of impotence varied inversely with high density lipoprotein cholesterol," stated the researchers.[11]

On the scale of oils which contribute to heart health, grapeseed oil is number one, followed by olive oil, then canola oil.[12] In addition to raising HDL and lowering LDL, which helps maintain the health of the arteries, grapeseed oil reduces platelet aggregation (keeps cells in the blood from sticking together; clustering contributes to heart disease) and helps to prevent high blood pressure caused by sodium excess.

The study results showed that LDL/HDL levels in the blood are an important indicator of health. Over the five-year period of the study, there were 34% fewer incidents of heart disease in the treated group compared to the placebo group and also fewer deaths (14 vs. 19).

The Heart Benefits of Olive Oil

Among the sources of **organic olive oil**, contact: Critelli Olive Oil Co. (CCOF certified), 1009 Factory Street, Unit A, Richmond, CA 94801; tel: 510-412-8990; fax: 510-412-8999. Spectrum Naturals, Inc. (QAI certified), 133 Copeland St., Petaluma, CA 94952; tel: 707-778-8900; fax: 707-765-1026. Sadeg Organic (OCIA certified), 909 Marina Village Parkway, Suite 236, Alameda, CA 94501; tel: 800-400-8851 or 510-521-6548; fax: 510-521-5106.

The ancient Greeks knew premium cooking oil when they tasted it, and today Italian, Greek, and Spanish olive oil processors who have been producing oil for generations take great pride in the quality of their oil. The olive tree (*Olea europaea*) was first domesticated around 6,000 B.C. in southern Europe, and olive oil has been a main ingredient in the Mediterranean diet ever since. In recent years, scientific studies have confirmed that olive oil is of considerable health benefit, especially for the heart. That's because it's very low in saturated fats (a major factor in heart disease) and high in omega-3 fatty acids and antioxidants, which are both essential for heart health.

The chief benefit of using high-quality olive oil is cardiovascular—it's good for your heart because, among commonly available vegetable oils (canola, peanut, corn, soybean, sunflower, safflower) and margarine and butter, it is the highest in *monounsaturated* fats. Studies have demonstrated that this type of fat is excellent for lowering blood cholesterol levels, especially of the harmful LDL variety. Olive oil is also an excellent source of antioxidants, heart-protective substances which must be replenished through the diet.

Saturated and Unsaturated Fat—In 1958, the "Seven Countries" study compared the heart disease rates with dietary content in 13,000 men in seven countries. Researchers found the lowest rate of heart disease on Crete, an island in Greece. Even though the *percentage* of fat in the diet (40%) was the same on Crete as in the country with the highest rate (Finland), the Cretan diet was naturally lower in *saturated* fats. It has since been dubbed the "Mediterranean" diet, and consists primarily of grains, vegetables, bread, and olive oil, with minimal animal protein.

In other words, the *type* of fat can make all the difference, because the Finns ate meat and dairy products, both high in saturated fats, while the Cretans derived much of their fat from olive oil, which is 77% monounsaturated. Saturated fats come mainly from animal sources (meat and butter), but palm and coconut oils are also high in saturated fats. "Saturated fats are the worst threats to the cardiovascular system," says Stephen T. Sinatra, M.D., author of *Optimum Health* and editor of *HeartSense* newsletter. "They are converted to cholesterol in the body and will raise cholesterol levels significantly if consumed in excess."

Conversely, unsaturated fatty acids have been found to lower total cholesterol by reducing LDL (the so-called bad cholesterol) without affecting the level of high-density lipoproteins (HDL, "good" cholesterol). The advantage of monounsaturated fats (olive, canola, and peanut oils) over polyunsaturated fats (corn, sesame, and safflower oils) is that they are less likely to oxidize (become rancid) during cooking. Olive oil also appears to preserve beneficial HDL levels and to exert a mild blood-thinning effect (which prevents clotting within arteries).

> **The chief benefit of using high-quality olive oil is cardiovascular—it's good for your heart because, among commonly available vegetable oils (canola, peanut, corn, soybean, sunflower, safflower) and margarine and butter, it is the highest in *monounsaturated* fats.**

"Given the documented evidence on the positive effects of monounsaturated fats on LDL and HDL levels, it seems likely that the Mediterranean diet, rich in olive oil, plays a significant role" in maintaining a higher level of cardiovascular health, says Dr. Sinatra. "Although it is best to use as little oil as possible, I wholeheartedly endorse the use of olive oil for salads and cooking."

Heart-Protective Antioxidants—Olive oil contains antioxidants, which protect against the development of atherosclerosis (a thickening or hardening of the arteries due to fatty deposits on arterial walls). In a recent study published in *Atherosclerosis*, researchers tested polyphenols (compounds with potential antioxidant properties) extracted from extra virgin olive oil, specifically hydroxytyrosol, oleuropein, and elenolic acid. These substances, it was hypothesized, blocked LDL oxidation.

Atherosclerosis can be caused by many factors, but a prime factor is the oxidation of LDL, according to Dr. Sinatra and a growing body of research. Oxidized LDL leads to the formation of cholesterol blockages. Oxidation, a chemical reaction in the body, can produce free radicals; these are molecules that damage arterial walls and red blood cells.

In the study, three olive oil compounds were incubated with samples of LDL along with copper sulphate, a substance which induces oxidation. To test the results, levels of vitamin E (an antioxidant) were measured periodically (at 30 minutes, one hour, three hours, and six hours) during incubation, as the loss of vitamin E correlates with the degree of oxidation.

Any substance that inhibits this process of oxidation will help prevent the development of atherosclerosis. These substances are called antioxidants and include nutrients such as vitamins E and C, selenium, and beta carotene, among others. Antioxidants are like "friendly guardians or bodyguards," explains Dr. Sinatra. "Sacrificing themselves in chemical reactions, they engulf free radicals before they can do their damage to the body."

The study results demonstrated that all three compounds inhibited free radical formation. They "markedly slowed the loss of vitamin E and retarded the onset of oxidative processes," the researchers concluded. In the control group (without the added compounds), vitamin E disappeared after 30 minutes. The samples incubated with the polyphenols showed 80% protection after 30 minutes and 60% after three hours; and there was still 40% of the original level of vitamin E after six hours incubation time. This antioxidative effect was present even with low concentrations of polyphenols.

The researchers estimated that among olive oil–consuming populations, the daily intake of polyphenols from olive oil alone was about 10 to 20 mg. They concluded that "these amounts of dietary antioxidants, consumed by population groups for several years, are able to reduce the mortality due to CHD [coronary heart disease]."[13]

A Vegetarian Diet Can Prolong Life by 44%

In case you've wondered if following a mostly vegetarian diet that emphasizes the consumption of fresh fruits and vegetables really has long-term health benefits, a new British study provides unarguable evidence that it does.[14] Researchers at the Cancer Epidemiology Unit at Radcliffe Infirmary in Oxford, England, tracked 4,336 men and 6,435 women over a 17-year period to see what effect healthy eating habits produced.

When initially surveyed, the 10,771 subjects described their daily lifestyle and dietary habits: 19% smoked, 43% were vegetarian, 62% ate whole-grain bread, 38% ate nuts or dried fruit, 38% ate raw salads, and 77% ate fresh fruits. The researchers concluded that following healthy eating practices, especially the daily consumption of fresh fruits, was responsible for a much lower death rate from heart and cerebrovascular disease in particular and all causes in general, compared to the general population.

Specifically, only 1,343 individuals died before reaching the age of 80, compared to the expected death rate of about 2,400 from the general population. In other words, a health-conscious diet accounted for a 44% reduction in early deaths. The differences in death rate were especially marked in the areas of cancer, diabetes, heart disease, and gastrointestinal diseases. The death rate from cancer for health-conscious people was only 63% that of the general population; for heart disease, it was 50%; stomach cancer, 48%; lung cancer, 30%; and diabetes, 27%. For those individuals who ate fresh fruit daily, there was a 24% lower premature death rate from heart disease, 32% less cerebrovascular disease, and 21% reduced mortality from all causes.

Lifestyle and Your Heart

There are numerous lifestyle factors aside from diet which have an impact on heart health. High stress levels, smoking, and lack of exercise are probably the greatest contributors to cardiovascular disease.

The Psychology of a Heart Attack

Anxiety increases the risk of sudden cardiac death by 4½ times, even among men free of chronic health problems, according to a 32-year study of 2,280 men, 21-80 years old, as reported in *Circulation* (November 1994). High anxiety is considered a twofold stronger risk factor than cigarette smoking.

Anxiety is a risk factor because it can contribute to the process of plaque buildup in the arteries. "When people are under stress, they form more free radicals, which cause a greater conversion of normal cholesterol into oxidized cholesterol (oxysterols)," says cardiologist W. Lee Cowden, M.D. "These oxysterols then build up in white blood cells and are carried to the site of damage in the arteries." He adds that stress also stimulates the release of adrenalin, which in turn has been shown to cause platelet aggregation (clustering) and

Eliminating the Need for a Heart Transplant

While conventional medicine often relies on the high-risk procedure of heart transplant in treating heart disease, this radical method can often be avoided. William Lee Cowden, M.D., reports the case of a 45-year-old physician who was suffering from pneumonia and an enlarged heart. When given an ejection fraction test (measuring the percentage of the blood contained in the ventricle that is ejected on each heartbeat), his heart was only ejecting 16% of its contents (60% is normal), and his doctor told him his only hope was to receive a heart transplant. When he came into Dr. Cowden's office, he could not walk across the room without becoming short of breath.

Dr. Cowden immediately put him on a detoxification program that included a vegetarian diet and a three-day vegetable juice fast with garlic. Dr. Cowden also had him follow a nutritional supplementation regimen including coenzyme Q10, vitamin C, magnesium, vitamin B complex, trace minerals, omega-3 fatty acids, lauric acid (an essential fatty acid), and the amino acid L-carnitine, as well as the antiviral herbs St. John's Wort, *Pfaffia paniculata*, and *Lomatium dissectum*.

Within three months, Dr. Cowden reports, the patient could jog ten miles a day and, upon repeating the ejection fraction test, his score was up to 30%. Now he works 60 hours a week and continues to jog ten miles daily.

increased blood viscosity (thickness).[15] Increases in blood viscosity can result in spontaneous clot formation. These can either adhere to arterial walls, initiating further plaque formation, or become lodged in narrowed arteries or capillaries, initiating a heart attack or stroke.

Researchers at Duke University Medical Center studied 126 people for five years and found that 27% of those who responded adversely to mental stress in a test situation, such as in public speaking or tight deadlines, later suffered serious heart problems. This means that if a person shows abnormal heart function in response to mental stress, it increases the risk of a future heart problem by two to three times, the researchers reported in the *Journal of the American Medical Association* (June 1996).

In a Danish study (*Circulation*, 1996), 730 men and women followed over a 27-year period showed that, regardless of gender, those with numerous symptoms of depression (such as hypochondria or low self-esteem) had a 70% increased risk of a major heart attack (myocardial infarction). Those who showed strong signs of depression at the beginning of the study were 60% more likely to die early from any cause.

Patients with ischemic heart disease (blood flow shortage to the heart) who had strongly negative thoughts had 1.6 times as many episodes of the disease and were 1.5 times more likely to die from it, a scientist from the U.S. Centers for Disease Control reported in November 1995. About 5% of the 26,000 deaths from this heart problem are due to a patient's negative expectations.

A study of 1,236 men and 538 women found that within the first 24 hours following the death of a loved one, close friends and family members have a 14-fold increased risk of heart attack. The risk of heart attack from grief remains eight times above normal on the second day, six times on the third day, and between two and four times above normal for the next month, according to *Family Practice News* (April 15, 1996).

Stress Reduction

Stress-reduction techniques and exercise have been shown to be highly effective in reversing heart disease. In a study conducted by Dean Ornish, M.D., an experimental group following a routine that combined a low-fat vegetarian diet, stress-management training, the elimination of smoking, and moderate exercise, had a 91% decrease in the frequency

Anxiety increases the risk of sudden cardiac death by 4½ times, even among men free of chronic health problems. High anxiety is considered a twofold stronger risk factor than cigarette smoking.

of angina, as opposed to a control group which experienced a 165% increase in the frequency of angina.[16]

Dr. Cowden also includes stress-reduction exercises as part of his treatment of cardiovascular patients. He believes that deep breathing and imaging techniques aimed at reducing stress should be conducted frequently throughout the day to reduce the output of adrenal hormones and lower the level of platelet aggregation. He encourages patients to do these techniques before meals and at bedtime, as they can not only reduce stress but can improve digestion. "Some of the nutrients we are giving as treatment have to be absorbed out of the gastrointestinal tract. If the gut is in a stressed state, it will not absorb those nutrients nearly as well as if it is in a relaxed state."

Smoking Your Way to Heart Disease

Heart disease specifically related to smoking takes the life of an estimated 191,000 Americans every year. This is 44% more people than are killed by smoking-related lung cancer.[17] In other words, smoking can be worse for your heart than for your lungs. It also endangers the heart health of those around you. An estimated 37,000 to 40,000 people are killed annually by cardiovascular disease caused by secondary smoke, according to the American Heart Association.

Recent research shows that habitual exposure to secondary smoke almost doubles the risk of heart attack and death in non-smokers. The level of risk (91% higher), determined in a ten-year study of 32,000 women, is far greater than scientists previously thought. The study also found that even occasional exposure produced a 58% higher risk. "The 4,000 chemicals in tobacco smoke just about do everything that we know that is harmful to the heart," Dr. Ichiro Kawachi, of the Harvard School of Public Health, said. "They will damage the lining of the arteries, increase the stickiness of your blood, and therefore increase the chances that you will develop clotting and develop a heart attack."[18]

Until recently, nicotine was thought to be the main culprit in blood vessel constriction, plaque buildup, and reduced blood flow to the heart, and, thus, the link between smoking and heart disease. Now, researchers have identified a substance that is elevated in the blood of smokers and which they believe is behind smoking's damaging effects on the cardiovascular system. Called advanced glycation endproducts (AGEs), these substances are created during the tobacco drying process. AGEs produce sugars which are absorbed from the lungs into the smoker's bloodstream. There, the sugars act like "molecular glue," attaching to arterial walls and eventually creating a blockage.[19]

Exercise is Essential for Heart Health

Research has clearly established exercise as a vital component in maintaining the health of your heart and preventing cardiovascular disease. "Even ten minutes of extra exercise per day can significantly reduce the risk of heart disease," says Dr. Cowden. However, many people have difficulty building a regular program of exercise into their lives. In the following section, **David Essel, M.S.**, provides some helpful tips to accomplish this.

Four Steps to Better Heart Fitness Through Exercise

As mentioned earlier, cardiovascular disease is the leading cause of death in the United States. The reasons for this are varied, but most experts believe the main cause has to do with daily lifestyle choices. The way we deal with stress, the foods we eat, and how we take care of our bodies through exercise—all have a health impact on our cardiovascular system.

It has been well documented for more than 30 years that exercise can have a dramatic effect on enhancing heart health. Yet, according to the U.S. Centers for Disease Control and Prevention, only 12%-18% of the U.S. population exercises frequently enough to receive these benefits. One of the reasons the other 82%-88% don't exercise enough is a belief that they do not have enough time to gain any substantial health benefits from exercise.

The fact is, you don't need that much time to benefit. **Here are four hints for how to approach an exercise program and build cardiovascular fitness into your life.**

1. Move at least a little. Set a goal to walk, swim, skate, jump rope, aerobic dance, run or ride a bike three times a week for 20 minutes if possible, but even a ten-minute walk is better than nothing.

2. Exercise can help you control or lose weight. This will likely have a positive effect on your cardiovascular health. Again, the amount of time you exercise is not the most important factor; that you exercise at all is what counts. In a study in the *American Journal of Cardiology*, physicians showed that there was no significant difference in weight loss between a group that walked nonstop for 30 minutes, three times per week, and those who broke a daily walk into three sessions of ten minutes each.

Therefore, if you are seriously short of time, set a minimum goal of three daily walking sessions of 10 minutes each.

Here's to Your Health: Drinking and the Heart

A number of studies have concluded that moderate alcohol consumption—of red wine in particular—can be beneficial to the heart by raising HDL cholesterol levels and reducing the likelihood of blood clots, which can result in a heart attack. A new study challenges red wine's position as the drink of choice. Coronary heart disease patients who drank liquor, wine, or beer all experienced a lowered risk, although wine and beer lowered it more than liquor.[20]

Before you start imbibing, you might want to consider the results of another recent study. University of Wisconsin-Madison researchers compared purple grape juice, white grape juice, and red wine in terms of their heart-protective effects. Purple grape juice was found to be as beneficial as red wine, and possibly more so.[21] Since alcohol consumption brings health risks along with its heart benefits, purple grape juice can provide a safe alternative.

"The 4,000 chemicals in tobacco smoke just about do everything that we know that is harmful to the heart," Dr. Ichiro Kawachi, of the Harvard School of Public Health, said. "They damage the lining of the arteries, increase the stickiness of your blood, and therefore increase the chances that you will develop clotting and develop a heart attack."

3. Increasing lean muscle tissue can im-prove your heart's health. A twice-weekly strength-training program using calisthenics, free weights, or exercise machines in which the major muscle groups of the body (chest, back, legs, etc.) are exercised for 1 to 3 sets of 8 to 12 rep-etitions, can increase lean muscle tissue. This allows the body to burn more calories during the day, thereby assisting in weight loss.

4. Keep to the program because exercise regularity is important. To stick with any program that enhances cardiovascular fitness, con-sider the following: Invite a friend to exercise with you one or several days each week. Schedule your exercise session in your daily planner so it has the same or higher priority as any other meeting for that day. Or use a walkman with your favorite music, book on tape, or motiva-tional audio to inspire (or entertain) you during your workout.

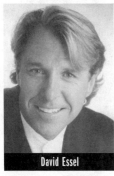

David Essel

David Essel, M.S., is a professional speaker and the host (through Westwood One Entertainment, Ft. Myers Beach, Florida) of the syndicated "positive talk" and lifestyle radio show, "David Essel—Alive!," heard in over 270 U.S. cities each weekend. To contact David: tel: 941-463-7702; fax: 941-463-4019; Internet: http://www.davidessel.com.

By following a regular exercise program, you may achieve a reduction in your blood pressure (if it was high), a reduction in the fatty substance triglyceride and LDL cholesterol levels (which can harm the heart), and an increase in HDL cholesterol (the kind that is beneficial to your system).

A regular exercise program could be one of the most important changes you make to improve your cardiovascular health. However, some peo-ple may find the prospect of moving from a sedentary to an active lifestyle daunting, even threatening. It need not be if you tailor your pro-gram to your likes and needs, move at your own speed, and respect your limits.

As people become more active, they also start to make healthier choices in the foods they eat and the way they handle stress. The benefi-cial combination created by this "trickle-down" effect may go far in reducing the number of cardiovascular-related deaths.

The Benefits of Exercise

Many studies provide evidence of the positive effects on the heart of regular exercise, including strengthening the heart muscle, improving blood flow, reducing high blood pressure, and raising HDL cholesterol levels while lowering

CAUTION
If you are in ill health or over the age of 40, check with your physician first.

LDL levels. The British Heart Foundation (BHF) reports that people who do not exercise are twice as likely to develop coronary heart disease as those who exercise on a regular basis. In addition, exercising moderately five times a week reduces your chances of dying from coronary heart disease. If people who exercise suffer a heart attack, their risk of dying from it is half that of those who do not exercise. The BHF recommends 30-minute exercise sessions that are aerobic in nature.[22]

Researchers at the University of Colorado in Boulder demonstrated that exercise is more important than advancing age as a factor in decreased heart function. Comparing older active women (average age of 61), older sedentary women (average age of 62), and young active women (average age of 29), the study showed that the heart health of the younger and older active women was almost the same, as measured by heartbeats per minute, amount of blood pumped with each beat, and the total blood volume pumped by the heart. The heart function of the older sedentary women, on the other hand, was significantly worse, with a six-beat-per-minute faster heartbeat, 24% less blood pumped with each beat, and a 23% lower total blood volume. In addition, the sedentary women were an average of 22 pounds heavier than the older, active women.

Researcher Bryan Hunt observed that this outcome lends weight to the view that "many changes in cardiovascular function typically attributed to aging are likely due to other factors such as age-related reduction in physical activity and increases in body fatness."[23]

As part of a cardiac rehabilitation program, resistive exercises can increase muscle strength and cardiovascular endurance, improve bone density and mineral content, facilitate a return to regular activities, and raise self-confidence.[24]

It is never too late to start exercising. In one study, a regular walking program produced a decrease in the heart rates of previously sedentary people in just 18 weeks.[25] The exercise need not be intensive aerobics. Tai chi, a slow, low-impact activity which never-

The British Heart Foundation (BHF) reports that people who do not exercise are twice as likely to develop coronary heart disease as those who exercise on a regular basis. If people who exercise suffer a heart attack, their risk of dying from it is half that of those who do not exercise.

theless increases the heart rate during practice, has been found to improve overall cardiovascular health.

Get Fit While Running in Place

It is common knowledge that exercising regularly can benefit your health in numerous ways, including losing weight and reducing your risk for cardiovascular disease, prostate cancer, and osteoporosis. But getting that regular exercise can be a problem. Your new year's resolution to join a gym fades quickly or inclement weather has a way of preventing that daily walk you promised yourself. Home exercise on a treadmill—used for walking or running in place—may be the answer.

A study by the Medical College of Wisconsin at Milwaukee[26] compared the effectiveness of the most common exercise machines: a treadmill, exercise cycle, rowing machine, cross-country skier, stair stepper, and combination cycle/upper body machine. The researchers found that "the treadmill machine induced higher rates of energy expenditure [measured by number of calories burned] and aerobic demands than the other exercise machines." Specifically, the treadmill produced the "greatest cardiorespiratory training stimulus during a given duration of exercise" and burned 700 calories/hour compared to 625 calories/hour for the stair stepper, and 500 calories/hour for the exercise bicycle.

In addition, the study measured the "rate of perceived exertion" (RPE) on the treadmill compared to the other exercise machines. RPE means how strenuous the subject felt the exercise was compared to how much energy was used in terms of calories burned.

The 13 subjects (eight men, five women) of the study were given a beginning fitness test and were then acclimated to the machines over a four-week period to establish their individual RPE values. The RPE value of an exercise

The following are a few **treadmill manufacturers**: Life Fitness, 10601 West Belmont Avenue, Franklin Park, IL 60131; tel: 800-877-3867 or 847-288-3300; fax: 847-288-3741. Precor Inc., 20001 North Creek Parkway, Bothell, WA 98041; tel: 800-4-PRECOR or 206-486-9292; fax: 206-486-3856. True Fitness Technology, Inc., 865 Hoff Road, O'Fallon, MO 63366; tel: 800-426-6570 or 314-272-7100; fax: 314-272-7148. Star Trac by Unisen, Inc., 14352 Chambers Road, Tustin, CA 92780; tel: 800-228-6635 or 714-669-1660; fax: 714-838-6286. Trotter Inc., 10 Trotter Drive, Medway, MA 02053; tel: 800-677-6544 or 508-533-4300; fax: 508-533-5500.

turned out to be a major factor in how strenuously a person exercised. In other words, how hard you think you're exercising determines how many calories you actually burn during the exercise. Treadmills came out on top, with a 40% greater energy expenditure, burning more calories at all levels of perceived exertion than the other exercise equipment.

Whatever your initial fitness level, treadmills can provide the kind of workout you need, from gentle to strenuous. Even a moderate program on the treadmill can help you control your weight, guard against heart disease, and reduce your cholesterol levels by providing a regular cardiovascular workout. It can also improve your muscle tone, reduce your stress level for greater emotional stability, and improve your mood and self-esteem.

Pedal Your Way to a Healthier Heart

A popular choice among types of home exercise equipment is the stationary bicycle because it is easy to use, can accommodate all fitness levels, takes up a small amount of space, and provides the exercise you need for good heart fitness.

That stationary bicycles can be beneficial for any fitness level is demonstrated by the fact that they are used in many physical rehabilitation programs. Stationary bicycles are gentle on the back and joints (hips, knees, and ankles, especially)

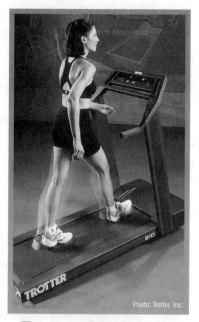

Photo: Trotter, Inc.

The researchers found that "the treadmill machine induced higher rates of energy expenditure [measured by number of calories burned] and aerobic demands than the other exercise machines." Specifically, the treadmill produced the "greatest cardiorespiratory training stimulus during a given duration of exercise."

It is never too late to start exercising. A regular walking program produced a decrease in the heart rates of previously sedentary people in just 18 weeks.

and, unlike running or walking, they provide a nonimpact workout that is nonetheless effective in strengthening the heart and lungs.

A recent French study (*Archives des Maladies du Coeur et des Vaisseaux*, 1996) compared fitness tests of elderly patients (over 65 years old) with a second group 65 years old and younger.[27] Exercise tests were conducted on stationary bicycles during each patient's period of hospital admission for heart surgery.

The results showed a 21% increase in power output and a 28% increase in duration of the elderly patients' exercise periods compared to 25% and 28%, respectively, in the younger group. In other words, the bikes helped both groups of heart patients exercise harder and longer. All patients showed significant improvement in fitness levels without any serious complications.

QUICK DEFINITION

Heart rate is the number of heartbeats (contractions of the ventricle chambers) per unit of time, usually expressed as beats per minute (bpm). **Maximum heart rate (MHR)** can be calculated by subtracting your age from 220 (e.g., a 50-year-old would have an MHR of 170); an individual's MHR will vary slightly from this figure depending on height and body type. Heart monitors on exercise equipment use **heart-rate training zones**, which are percentages of the maximum heart rate. Zone 1 is the easiest at 65% of MHR. Zone 2 is 65%-72%, or basic aerobic endurance. Zone 3 is 73%-80% of MHR, or higher aerobic capacity. Zones 4 (84%-90% of MHR) and 5 (91%-100% of MHR) are the most strenuous; as lactic acid builds up in the muscles, these can only be maintained for short periods.

How Exercise Helps the Heart—One way exercise improves cardiovascular fitness is by increasing the maximum cardiac output. This is the amount of blood pumped by the heart during a heartbeat. Since the maximum heart rate while exercising doesn't change (or may actually lower with continued training), the increase in the amount of blood pumped is due to physiological changes, enabling the heart to work more efficiently by pumping more blood with each beat. This means that your heart rate while at rest will also be lower (a good indicator of your fitness level).

Oxygen consumption—how efficiently your muscles use oxygen—is another measure of cardiovascular fitness. As muscles develop and strengthen through exercise, more capillaries form to supply blood to the muscles; the muscle fibers become more active and can extract more oxygen from the blood with each heartbeat. The increased cardiac output and greater lung capacity that result from regular exercise also support greater oxygen use. When the muscles are not extracting enough oxygen, they deplete their own stores of carbohydrates and lactic acid builds up in the fibers, leading to fatigue and diminished performance.

One of the easiest ways to measure your cardiovascular

fitness—whether or not your heart and muscles are operating at capacity—is by your heart rate. If, after exercising strenuously for ten to 12 minutes, your heart rate is within ten bpm (beats per minute) of the ideal maximum heart rate for your age, then you are probably processing oxygen optimally.

This is why many stationary bikes use heart rate monitors to tailor workout programs to heart rate training "zones." These zones are based on percentages of your maximum heart rate and help you measure your fitness level and set training goals. Using a stationary bike is one of the best ways to get an intense cardiovascular workout because you can focus on heart-rate training without the distractions of road biking.

For those looking for an effective way of recovering from severe congestive heart failure, a regular workout on an exercise bicycle (or treadmill) can be of considerable benefit. German researchers found that 18 patients hospitalized with this condition experienced improvements in

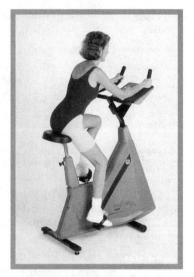

For those looking for an effective way of recovering from severe congestive heart failure, a regular workout on an exercise bicycle (or treadmill) can be of considerable benefit.

their breathing capacity and a reduction in the symptoms of congestive heart failure after only three weeks of specialized exercising.[28] Specifically, they used an exercise bicycle for 15 minutes five times weekly, did treadmill walking for ten minutes, and practiced other exercises for 20 minutes three times weekly.

Lose Weight While Pedaling in Place—Using a stationary bike can also assist weight loss by burning calories. As with other forms of aerobic exercise, there is an additional weight-control benefit from exercising regularly. It increases your basal metabolism rate (BMR). This is the number of calories used by the body at complete rest to maintain basic life processes such as respiration and circulation. It's a bit like gasoline consumption while your car is idling.

Even a moderate exercise schedule—30-40 minutes, three to four times per week—can raise your BMR. Even better, the physiology is such that you burn additional calories for approximately 12 hours immediately after exercise because of having elevated your BMR. This can amount to as much as 15% of the calories burned during your workout, a significant number when you're trying to lose weight.[29]

Stopping a Heart Attack with Your Hands

There are particular locations on your body called "Energy Sphere Points"—when you press on them with your fingers, you can stop a heart attack, seizure, or asthma fit, or give yourself a whole body energy massage, says Glenn King, director of the Glenn King Institute for Better Health in Dallas, Texas.

King is the foremost U.S. practitioner of a little-known Asian art called *Ki-Iki-Jutsu*, which means, literally, "breath of life art." More practically, it's a finger-delivered form of therapy that "allows the body by its own tremendous power to heal itself by unconstricting any stagnation or blockage of the natural energy circulatory patterns," King explains.

Subtle bodily energy (known in Chinese medicine as *Qi*, and presented by King as *Ki*) flows along regular pathways throughout the body. Press on the right points and you can treat seizures (as King experienced personally), chronic pain, insomnia, depression, migraines, memory loss, lymph disorders, and other more serious health conditions.

■ Stopping a Heart Attack—If you are witnessing someone having a heart attack, place your hand on the person's fifth thoracic vertebra (the twelfth vertebra down from the top of the neck, see illustration, p. 68) and with your other hand hold the little finger of the person's left hand. "This prompt action has consistently stopped heart attacks in progress," states King. This process can shift a person from being on the verge of entering cardiac arrest into a state of no sign of heart arrhythmia, pain, or discoloration within two minutes, on average, King says, adding that these results have been confirmed by cardiologists.

■ Whole-Body Energy Tonic—Use this simple exercise to revitalize the circulation of energy throughout your body, relax tension,

To contact some specific manufacturers of **stationary bicycles:** Fitness Master, 504 Industrial Boulevard, Waconia, MN 55387; tel: 800-328-8995 or 612-442-4454; fax: 612-442-5655. Tectrix, 68 Fairbanks, Irvine, CA 92718; tel: 800-767-8082 or 714-380-8082; fax: 714-380-8710; www.tectrix.com. Cateye Ergocisers (Fuji America), 118 Bauer Drive, Oakland, NJ 07436; tel: 800-631-8474 or 201-337-1700; fax: 201-337-1762. Life Fitness, 10601 W. Belmont Avenue, Franklin Park, IL 60131; tel: 800-877-3867 or 847-288-3300; fax: 847-288-3707.

CAUTION

These are emergency, first-aid techniques; they are not curative. If you have any of these conditions, consult a qualified health practitioner for professional long-term treatment.

Original material supplied by **Glenn King,** Glenn King Institute for Better Health, 3530 Forest Lane, Suite 60, Dallas, TX 75234; tel: 214-902-9266; fax: 214-902-0091.

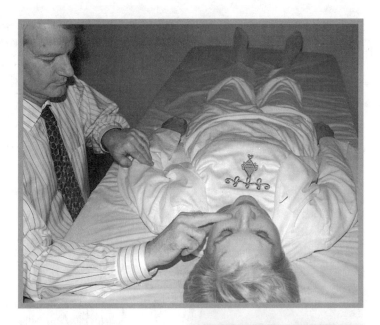

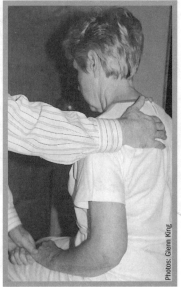

Glenn King demonstrates *Ki-Iki-Jutsu* techniques for stopping a heart attack and addressing related heart conditions such as arrhythmia, fibrillation, and angina.

Photos: Glenn King

promote mental alertness, and improve sleep, King advises. Only light finger contact, not pressure, is required. Use the finger pads of your index, middle, and ring fingers. Lie down on a comfortable surface. The sequence of eight steps should take about 24 minutes.

Step 1: Place your right hand on the top center of your head; place your left hand between the eyebrows. Hold for 3 minutes. *Keep your right hand in this location until you reach step 8.*

Step 2: Place your left hand at the tip of your nose; hold for 3 minutes.

67

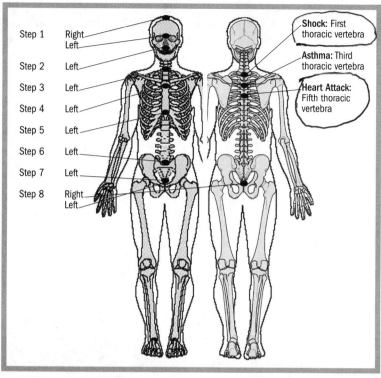

Step 1 Right
        Left

Step 2 Left

Step 3 Left

Step 4 Left

Step 5 Left

Step 6 Left

Step 7 Left

Step 8 Right
        Left

Shock: First thoracic vertebra

Asthma: Third thoracic vertebra

Heart Attack: Fifth thoracic vertebra

Location of *Ki-Iki-Jutsu* treatment points

Step 3: Place your left hand at the center of your collarbone; hold for 3 minutes.

Step 4: Place your left hand at the center of your chest; hold for 3 minutes.

Step 5: Place your left hand at the bottom of your sternum; hold for 3 minutes.

Step 6: Place your left hand at your navel; hold for 3 minutes.

Step 7: Place your left hand at the top center of your pubic bone; hold for 3 minutes.

Step 8: Place your right hand at the tip of your tail bone or coccyx; hold for 3 minutes.

Eating onions and apples and drinking black tea can also contribute to heart health. These items contain high concentrations of quercetin, a bioflavonoid, and are inversely associated with coronary heart disease mortality rates. In other words, the more onions, apples, and black tea you consume, the lower your risk of dying from heart disease. A recent study found that men in the highest third dietary level of the bioflavonoid quercetin had a 53% lower risk of coronary heart disease than those in the lowest third.

Scrubbing the Arteries Naturally

HOW CHELATION THERAPY CAN HELP PREVENT AND TREAT HEART DISEASE

THERE IS MOUNTING EVIDENCE that chelation therapy offers an alternative to the hundreds of thousands of bypass surgeries and angioplasties performed each year. In this therapy, the nontoxic synthesized chemical EDTA (ethylene-diamine-tetra-acetic acid) is given intravenously to remove plaque and calcium deposits from the arterial walls and then the unwanted material is excreted through the urine.

Beginning in the 1940s, the U.S. Navy used EDTA to safely and successfully treat lead poisoning. EDTA was also traditionally used to remove calcium from pipes and boilers. Norman Clarke, Sr., M.D., Director of Research at Providence Hospital in Detroit, Michigan, hypothesized that because calcium plaque is a prominent component in atherosclerosis, EDTA would be an effective treatment for heart conditions. His experiments confirmed his theory, and angina patients treated by Dr. Clarke reported dramatic relief from chest pain. For many patients, memory, sight, hearing, and sense of smell improved, and most reported increased vigor.[1]

In a study completed in 1989, every patient suffering from a vascular disease who was treated with chelation therapy showed a measurable improvement midway through the course of treatment.[2] A second study showed that 88% of the patients receiving chelation therapy exhibited improved blood flow to the brain.[3]

Charles Farr, M.D., Ph.D., of Oklahoma City, Oklahoma, co-founder of the American Board of Chelation Therapy, reports that during the past 20-plus years, he has given more than 500,000 chelation treatments to over 20,000 patients, 60% to 70% of which were for some form of cardiovascular disease or circulatory problems. He reports very positive results in 70% to 80% of the cases. "Many of our patients who were originally scheduled to have bypass surgery or angioplasty continue to be healthy today, some 10 to 15 years past the time they were supposed to die if they did not have the surgery." According to Dr. Farr, chelation is remarkably effective in removing arterial plaque and dissolving clots, as well as in softening up and dilating the blood vessels and allowing nutrients to get to damaged tissues.

> **"Many of our patients who were originally scheduled to have bypass surgery or angioplasty continue to be healthy today, some ten to 15 years past the time they were supposed to die if they did not have the surgery," reports Charles Farr, M.D., Ph.D.**

Dr. Farr reports the case of a man who had several episodes of cardiovascular disease and who had been told by his doctor that he would die if he did not have immediate bypass surgery. Deciding against surgery, the man, who was unable to walk, went to Dr. Farr and, despite the protests of his family, began chelation therapy. Within 45 days, he had gone back to his job of running a construction company and continued to work for many years.

Researchers L. Terry Chappell, M.D., and John P. Stahl, Ph.D., recently reviewed the results of 19 studies evaluating the effectiveness of EDTA chelation therapy on 22,765 patients. They found that 87% registered clinical improvement according to objective tests. In one study, 58 out of 65 bypass candidates and 24 of 27 people scheduled for limb amputation were able to cancel their surgery after chelation therapy. The analysis provides "very strong evidence that EDTA is effective in the treatment of cardiovascular disease," state Chappell and Stahl.[4]

Efrain Olszewer, M.D., and James P. Carter, M.D., reviewed the cases of 2,870 patients with hardening of the arteries and other age-associated diseases who were treated with EDTA chelation therapy and vitamin/mineral supplementation between 1983 and 1985 at the

In one study, 58 out of 65 bypass candidates and 24 of 27 people scheduled for limb amputation were able to cancel their surgery after chelation therapy.

Clinica Tuffik Mattar in Sao Paulo, Brazil. According to their results, marked improvement occurred in 76.9% of patients with ischemic heart disease (coronary artery blockage) and 91% of patients with peripheral vascular disease. In addition, 75% of all patients had reductions in vascular symptoms and, overall, 89% had benefits rated as "good."[5]

Chelation therapy can also relieve chest pain, according to a study involving 18 patients, 45-73 years old, with heart disease, conducted by H. Richard Casdorph, M.D. (*Journal of Advancement in Medicine*, 1989). After 20 chelation infusions, "all patients improved clinically and in all but two there was a complete subsidence of angina during the course of chelation therapy," said Dr. Casdorph.

Chelation Therapy Success Stories

Before we explain in more detail how chelation works, let's look at some actual case studies of successfully treating heart disease with chelation therapy. Michael B. Schachter, M.D., director of the Schachter Center for Complementary Medicine in Suffern, New York, sees many patients who have heart disease and has found chelation extremely useful. Here are two of his cases:

David, 50, had three angioplasties during a six-month period. This kept the veins open twelve, eight, and ten weeks, respectively. When his cardiologist recommended a fourth angioplasty, he chose chelation therapy instead. On his first visit to Dr. Schachter, four months after his last angioplasty, David could walk only two city blocks without severe chest pains. After 24 EDTA infusions, he could walk for 60 to 90 minutes three times weekly with little or no discomfort, and his cardiac-medication use had been reduced by 50%.

Dr. Schachter's anti-cancer protocols are featured in *An Alternative Medicine Definitive Guide to Cancer* (Future Medicine Publishing, 1997); to order, call 800-333-HEAL.

Ending 11 Years of Angina

William began suffering from angina pectoris at the age of 25. By 29, bearing a clinical diagnosis of coronary artery disease, William had undergone three balloon angioplasties (which produced short-term improvement, for, respectively, one, three, and 18 months) and a quintuple heart bypass, then, four years later, a heart attack. Following these poor results with conventional medicine, William, then 33, was referred to the Schachter Center for an alternative approach.

Dr. Schachter started William on a comprehensive program including EDTA chelation therapy, nutritional supplements, an exercise regimen, and dietary changes. William's intravenous chelation, administered over a 3½ hour period, consisted of the basic EDTA solution and support nutrients such as ascorbic acid, magnesium sulfate, pantothenic acid, potassium chloride, and heparin (a blood thinner), among others. He would receive chelation once weekly for 30 months, then twice monthly for ten months, then once a month indefinitely.

William also began an intensive daily nutritional supplementation program including:

- potassium (99 mg, 4X)
- vitamin C (1,000 mg, 2X)
- vitamin E (400 IU, 4X)
- coenzyme Q10 (60 mg, 2X)
- Ultra Preventive (a multivitamin/ mineral, 2 tablets, 3X)
- L-carnitine (250 mg, 2X)
- L-taurine (500 mg, 2X)
- beta carotene (25,000 IU, 1X)
- amino acid capsules (3X)
- vitamin B6 (250 mg, 1X)

To replace the good minerals which are removed along with the toxins in EDTA chelation, William took extra minerals in the form of:

- Tri-Boron Plus (3X) which includes calcium (1,000 mg)
- magnesium (500 mg)
- zinc (25 mg)
- copper (2 mg)
- manganese (10 mg)
- boron (3 mg).

His program also included:

- selenium (250 mcg, 2X)
- zinc picolinate (1X)
- copper (4 mg, 1X)

Finally, Dr. Schachter gave William

Is EDTA Chelation Therapy Cost-Effective?

A recent Danish study says yes. Of 470 cardiovascular patients treated with EDTA chelation therapy, 85% improved. Of 72 patients on a waiting list for coronary bypass surgery, 65 did not require bypass following chelation. Of 30 patients referred for leg amputation, only three required amputation. Aside from the reduced human suffering, the estimated cost savings to the Danish government was $3 million. If EDTA chelation therapy were widely used in the U.S., the estimated cost savings for coronary artery bypass surgery alone would be $8 billion a year.

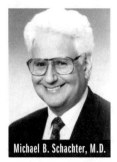

Michael B. Schachter, M.D.

"It was the *combination* of chelation, supplementation, exercise, and diet that gave him such beautiful results," Dr. Schachter says. "I don't think he would have done as well if any one of these four components had been left out."

Ultra GLA (high-potency borage oil rich in gamma linolenic acid, which is important for balancing the essential fatty acids in patients with cardiovascular disease), lecithin capsules (1,350 mg, 4X), lysine (500 mg, 6X), grapeseed extract (50 mg, 1X), and pine bark pycnogenol (50 mg, 1X).

Regarding exercise, the third component of Dr. Schachter's approach, William underwent a cardiac rehabilitation program. His heart rate was monitored as he exercised on a treadmill. As the chelation therapy and nutrient program began to have an effect, William was able to exercise longer and harder without any evidence of heart strain. In medical jargon, his cardiogram showed he had a "negative heart stress test." In fact, William was able to exercise for between 90 and 120 minutes four days a week using aerobic, circuit, and weight-training equipment.

Lastly, Dr. Schachter recommended that William make major dietary changes. These included a low- to moderate-fat, high-fiber diet of whole grains, fruits, and vegetables, with modest amounts of nuts, seeds, fish, and organic chicken, and restricted intake of eggs and dairy products. He was also advised to avoid tobacco smoke, alcohol, sugar, white flour, "junk food," caffeine, artificial sweeteners, preservatives, food additives, pesticides, chlorinated water, fluoride in all forms (including toothpaste), margarine, and aluminum cookware, says Dr. Schachter. This same dietary regimen, he adds, is often given to Schachter Center patients with cancer.

William fared excellently under this fourfold plan, reports Dr. Schachter. It's interesting to note that six years before starting the Schachter program, William had started taking vitamins, watching his weight, and controlling his cholesterol, but this had failed to improve his condition. "It was the *combination* of chelation, supplementation, exercise, and diet that gave him such beautiful results," Dr. Schachter says. "I don't think he would have done as well if any one of these four components had been left out."

"I feel healthier and have a sense of well-being and security that was not there after the bypass," says William. In Dr. Schachter's words, William's treatment resulted in "subjective and objective improvement and full recovery so that he now works full-time and frequently outperforms his law enforcement colleagues in physical endurance activities. He has had no heart attacks in four years and his stress tests keep improving rather than getting worse, as is usual with this disease."

Ironically, William's insurance company refused to reimburse him for the chelation therapy despite the clinical proof of its efficacy. "Yet they loved paying for his dramatic heart surgeries that didn't help him," notes Dr. Schachter. During the course of William's treatments at the Schachter Center, his cardiologist, whom he was still seeing every six months, took him off all his conventional heart drugs except for lovastatin for cholesterol management.

To a large extent, Dr. Schachter's views on complementarity highlight his attitude about how to approach most health problems: "I believe that in many cases, patients who select *only* the alternative program and leave out the more

To contact **Michael Schachter, M.D.:** Schachter Center for Complementary Medicine, 2 Executive Boulevard, Suite 202, Suffern, NY 10901; tel: 914-368-4700; fax: 914-368-4727. Dr. Schachter is coauthor of the forthcoming book, *An Alternative Medicine Definitive Guide to the Prostate* (Future Medicine Publishing).

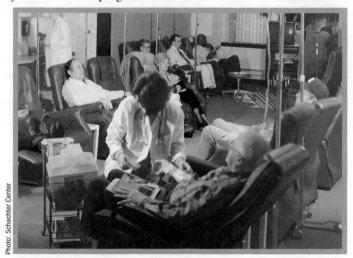

Photo: Schachter Center

Chelation therapy, given intravenously over a 1½- to 3-hour period, is a bit like *gently* scrubbing the inside of approximately 60,000 miles of arteries, veins, and capillaries to remove the deposits that have thickened and hardened the blood vessel walls, blocking blood flow.

The main way chelation reverses atherosclerosis is by removal of calcium plaque. Unabsorbed calcium floating in the bloodstream can build up in the tissues and joints and lead to the formation of plaque lesions on the inner walls of the arteries, making them thick and hardened, producing atherosclerosis.

destructive conventional treatment will do better."

Severe Angina Reversed in Three Months

Guillermo Asis, M.D., of the Marino Center for Progressive Health in Cambridge, Massachusetts, reports similar success treating angina with chelation, as illustrated by the following case study.

Albert, 70, had suffered with severe angina for almost ten years. He had an average of ten searing chest pains daily. In an attempt to correct this, his conventional physicians had performed 14 balloon angioplasties and one heart bypass surgery. By the time Albert came to Dr. Asis, Albert's doctors had essentially written him off as untreatable. They had advised him to take as much nitroglycerin as he needed to get pain relief.

To contact **Guillermo Asis, M.D.**: The Marino Center for Progressive Health, 2500 Massachusetts Avenue, Cambridge, MA 02140; tel: 617-661-6225; fax: 617-492-2002; Internet: www.allhealth.com. **Vitality Plus** is available from the Marino Health Store; tel: 800-456-LIFE or 617-661-6124.

"It was a serious case," says Dr. Asis. "His doctors literally did not know what else to do for Albert." However, in the view of Dr. Asis, Albert was medically treatable.

He put Albert on a once-weekly program of chelation therapy to improve his circulation and heart function. For approximately 3 hours per session, Albert sat comfortably in Dr. Asis' office receiving an intravenous infusion of EDTA, the prime substance used in chelation therapy.

In addition, Dr. Asis gave Albert "a very aggressive" multivitamin supplement called Vitality Plus (with high levels of the B vitamins, zinc, and copper) which he took six times daily. Albert also began taking magnesium aspartate (400 mg, four times daily) and zinc picolinate (50 mg daily). The reason for these two supplements is that the chelation process unavoidably flushes these minerals out of the body, so adequate levels of both must be restored, says Dr. Asis. Albert started taking grapeseed extract (50 mg, twice daily, as an antioxidant to help remove free-radical poisons) and selenium (200 mcg, twice daily, an antioxidant known to benefit the heart).

Within eight weeks, Dr. Asis was able to take Albert off all conventional heart medications. Even better, his angina symptoms were dramatically improved—Albert experienced only one incident of chest pain per month. Albert received a total of 12 chelation treatments. By the end of the three-month treatment, "virtually all of Albert's symptoms and discomfort were gone and he continues to do very well," says Dr. Asis.

Understanding Chelation Therapy

Chelation (key-LAY-shun) comes from the Greek word *chele* meaning "to claw" or "to bind." EDTA circulates through the blood vessels and binds to ("chelates") excess amounts of calcium, iron, copper, lead, or

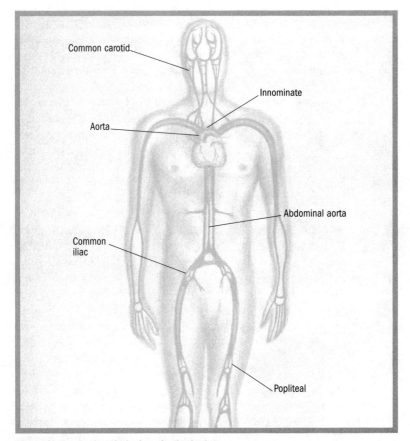

Sites of atherosclerotic lesions in the body

EDTA is nearly three-and-a-half times less toxic than common aspirin and 300 times safer than bypass surgery. Chelation therapy has been used safely on more than 500,000 patients in the United States for the past 40 years, without a single death attributable to EDTA when the American College for Advancement in Medicine (ACAM) protocol is followed.

other heavy metals; the EDTA along with the bound substance is then eliminated in urine.

The main way in which chelation reverses atherosclerosis is by removal of calcium plaque. Unabsorbed calcium floating in the bloodstream can build up in the tissues and joints and lead to the formation of plaque lesions on the inner walls of the arteries, making them thick and hardened, producing atherosclerosis. Calcium acts as a kind of glue that holds the plaque lesions together. These limit the amount of blood flow, reduce the supply of oxygen to body organs, and increase the risk of inappropriate blood clotting. The plaque lesions and the subsequent reduced oxygen supply can lead to heart attacks, coronary heart disease, and chest pain.

If you take an average 80-year-old man and examine his aorta, says Garry F. Gordon, M.D., D.O., a chelation pioneer and co-founder in 1973 of the American College for Advancement in Medicine, now in Laguna Hills, California, you will probably see evidence of 140 times more calcium than he had at age ten. "The abdominal artery shows a 50-fold increase, and the coronary

The aorta (the heart's major artery). The aorta of a typical 80-year-old man will probably show signs of 140 times more calcium than that of a 10-year-old; consequently, there will be greatly reduced blood flow.

Copyright © 1989-97 by TechPool Studios, Inc. USA

artery shows a 30-fold increase. This means you're gradually turning to stone in all your arteries. However, we can document that calcium accumulation in the arteries is totally reversible by enough chelation."

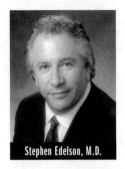

Stephen Edelson, M.D.

"Free radical pathology, it is now believed, is the underlying process triggering the development of most age-related ailments," says Dr. Edelson.

EDTA is closely related to vinegar, or ordinary acetic acid, says Dr. Gordon. "It's actually a weak acid; if you put an eggshell in vinegar, it will dissolve. In the same way, EDTA will take calcium off your arteries. Because EDTA ties up calcium so avidly, it was used by blood banks for 15 years to prevent blood from clotting. Once you tie up calcium, blood cannot clot." At the same time, EDTA does not deplete the body of calcium. By a surprising biochemical mechanism, chelation therapy actually stimulates bone growth and can help prevent osteoporosis. People do not die from atherosclerosis, says Dr. Gordon, but from *preventable* complications of blood vessel spasm (preventable by adequate magnesium intake), irregular heart rhythms (preventable by sufficient mineral intake), or blood clots.

Much of the long-term benefit of chelation therapy derives from its ability to slow down free-radical activity and undo the underlying cause of arterial blockage, says Dr. Gordon. "Damaging free radicals are increased by the presence of heavy metals and act as a chronic irritant to blood vessel walls and cell membranes." This free-radical activity is stimulated by excess heavy metals and minerals in the blood and plays a major role in the development of heart disease. "EDTA removes those metallic irritants, allowing leaky and damaged cell walls to heal."

According to Stephen F. Edelson, M.D., a progressive alternative physician who uses chelation therapy in his practice in Atlanta, Georgia, EDTA's ability to bind with and remove metals, such as iron, copper, lead, mercury, and cadmium, may be a more important factor in reducing heart disease than its effect on calcium plaque. These metals are powerful triggers of excessive free-radical reactions, Dr. Edelson explains. "Free radical pathology, it is now believed, is the underlying process triggering the development of most age-related ailments."

EDTA is nearly three-and-a-half times less toxic than common aspirin[6] and 300 times safer than bypass surgery. Chelation therapy has been used safely on more than 500,000 patients in the United States for the past 40 years, without a single death attributable to EDTA when the American College for Advancement in Medicine (ACAM) protocol is followed.[7] This makes it one of the safest therapies in modern medicine.

However, EDTA, the drug used during the infusions, has yet to receive FDA (Food and Drug Administration) approval for anything other than lead and heavy-metal toxicity. Still, there are over 1,000 physicians who recommend and use chelation therapy for cardiovascular disease and related health problems. Following the treatment protocol set by the American College of Advancement in Medicine and the American Board of Chelation Therapy, FDA-approved studies are currently underway to establish the safety of EDTA.

How Chelation Therapy is Administered

Chelation therapy is performed on an outpatient basis, is painless, and takes approximately 1½ to 3½ hours. For optimal results, physicians who use chelation therapy recommend 20 to 30 treatments given at an average rate of one to three per week, with patient evaluations being made at regular intervals.[8] There is no need to worry about a buildup of EDTA in the body. Chelation therapists state that within 24 hours 99% of the infused EDTA has been excreted.

The patient reclines comfortably while receiving an intravenous solution of EDTA with vitamins and minerals. To monitor the patient's progress, James Julian, M.D., of Los Angeles, California, recommends that the following tests be taken before, during, and after chelation:

- blood pressure and circulation
- cholesterol and other blood components
- pre- and post-vascular
- blood sugar and nutritional
- kidney and organ function
- tissue minerals, if indicated

A whole foods, low-fat diet and appropriate exercise are normally recommended as part of a full treatment program. According to Dr. Gordon, a carefully tailored program of vitamin and nutritional supplements should also be part of the treatment, and can include ascorbic acid (vitamin C), heparin, selenium, chromium, copper, zinc, and manganese. Smoking is strongly discouraged and alcohol should be consumed only in moderation. The cost per treatment can vary, depending in part on the nutritional ingredients the doctor chooses to use.

Conditions Benefited by Chelation Therapy

EDTA chelation therapy has proven safe and effective in the treatment and prevention of ailments linked to atherosclerosis, such as coronary artery disease (which can cause a heart attack), cerebrovascular disease (which can produce a stroke), peripheral vascular disease (leading to pain in the legs and, ultimately, gangrene), and arterial blockages from atherosclerosis elsewhere in the body.

Warren Levin, M.D., of New York City, once administered chelation therapy to a psychoanalyst on the staff of a major New York medical center. "He was in his fifties and looked remarkably healthy, except that he was in a wheelchair," says Dr. Levin. "He had awakened that morning to discover his lower leg was cold, numb, mottled, and blue, with two black-looking toes. He rushed to his hospital and consulted the chief of vascular surgery, who recommended an immediate amputation above the knee. He asked this world-renowned surgeon about the possibility of using chelation in this situation, and was told, 'Don't bother me with that voodoo.'

"The ailing man decided to get a second opinion. This physician also urged him to have an immediate amputation. When asked about chelation therapy, the second doctor's response was, 'You can try it if you want, but it's a waste of time.'

"Through his own tenacity, the psychoanalyst showed up in my office. We started emergency chelation and after approximately nine treatments—one taken every other day—he was pain-free and picking up. After approximately 17 chelation treatments, he was walking on the leg again. He never had an amputation, and he lived the rest of his life without any further complications."

Anecdotal stories of patient success tend to mean little to medical researcher Morton Walker, D.P.M. "But," he writes, "what must an investigative medical journalist do when exposed to story after story of potentially imminent death, blindness, amputation, paralysis, and other problems among people, and upon visiting those people to check their stories, finds them presently free of all signs of their former health problems? About 200 individuals who were victims of hardening of the arteries are ... [now] vibrant, productive, youthful looking, vigorous, full of zest, and enthusiastically endorse chelation therapy as the cause of their prolonged good health. I have turned up not a single untruth."[9]

Medical journalists Harold and Arline Brecher, who have written extensively about chelation therapy, note that physicians who use it not only advise it for their patients, but use it for themselves, unlike many of their orthodox colleagues. "We have yet to find a physician who offers chelation to his patients who does not chelate himself, his family, and friends," they report.

One study documented significant improvement in 99% of patients suffering from peripheral vascular disease and blocked arteries of the legs. Twenty-four percent of those patients with cerebrovascular and other degenerative cerebral diseases also showed marked improvement, with an additional 30% having good improvement. Overall, nearly 90% of all treated patients had marked or good improvement as a result of chelation therapy.[10]

A double-blind study in 1989 revealed that every patient suffering from peripheral vascular disease who was treated with chelation therapy showed a statistically significant improvement after only ten treatments.[11] In another study published in 1989, 88% of the patients receiving chelation therapy showed improvement in cerebrovascular blood flow.[12]

Other documented benefits of chelation therapy include:

- normalization of 50% of cardiac arrhythmias[13]
- improved cerebrovascular arterial occlusion[14]
- improved memory and concentration when diminished circulation is a cause[15]
- improved vision (with vascular-related vision difficulties)[16]
- significantly reduced cancer mortality rates (as a preventive)[17]
- protection against iron poisoning and iron storage disease[18]
- detoxification of snake and spider venoms[19]

According to Elmer Cranton, M.D., of Troutdale, Virginia, chelation therapy has a profound effect on overall health. "In my clinical experience there is no doubt that intravenous EDTA chelation therapy to some extent slows the aging process," says Dr. Cranton. "Allergies and chemical sensitivities also seem to improve somewhat due to a better functioning of the immune system. All types of arthritis and muscle and joint aches and pains seem to be more eas-

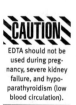

CAUTION

EDTA should not be used during pregnancy, severe kidney failure, and hypoparathyroidism (low blood circulation).

Angioplasty and Bypass
Surgery Do Not Extend Life

In 1992, Nortin Hadler, M.D., Professor of Medicine at the University of North Carolina School of Medicine, wrote that none of the 250,000 balloon angioplasties performed the previous year could be justified, and that only 3%-5% of the 300,000 coronary artery bypass surgeries done the same year were actually required. Yet a cost comparison study prepared for the Great Lakes Association of Clinical Medicine in 1993 estimated that $10 billion was spent in the United States in 1991 on bypass surgery alone.[20] At a symposium of the American Heart Association, Henry McIntosh, M.D., stated that bypass surgery should be limited to patients with crippling angina who do not respond to more conservative treatment.[21]

Elmer Cranton, M.D., of Troutdale, Virginia, estimates chelation therapy can help avoid bypass surgery in 85% of cases. He points out that during all the time that chelation therapy has been administered according to established protocol, not one serious side effect has been reported.

A study reported in the *New England Journal of Medicine* demonstrated the ineffectiveness of most angioplasty and bypass surgery procedures to extend life following a heart attack. Scientists at the University of Toronto in Ontario, Canada, studied the death rates for 224,258 U.S. and 9,444 Canadian heart patients. They found that at the end of one year following the heart attack, the death rate was 34% in both countries. The crucial difference, however, is that whereas 12% of U.S. heart attack patients received angioplasty, only 1.5% of Canadian heart patients did; further, while 11% of American heart patients have bypass surgery, only 1.4% of Canadians do.

U.S. patients are also far more likely to have coronary angiography (catherization of heart arteries) than Canadians, 34.9% to 6.7%. The only benefit to the various invasive heart procedures was a slight improvement in 30-day survival rates for Americans, 22.3%, compared to 21.4% for Canadians, a difference that disappeared after 12 months when the mortality rates evened out. The wastefulness and ineffectiveness of these invasive procedures are clearly appreciated in light of the following statistics. Between 1980 and 1992, the rate of coronary angiography in the U.S. grew by 163%, percutaneous coronary revascularization increased by 5946%, and coronary artery bypass surgery increased by 102%.

Comparatively, American patients receive these procedures, within 30 days of a heart attack, at a far higher rate than Canadians: angiography 5.2 times as often; angioplasty, 7.7 times; bypass surgery, 7.8 times. "The strikingly higher rates of use of cardiac procedures in the United States, as compared with Canada, do not appear to result in better long-term survival rates for elderly U.S. patients with acute myocardial infarction [heart attack]," the study directors concluded.[22]

Catheterization After Heart Attacks *Reduces* Lifespan

New data released by William E. Boden, M.D., of the Veterans Affairs Upstate Health Care System in Syracuse, New York, shows that heart surgery (specifically, catheterization, or angiography) given immediately following mild heart attacks does not extend the life of the heart patient. Dr. Boden tracked the health status of 920 heart attack patients for 30 months. Out of this group, 458 received a post–heart attack "conservative strategy," consisting of medications and treadmill and thallium tests as a way of monitoring their condition; the other 462 patients, who received "invasive therapy," underwent catheterization, which was followed by bypass or angioplasty for 45% of these patients.

Dr. Boden found that, within nine days, 21 of the invasive therapy group died, compared to six in the conservative strategy group. After 30 months, 80 patients from the invasive therapy group had died compared to only 59 in the conservative strategy group. This means catheterization, followed in almost half the cases by bypass or angioplasty, *increased* the death rate of heart attack survivors by 36%.[23]

According to Julian Whitaker, M.D., catheterization "leads to a dramatic increase in the use of bypass surgery and angioplasty because physicians then try to open up observed blockages to prevent future heart attacks or death." In catheterization, a catheter is threaded through arteries of the heart; a dye is injected, enabling the arteries to be tracked by X ray to pinpoint blockages in those arteries.[24]

---

ily controlled after chelation, although it is not a cure. In most cases, the progression of Alzheimer's disease will be slowed, and in some cases the improvement is quite remarkable and the disease does not seem to progress. Macular degeneration, a major cause of visual loss in the elderly, is often improved and almost always arrested or slowed in its progression by chelation therapy."

Chelation Therapy vs. Bypass Surgery and Angioplasty

Chelation therapy could save billions of dollars each year by preventing unnecessary coronary bypass surgeries, angioplasties, and other expensive procedures related to vascular disorders.

Each year nearly 300,000 bypass surgeries and 250,000 angioplasties are performed in the United States. Furthermore, nearly 20,000 deaths occur annually as a result of these procedures.[25] The risks of bypass surgery are obvious and, since the benefits are not long-lasting, many people have multiple bypass operations.

Angioplasty is a fairly brutal way of mechanically scrubbing the inside of arteries with an inflated balloon catheter to flatten deposits that have thickened to the point of being dangerous to health. The balloon expands the artery, allowing more blood to pass. The goal is to prevent heart disease and reduce the risk of

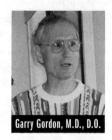

Garry Gordon, M.D., D.O.

"I firmly believe that an oral chelation program can do more for your overall longevity than you can do even with the most prudent lifestyle possible, because of the continuous nutritional protection chelation offers against a stressful and polluted world," says Dr. Gordon.

heart attack. According to cardiologist W. Lee Cowden, M.D., there is an 80% chance of a person's arteries blocking again within one year of undergoing angioplasty.

Oral Chelation

There are a variety of substances that act as oral chelating agents, according to Dr. Gordon. "Oral chelation is a well-documented, firmly established medical practice," he says. He points out that penicillamine, a drug used to treat heavy-metal poisoning, rheumatoid arthritis, and Wilson's disease (a rare metabolic disorder resulting in an excess accumulation of copper in the liver, red blood cells, and the brain), works in a fashion similar to EDTA. "Some of the benefits derived from penicillamine in the treatment of rheumatoid arthritis are undoubtedly related to the control and removal of excess free radicals.

"Oral chelation is an insurance policy to guarantee that you stay alive long enough to take intravenous chelation when and if you choose to," observes Dr. Gordon. "The oral approach has several major advantages, including convenience, potential long-term continuous health maintenance, and low cost. Its primary shortcoming is that it will take longer and require much more in quantity to get the same benefits as intravenous chelation."

Dr. Gordon notes that for years he has given his cardiac patients 800 mg daily of oral EDTA, of which he estimates only 3%-8% is absorbed compared to 100% of intravenous EDTA. This means it will take about 5 to 8 weeks of daily oral EDTA chelation to get the same effects of a single four-hour intravenous chelation, says Dr. Gordon.

Dr. Gordon also uses many nutritionally-based substances as oral chelators, such as garlic, vitamin C, carrageenan, zinc, and certain amino acids like cysteine and methionine. "Cysteine, for instance, is very effective in the treatment of nickel toxicity," he says, "and it seems to also increase glutathione in the body, which in turn helps to control free radicals." Dr. Gordon recently introduced his own oral chelation product called Garlic-EDTA Chelator™ (each capsule contains 400 mg garlic and 100 mg EDTA).

In his patients who use oral chelation formulas, Dr. Gordon has consistently observed a reduction of serum cholesterol by an average of 20% or more, which he feels significantly decreases the likelihood of atherosclerosis. "The thousands of patients who visit my clinic each year and follow our recommended oral chelation program have all successfully avoided strokes, and heart attack rates were also greatly diminished," he says. "We've never had more than two heart attacks per year among all of our patients, even among those with a history of severe heart disease. I firmly believe that an oral chelation program can do more for your overall longevity than you can do even with the most prudent lifestyle possible, because of the continuous nutritional protection chelation offers against a stressful and polluted world."

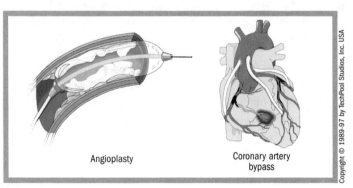

Angioplasty   Coronary artery
                                    bypass

Copyright © 1989-97 by TechPool Studios, Inc. USA

Angioplasty is a surgical procedure to open partially-blocked blood vessels. Also known as balloon angioplasty, this procedure inserts a balloon-tipped catheter into the clogged blood vessel, where the balloon is inflated, flattening the plaque causing the blockage against the vessel wall and increasing blood flow.

Coronary artery bypass is a surgical procedure which creates a pathway around a blocked blood vessel. One to five vein grafts (usually from the patient's leg) are attached from the aorta to a point on a coronary artery past the obstruction.

Cardiologist W. Lee Cowden, M.D., argues that a precise combination of nutritional substances and dietary factors can "cause the body to spontaneously, naturally break down the plaque, pull it off the arterial walls, and produce an effect that is equivalent to the chelation process."

Dr. Gordon does not recommend oral chelation as a substitute for intravenous chelation therapy, however. "There is a significant difference in both the rapidity and degree of benefits achieved with intravenous chelation over any currently available oral chelation agents," he says. "And the intravenous approach is clearly the proper choice for patients who have only a few months to get well before facing surgery or worse." But for patients whose conditions are not as drastic, as well as for those who want to optimally safeguard themselves against free radicals and plaque buildup, Dr. Gordon views oral chelation as an effective, noninvasive, inexpensive choice.

However, in Dr. Gordon's view, EDTA-based oral chelation can provide "automatic protection against the clotting process, as well as lowering a patient's lead level, so that they will have a higher functioning immune system, higher IQ, and better coordination."

When platelets, the factors in blood that produce clotting, become "sticky," they tend to clump together or aggregate, and this sets up conditions for excessive and unwanted blood clotting, explains Dr. Gordon. This in turn promotes the formation of vessel-thickening plaque and an increased risk of heart attack and stroke. While conventional drugs such as aspirin and coumadin are given to circumvent this problem, Dr. Gordon notes, these approaches are "dangerous and far less effective" than a comprehensive oral chelation approach.

Dr. Gordon also notes that intravenous chelation cannot provide 24-hour-a-day protection against the main causes of sudden death from heart problems and that this is where oral chelation finds its niche. "Continuous protection is afforded by an oral chelation program," Dr. Gordon says. He claims that "in the last 14 years, new heart attacks and/or strokes have been virtually nonexistent in my patients on this oral chelation program."

Garlic, taken alone, is an excellent chelator of metals such as lead and mercury, says Dr. Gordon. "Now, if you add EDTA to it, you get more removal of lead, but you also enhance the garlic's anti-platelet [anti-blood-clotting] activity. Through this combined action, since

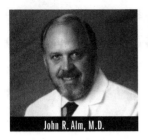

Six weeks after starting the TriCardia+ program, Colin's heart "spontaneously converted to a normal rhythm and has stayed that way for three months," Dr. Alm reports.

John R. Alm, M.D.

EDTA binds with the calcium that is required for blood to clot, you can protect yourself far more effectively against a blood clot, even more so than any aspirin dose you might take."

As a supplement to oral chelation with EDTA, Dr. Gordon recommends OC Packs, a heart nutrient program he originally customized for his patients in the early 1980s. These nutrients represent an "important part of the insurance policy" to prevent death from heart disease, says Dr. Gordon.

A Pill Instead of Angioplasty

John R. Alm, M.D., a physician practicing in Vista, California, views oral chelation as a viable way of "roto-rootering" the cardiovascular system and of detoxifying the liver and kidneys, the system's main filters. Dr. Alm works with the new Cardio-Care line of oral chelation products including Buffer-pH+, TriCardia+, and Systemex. This is a three-step, three-month program designed by Växa International, a maker of homeopathic formulas based in San Diego, California. The concept here is to detoxify, balance, and nourish the cardiovascular system, says Dr. Alm, who is a member of Växa's medical advisory board.

First, Buffer-pH+ helps to restore a more alkaline pH in the body. An acid pH is regarded as the "seed-bed of degenerative disease," including most forms of heart disease. Most people are in a constant state of acidosis, in which their system is overly acidified, primarily from a faulty diet, explains Dr. Alm. This in turn leads to a kind of "corrosion" of the blood vessel linings; in a curious way, hardening of the arteries may emerge as the "body's protective reaction" to this acidic state, Dr. Alm speculates.

"In an acid environment, heavy metals tend to bind with cholesterol which then adheres to vessel linings and attracts fibrin [blood-clotting protein] and other debris, building layer upon layer, eventually becoming a cement of plaque blocking arteries." This decreases blood flow which further acidifies the body's tissues.

However, when the pH is balanced again, heavy metals remain free and unbonded, while those that were previously bonded are easier to remove with EDTA in the program's second element, TriCardia+, says Dr. Alm.

TriCardia+ contains 32 amino acids including EDTA, plus home-opathic ingredients, lipids, enzymes, and herbal ingredients. The product is intended to remove plaque and debris from the circulatory system using EDTA with other orally-delivered chelating agents, says Dr. Alm. Systemex, the third element in Växa's Cardio-Care program, is a liquid meal-replacement formula designed to nutritionally support the cardiovascular system. The formula is fat-free and lactose-free and contains proteins, complex carbohydrates, essential fatty acids, amino acids, and 36 vitamins and minerals.

A reasonable question often raised is whether oral EDTA is absorbed as well as that taken intravenously. According to Gregory C. D. Young, Ph.D., Växa president, "Assimilation of EDTA is effective when it is taken either intravenously or orally." Dr. Young states that, even though EDTA is a synthetic amino acid, "in free form it biochemically behaves and is absorbed in exactly the same way as other free-form (or unbound) amino acids." It bypasses the digestive system entirely and, owing to its small molecular size, enters the bloodstream through the first segment of the small intestine, says Dr. Young. He estimates that, just as with other free-form amino acids, about 80% of oral EDTA is assimilated by the body in the first 20 minutes, the rest following within 90 minutes.

"The notion that EDTA is not absorbed, is in some way destroyed, or suffers from diminished potency when given orally, is unfounded and contradicts the experience of the U.S. Navy in the late 1940s," says Dr. Young. "At that time thousands of sailors benefited from simple oral administration of EDTA for lead toxicity."

Until further definitive research is performed or made public, absorption rates for oral EDTA will have to be placed *somewhere* between Dr. Gordon's 3%-8% and Dr. Young's 80%-100%. Växa's Cardio-Care program has not been on the market long enough—it was introduced in late 1996—for there to be much clinical evidence supporting its claims. However, Dr. Alm offers the following case report showing good results using this approach.

Colin, 74, had chronic high blood pressure and a 20-year history of arrhythmia, and had suffered a series of

QUICK DEFINITION

The term **pH**, which means "potential hydrogen," represents a scale for the relative acidity or alkalinity of a solution. Acidity is measured as a pH of 0.1 to 6.9, alkalinity is 7.1 to 14, and neutral pH is 7.0. The numbers refer to how many hydrogen atoms are present compared to an ideal or standard solution. Normally, blood is slightly alkaline, at 7.35 to 7.45; urine pH can range from 4.8 to 7.5, although normal is closer to 7.0.

Dr. Cowden's Daily Oral Nutritional Chelation Program for Brandon

- Vitamin E: 2,000 IU
- Vitamin C: to bowel tolerance (slightly less than the amount that produces diarrhea)
- Bioflavonoids (vitamin C helpers): 2,000 mg
- Grapeseed extract: 200 mg
- EPA (eicosapentaenoic acid): 1,200 mg
- DHA (docosahexaenoic acid): 400 mg
- Fish oils: 400 mg
- Lysine (amino acid): 4,000 mg
- Proline (amino acid): 4,000 mg
- L-taurine (amino acid): 2,000 mg
- Hawthorn berry: 1 capsule, 3X
- *Ginkgo biloba*: 40 mg, 3X
- Cool Cayenne: to bowel tolerance (the amount that causes slight rectal burning on defecation)
- Super Garlic: 3X
- Chorella: 6 capsules, 2X
- Magnesium: 300 mg, 3X
- Vitamin B6: 100 mg
- Vitamin B complex: B1 (thiamine), 100 mg; B2 (riboflavin), 100 mg; B3 (niacin), 100 mg; B5 (pantothenic acid), 100 mg; B6 (pyridoxine), 100 mg; choline, 100 mg; inositol, 100 mg; PABA (para-aminobenzoic acid), 100 mg; B12, 100-400 mcg; folic acid, 400 mcg

strokes after being put on a blood-thinning drug. The strokes produced a partial paralysis and considerable weakness of his right arm and leg, says Dr. Alm. Six weeks after starting the TriCardia+ program, Colin's heart "spontaneously converted to a normal rhythm and has stayed that way for three months," Dr. Alm reports.

Obviously more clinical evidence will be required before it is known for certain if the persuasive theory behind Växa's oral chelation program is borne out.

Chelating Brandon with Diet and Nutritional Substances

Cardiologist W. Lee Cowden, M.D., of the Conservative Medicine Institute in Richardson, Texas, believes that oral EDTA is not "particularly effective" for arterial plaque. But he argues that a precise combination of nutritional substances and dietary factors can "cause the body to spontaneously, naturally break down the plaque, pull it off the arterial walls, and produce an effect that is equivalent to the chelation process."

As evidence, Dr. Cowden cites the case of Brandon, 57, who had severe disease in three coronary arteries. His physicians were strongly urging him to undergo angioplasty and even Dr. Cowden, a long-time advocate of progressive alternatives in medicine,

Patients interested in chelation therapy should choose a doctor who follows the protocol of the American Board of Chelation Therapy or the American College for Advancement in Medicine.

regarded Brandon's condition as dangerous. "I've never had anyone in my office so close to having a heart attack without yet having one," he comments. An echocardiogram revealed that 60% of one heart quadrant was immobilized and the rest was working poorly. Despite the risk, Brandon refused to be hospitalized and asked Dr. Cowden for home-care strategies.

Dr. Cowden put Brandon on a strict vegetarian diet, emphasizing mostly raw fresh foods, whole grains, and beans. Brandon avoided dairy products, red meats, chicken, and turkey, and only occasionally ate fish. The living enzymes in the raw foods probably helped to remove arterial plaque, says Dr. Cowden. Brandon's dietary changes were complemented with several key supplements (see "Dr. Cowden's Daily Oral Nutritional Chelation Program for Brandon," p. 90).

In addition, Dr. Cowden had Brandon wear the negative pole of a small 1,000-gauss magnet against his left chest during all his waking hours. "The magnet dilates blood vessels and increases the blood flow to the coronary arteries," Dr. Cowden says. He emphasizes the importance of using only the negative pole; the positive pole, when placed against the chest, could restrict blood supply and produce a heart attack.

Brandon followed the program faithfully for nine days, then came to Dr. Cowden for another evaluation. "He climbed up the stairs to my office without any chest discomfort," reports Dr. Cowden. "On the heart stress test, performed on a treadmill, Brandon went over 11 minutes, which is probably as far as I could have gone that day. He showed no abnormalities on his electrocardiogram. This means that after nine days we reversed about 90% of his advanced triple-vessel coronary disease. He returned to work the next day and was very healthy." A dental factor (mercury amalgams or infection), which Brandon could not afford to address at the time, probably accounted for the remaining 10% improvement that he failed to achieve, Dr. Cowden adds.

Dr. Cowden cites another case from his practice illustrating how nutritional substances can reverse the symptoms of heart disease. Louisa, 45, had a 75% blockage in the carotid artery in her neck and

A free radical is an unstable molecule with an unpaired electron that steals an electron from another molecule and produces harmful effects. Free radicals are formed when molecules within cells react with oxygen (oxidize) as part of normal metabolic processes. Free radicals then begin to break down cells, especially if there are not enough free-radical quenching nutrients, such as vitamins C and E, in the cell. While free radicals are normal products of metabolism, uncontrolled free-radical production plays a major role in the development of degenerative disease, including cancer and heart disease. Free radicals harmfully alter important molecules, such as proteins, enzymes, fats, even DNA. Other sources of free radicals include pesticides, industrial pollutants, smoking, alcohol, viruses, most infections, allergies, stress, even certain foods and excessive exercise.

For more on the health effects of **mercury amalgams**, see Chapter 4: The Dental Connection, pp. 94-105.

For more information about **chelation therapy**, contact: American College for Advancement in Medicine, 23121 Verdugo Drive, Suite 204, Laguna Hills, CA 92653; tel: 714-583-7666 or 800-532-3688. For **TriCardia+, Systemex**, and **Buffer-pH+**, contact: Växa International, Inc., 10307 Pacific Center Court, San Diego, CA 92121; tel: 800-248-8292 (reference RS# 30181-3) or 619-625-8292; fax: 619-625-8272; website: www.vaxa.com/vaxa/vaxa.html. For **John R. Alm, M.D.**, contact: Pacific Immediate Care, 1900 Hacienda Drive, Vista, CA 92083; tel: 760-940-2011; fax: 760-940-0359. For **Garry F. Gordon, M.D., D.O.**: Get Healthy, 901 Anasazi Road, Payson, AR 85541; tel: 520-472-9086; fax: 520-474-1297; e-mail: drgary@netzone.com. For **Garlic-EDTA Chelator™**, contact: Life Enhancement Products, Inc., P.O. Box 751390, Petaluma, CA 94975; tel: 800-543-3873 or 707-762-6144; fax: 707-769-8016. For **Stephen F. Edelson, M.D.**: Environmental and Preventive Health Center of Atlanta, 3833 Roswell Road, Suite 110, Atlanta, GA 30342; tel: 404-841-0088; fax: 404-841-6416. For Dr. Cowden's oral nutritional chelation program [from sidebar] available as **Master-Chel**, contact: Health Restoration Systems, Inc., P.O. Box 832267, Richardson, TX 75083; tel: 972-480-8909; fax: 972-480-8807. For **William Lee Cowden, M.D.**: Conservative Medicine Institute, P.O. Box 832087, Richardson, TX 75083; fax: 214-238-0327. For **Super Garlic**, contact: Metagenics West, Inc., 12445 East 39th Avenue, Suite 402, Denver, CO 80239; tel: 303-371-6848 or 800-321-6382; fax: 303-371-9303.

was told that, unless she had surgery to correct it, she was likely to have a stroke. Dr. Cowden put her on Brandon's nutritional program and after three months a new ultrasound scan of her carotid artery revealed it was only 22% blocked with plaque.

How to Find the Right Doctor

Patients interested in chelation therapy should choose a doctor who follows the protocol of the American Board of Chelation Therapy or the American College for Advancement in Medicine (ACAM).

■ Prior to chelation, a complete physical examination that includes a heart function test, hair mineral analysis, electrocardiogram, stress test, and doppler flow analysis should be conducted. Kidney function must also be checked.

■ EDTA dosage should be individualized for each patient according to age, sex, weight, and kidney function, and should be administered slowly over a period of three or more hours.

■ Treatments should be administered by well-trained staff members who are readily available to deal with any symptoms that might occur during the process, such as weakness or dizziness from low blood sugar levels.

If a patient decides to have chelation therapy, it should be performed by a doctor with several years of experience, who has completed the training conducted by ACAM. If the therapy is administered by a nurse or nonphysician, a qualified physician must be on the premises at all times during the procedure.

Scientists at the
University of Toronto in Ontario, Canada,
studied the death rates for 224,258 U.S.
and 9,444 Canadian heart patients.
They found that at the end of one year
following the heart attack, the death
rate was 34% in both countries.
The crucial difference, however, is that
whereas 12% of U.S. heart attack
patients received angioplasty, only 1.5%
of Canadian heart patients did;
further, while 11% of American heart
patients have bypass surgery,
only 1.4% of Canadians do.

The Dental Connection

PROBLEMS WITH YOUR TEETH CAN AFFECT YOUR HEART—AND HOW TO REVERSE THEM

THERE IS A GROWING RECOGNITION among alternative dentists and physicians that dental health has a strong impact on the health of the body. European researchers estimate that perhaps as much as half of all chronic degenerative illness (including heart disease) can be linked either directly or indirectly to dental problems and the traditional techniques of modern dentistry used to treat them. The well-publicized dangers associated with the use of silver/mercury fillings (amalgams) are only the tip of the iceberg as far as the negative impact that dentistry can have on a person's health.

"One of the big problems in the United States," says Gary Verigan, D.D.S., of Escalon, California, "is that dentists are trained to practice with only the most meager of diagnostic equipment. These instruments, consisting primarily of X rays, are incapable of detecting enough about the tooth and its surrounding environment, giving the dentist only a superficial understanding of the problem and the impact it may be having on the patient's health. People often go through many doctors and therapies in search of answers for their problems, never realizing that their chronic conditions may be traceable to dental complications."

In contrast, biological dentistry treats the teeth, jaw, and related structures with specific regard to how treatment will affect the entire body. According to Hal Huggins, D.D.S., of Colorado Springs, Colorado, a pioneer in this field, "Dental problems such as cavities, infections, toxic or allergy-producing filling materials, root canals,

Dr. Huggins reports the improvement or disappearance of many cardiovascular problems including angina, unidentified chest pains, and tachycardia (rapid heartbeat for no apparent reason) after removing toxic dental amalgams.

and misalignment of the teeth or jaw can have far-reaching effects throughout the body."

How Dental Problems Contribute to Illness

"Dental infections and dental disturbances can cause pain and dysfunction throughout the body," states Edward Arana, D.D.S., former president of the American Academy of Biological Dentistry, "including limited motion and loose tendons, ligaments, and muscles. Structural and physiological dysfunction can also occur, impairing organs and glands."

Dr. Arana cites several major types of dental problems that can cause illness and dysfunction in the body:

- infections under and around teeth
- problems with specific teeth related to the acupuncture meridians and the autonomic nervous system
- root canals
- toxicity from dental restoration materials
- incompatability to dental restoration materials (evidenced by the body's negative reaction)
- temporomandibular joint syndrome (TMJ), a painful condition of the jaw, usually caused by stress or injury

Some of the more common causes of these dental problems are unerupted teeth (teeth that have not broken through the gum), wisdom teeth (both impacted and unimpacted), amalgam-filled cavities and root canals, cysts, bone cavities, and areas of bone condensation due to inflammation in the bone. These conditions can be diagnosed using testing methods such as blood tests, applied kinesiology, electroacupuncture biofeedback, and, in some cases, X rays. A thorough review of the patient's medical and dental histories is also essential.

Infections Under the Teeth

Pockets of infection can exist under the teeth and be undetectable on

QUICK DEFINITION

Biological dentistry stresses the use of nontoxic restoration materials for dental work and focuses on the unrecognized impact that dental toxins and hidden dental infections can have on overall health. Typically, a biological dentist will emphasize the following: the safe removal of mercury amalgams; in many cases, either the avoidance or removal of root canals; the investigation of possible jawbone infections (cavitations) as a "dental focus" or source of bodywide illness centered in the teeth; and the health-injuring role of misalignment of teeth and jaw structures.

Electroacupuncture Biofeedback

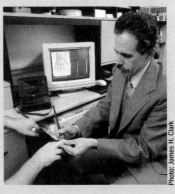

Photo: James H. Clark

Developed in the 1940s by Reinhold Voll, M.D., of Germany, electroacupuncture biofeedback makes use of the acupuncture meridian system to screen for infections and dysfunctions in the body. Today it is employed as a screening tool by alternative health practitioners worldwide, including biological dentists. As employed in biological dentistry, it involves placing an electrode on an individual tooth, then applying a small electrical current and recording the response. Any deviation from the normal reading indicates that there is an infection or disturbance in the vicinity of that particular tooth.[1]

This deviation can also indicate a similar unhealthy state in the organ that shares the same meridian as the tooth. Any determinations using electroacupuncture biofeedback should always be confirmed by a physician.

X rays. This is particularly true for teeth that have had root canals, as it is very difficult to eliminate all the bacteria and toxins from the roots during this procedure. These infections may persist for years without the patient's knowledge.

When infections are present, toxins can leak out and depress the function of the immune system, leading to chronic degenerative diseases throughout the body. Once the infection is cleared up, many of the symptoms of disease will disappear. Some dentists use applied kinesiology testing to identify these hidden infections. Applied kinesiology employs a simple strength resistance test on a specific indicator muscle that is related to the organ or part of the body that is being tested. If the muscle tests strong, maintaining its resistance, it indicates health. If it tests weak, it can mean infection or dysfunction.

Relationship Between Specific Teeth and Illness
In the 1950s, Reinhold Voll, M.D., of Germany, discovered that each tooth in the mouth relates to a specific acupuncture meridian. Using his electroacupuncture biofeedback technique (see sidebar), he found that if a tooth became infected or diseased, the organ on the same meridian could also become unhealthy. He found that the opposite held true as well, that dysfunction in a specific organ could lead to a

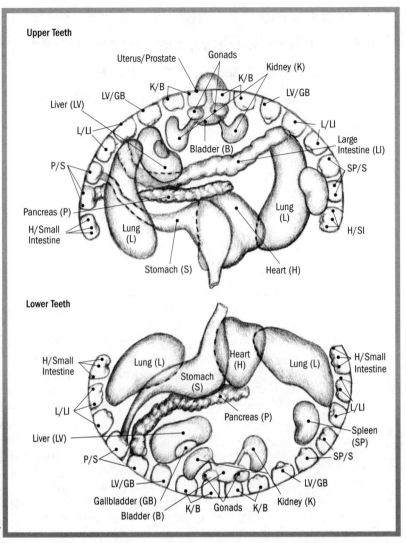

Used with permission from "The Micro-Acupuncture Systems III: The Principles and Systems of Micro-Acupuncture," Ralph Alan Dale, *The International Journal of Chinese Medicine* 1:4 (1984).

Organ and tooth correspondences on acupuncture meridians in the mouth

problem in the corresponding tooth. For example, Harold Ravins, D.D.S., of Los Angeles, California, has observed that people who hit their front teeth too hard often have kidney disturbances, as there is a specific relationship between the kidneys and the front teeth.

Ernesto Adler, M.D., D.D.S., of Spain, reports that many diseases can be caused by the wisdom teeth, which have a relationship to

The late Weston Price, D.D.S., former director of research for the American Dental Association, made the astonishing claim that if teeth that have had root canals are removed from patients suffering from heart disease, the disease will resolve in most cases.

Acupuncture meridians are specific pathways in the human body for the flow of life force or subtle energy, known as *qi* (pronounced *CHEE*). In most cases, these energy pathways run up and down both sides of the body, and correspond to individual organs or organ systems, designated as Lung, Small Intestine, Heart, and others. There are 12 principal meridians and eight secondary channels. Numerous points of heightened energy, or *qi*, exist on the body's surface along the meridians and are called acupoints. There are more than 1,000 acupoints, each of which is potentially a place for acupuncture treatment.

almost all organs of the body. When wisdom teeth are impacted, Dr. Adler points out, they press upon the nerves of the mandible (the large bone that makes up the lower jaw), which can result in disturbances in other areas of the body, including heart problems, stammering, epilepsy, pain in the joints, depression, and headaches. He adds that the upper wisdom teeth can cause calcium deficiency, resulting in muscle cramps.

Root Canals as a Cause of Illness

The late Weston Price, D.D.S., M.S., F.A.C.D., former director of research for the American Dental Association, made the astonishing claim that if teeth that have had root canals are removed from patients suffering from kidney and heart disease, these diseases will resolve in most cases. Moreover, implanting these teeth in animals results in the animals developing the same kind of disease found in the person from whom the tooth was taken. Dr. Price found that toxins seeping out of root canals can cause systemic diseases of the heart, kidney, uterus, and nervous and endocrine systems.[2]

Michael Ziff, D.D.S, of Orlando, Florida, points out that research has demonstrated that 100% of root canals result in residual infection. This may be due to the imperfect seal that allows bacteria to penetrate. The oxygen-lacking environment of a root canal can cause the bacteria to undergo changes, adds Dr. Huggins, producing potent toxins that can then leak out into the body. Nutrient materials are also able to seep into the root canal through the porous channels in the tooth, allowing this bacterial growth to flourish.

According to Dr. Ziff, however, there are cases where root canal teeth should not be pulled. It can be difficult to chew without certain teeth intact, and problems can arise if the teeth surrounding the extracted one become misaligned. "The best approach is a conservative one," says Dr. Ziff. "Try other measures first and only remove the tooth as a last resort."

Toxicity from Dental Restoration Materials

"Dental amalgam fillings can release mercury, tin, copper, silver, and sometimes zinc into the body," says Dr. Arana. All of these metals have various degrees of toxicity and when placed as fillings in the teeth can corrode or disassociate into metallic ions (charged atoms). These metallic ions can then migrate from the tooth into the root of the tooth, the mouth, the bone, the connective tissues of the jaw, and finally into the nerves. From there they can travel into the central nervous system, where the ions will reside, permanently disrupting the body's normal functioning if nothing is done to remove them.

Other types of metal-based dental restorations can similarly release toxic metals into the body. According to David E. Eggleston, D.D.S., of the Department of Restorative Dentistry at the University of Southern California in Los Angeles, a patient undergoing dental work developed kidney disease due to nickel toxicity from the dental crowns that were being placed in the patient's mouth. As each successive crown was placed, the disease intensified, verified by blood and urine tests, and physical examinations. Once the nickel crowns were removed, the patient gradually became symptom-free.[3]

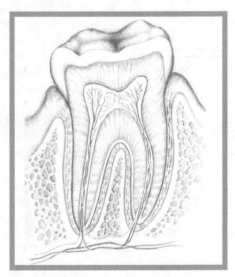

Mercury Dental Amalgams

While all metals used for dental restoration can be toxic, the most harmful are the mercury dental amalgams (silver/mercury) used for fillings. According to Joyal Taylor, D.D.S., formerly of Rancho Santa Fe, California, "These so-called 'silver fillings' actually contain 50% mercury and only 25% silver."

Mercury has been recognized as a poison since the

Cross section of a tooth. **The trouble with root canals is that bacteria become trapped within the literally three miles of microscopic dentin tubules inside a single-root tooth and from here can infect the rest of the body.**

Mercury has been recognized as a poison since the 1500s, and yet mercury amalgams have been used in dentistry since the 1820s. They are still being used today even though the Environmental Protection Agency (EPA) declared scrap dental amalgam a hazardous waste in 1988.

To contact **Joyal Taylor's practice,** now under the direction of former colleague Grant Lawton, D.D.S.: P.O. Box 2184, 16095 Avenita de Acacias, San Diego, CA; tel: 619-596-7626; fax: 619-756-7843.

For more on the **hazards of mercury fillings,** see Chapter 1: What Causes Heart Disease?, pp. 40-42.

1500s, and yet mercury amalgams have been used in dentistry since the 1820s. They are still being used today even though the Environmental Protection Agency (EPA) declared scrap dental amalgam a hazardous waste in 1988. Even the American Dental Association, which has so far refused to ban amalgams, now instructs dentists to "know the potential hazards and symptoms of mercury exposure such as the development of sensitivity and neuropathy," to use a no-touch technique for handling the amalgam, and to store it under liquid, preferably glycerin or radiographic fixer solution, in unbreakable, tightly sealed containers.[4]

For some dentists, such as Richard D. Fischer, D.D.S., of Annandale, Virginia, these measures are not enough. Since becoming aware of the health risk amalgams pose, he has refused to work with them and has had his own silver fillings removed. "I don't feel comfortable using a substance designated by the EPA to be a waste disposal hazard," he says. "I can't throw it in the trash, bury it in the ground, or put it in a landfill, but they say it's okay to put it in people's mouths. That doesn't make sense."

According to the German Ministry of Health, "Amalgam is considered a health risk from a medical viewpoint due to the release of mercury vapor."[5] Everyday activities such as chewing and brushing the teeth have been shown to release mercury vapors from amalgams.[6] Amalgams can also erode and corrode with time (ideally they should be replaced after seven to ten years), adding to their toxic output. Studies by the World Health Organization show that a single amalgam can release 3 to 17 mcg of mercury per day,[7] making dental amalgam a major source of mercury exposure.[8]

Since mercury is a cumulative poison, building up in the body with repeated exposure,[9] its effects can be devastating. It can prevent nutrients from entering the cells and wastes from leaving. Mercury can bind to the DNA (deoxyribonucleic acid) of cells as well as to the cell membranes, distorting them and interfering with normal cell

> **"I don't feel comfortable using a substance designated by the Environmental Protection Agency to be a waste disposal hazard. I can't throw it in the trash, bury it in the ground, or put it in a landfill, but they say it's okay to put it in people's mouths. That doesn't make sense"—Richard D. Fischer, D.D.S.**

functions.[10] Mercury poisoning can also lead to symptoms such as anxiety, depression, confusion, irritability, insecurity, and the inability to concentrate. It can cause kidney disease and cardiac and respiratory disorders. Mercury poisoning often goes undetected for years because the symptoms presented do not necessarily suggest the mercury as the initiating cause.

CAUTION

If you decide to replace your mercury amalgam fillings, it is essential that you have the procedure performed only by a dentist expert at mercury amalgam removal. Mercury vapor is released in the process and the proper steps must be taken to prevent poisoning from this vapor or from filling fragments.

A recent study, directed by Dr. Huggins and sponsored by the Adolph Coors Foundation, showed that mercury filling emissions affected blood hemoglobin levels (the oxygen and iron-carrying molecule), cellular energy production, and white-blood and natural-killer cell activity (our immune system's key agents against infection and disease, including cancer).[11]

Dr. Huggins reports the improvement or disappearance of many cardiovascular problems, including angina, unidentified chest pains, and tachycardia (rapid heartbeat for no apparent reason), after removing toxic dental amalgams. Though the ideal replacement for mercury amalgams has not yet been found, there are some less toxic alternatives that biological dentists are working with. The best one so far is the so-called composite amalgam, which is a combination of metals that are less toxic than mercury and slower to break down.

Biological Treatment of Dental Problems

Biological dentists treat dental problems in a variety of ways. They emphasize the conservation of all healthy tooth material and employ the latest techniques of bioenergetic medicine, including neural therapy, oral acupuncture, cold laser therapy, complex homeopathy, mouth balancing, and nutrition.

Neural Therapy

According to neural therapy, the body is charged with electricity or

Dr. Huggins reports the improvement or disappearance of many cardiovascular problems, including angina, unidentified chest pains, and tachycardia (rapid heartbeat for no apparent reason), after removing toxic dental amalgams.

biological energy. This energy flows throughout the body, with every cell possessing its own specified frequency range. As long as this energy flow is unimpeded and stays within its normal range, the body will remain healthy. However, if this balance breaks down, disruptions in the normal function of cells can occur, eventually leading to chronic disorders.

When injury, inflammation, or infection is present in the mouth, there is usually a corresponding blockage in the body's normal energy flow. Injection of a local anesthetic, such as procaine around the tooth to remove the energy blockage, will often resolve the problem. Dr. Adler cites the example of a sports instructor suffering from "tennis elbow." When Dr. Adler injected the man's two upper right premolars with procaine, the instructor received immediate relief from his pain.

Oral Acupuncture

Oral acupuncture, according to Jochen Gleditsch, M.D., D.D.S., of Munich, Germany, has been taught to dentists since 1976, and its use is expanding rapidly. It involves the injection of either saline water, weak local anesthetics, or sterile complex homeopathics into specific acupuncture points of the oral mucous membrane. It can also be combined with neural therapy.

Both Dr. Arana and Dr. Ravins use oral acupuncture to relieve pain during dental procedures with great success. Some dentists also use it to relax patients before any dental procedure. Toothache, tooth sensitivities, jaw pain, gingivitis, and other local problems often respond to oral acupuncture.

Cold Laser Therapy

Cold laser therapy is an alternative form of acupuncture that is especially useful for treating patients who object to the use of needles. The "cold laser" gets its name from the fact that its power output and the light spectrum it uses are incapable of causing any thermal damage to the body's tissues. This therapy kills bacteria, aids in wound healing, reduces inflammation, and helps to rebalance the flow of energy in the body's meridian system.

Selected Health Symptom Analysis of 1,569 Patients Who Eliminated Mercury-Containing Dental Fillings[12]

The following represents a summary of 1,569 patients in six different studies evaluating the health effects of replacing mercury-containing dental fillings with non-mercury fillings. The data was derived from the following sources: 762 Patient Adverse Reaction Reports submitted to the FDA by patients; and 807 patients reports from Sweden, Denmark, Canada, and the United States.

% of Total Reporting	Symptom	Number Reporting	Number Improved or Cured	% of Cure or Improvement
14	Allergy	221	196	89
5	Anxiety	86	80	93
5	Bad temper	81	68	84
6	Bloating	88	70	80
6	Blood pressure problems	99	53	54
5	Chest pains	79	69	87
22	Depression	347	315	91
22	Dizziness	343	301	88
45	Fatigue	705	603	86
15	Intestinal problems	231	192	83
8	Gum problems	129	121	94
34	Headaches	531	460	87
12	Insomnia	187	146	78
10	Irregular heartbeat	159	139	87
8	Irritability	132	119	90
17	Lack of concentration	270	216	80
6	Lack of energy	91	88	97
17	Memory loss	265	193	73
17	Metallic taste	260	247	95
7	Multiple sclerosis	113	86	76
8	Muscle tremor	126	104	82

Homeopathy in Biological Dentistry

According to Dr. Fischer, "Homeopathic first-aid remedies can help alleviate the pain or discomfort of dental emergencies, at least temporarily, until proper dental care can be received. They are not intended to replace regular dental care, but rather to serve as a safe and effective complement."

Mouth Balancing

Dr. Ravins specializes in "balancing" the mouth to improve a wide range of health problems. He believes that structural deformities of the skull influence the entire body. "With the new computerized technology, I can diagnose muscle dysfunction and pick up vibrations from the jaw and movement of the mandible," he says. Often the misalignment has been caused by a prior accident. By analyzing this data and making special orthopedic braces to be worn in the mouth, Dr. Ravins can realign the jaw and remove pain and other symptoms such as headaches, shoulder pain, back problems, and even some eye problems.

Nutrition

Dr. Huggins, like many other biological dentists, makes nutritional supplementation part of his overall protocol for dealing with dental conditions, especially for the patient recovering from mercury amalgam toxicity. According to Dr. Huggins, the basic supplementation program aids in the excretion of mercury from the cells, prevents the exacerbation of further symptoms, and provides the patient with a nutrient base for rebuilding damaged tissues.

Among the nutrients Dr. Huggins uses are magnesium, selenium, vitamin C, vitamin E, and folic acid, along with digestive enzymes. He cautions, however, that the nutrients need to be used in specific ratios, and that supplementation done without proper consultation can actually create further imbalances in the patient's system.

A proper diet is also important for patients suffering from mercury toxicity. Dr. Huggins recommends the avoidance of cigarettes, sugar, alcohol, caffeine, chocolate, soft drinks, refined carbohydrates, milk, cheese, margarine, fish, and excess liquids with meals.

The Politics of Dentistry

Although many new techniques of biological dentistry are available, only 2,000 to 3,000 dentists across the United States are using them in practice. This is due to a deliberate effort by the American Dental Association (ADA) to suppress such practices, even to the point of rescinding the licenses of practitioners using them. Electroacupuncture biofeedback testing by dentists is not allowed in some states and dentists may lose their license for using it, despite its proven effectiveness for screening hidden infections under teeth. For this reason, most dentists are forced to use other methods for detecting hidden infections and other dental problems. Dental acupuncture is also banned in some states.

In 1987, the ADA wrote a provision into their code to declare the removal of clinically serviceable mercury amalgams from patients' teeth to be unethical, according to Dr. Ziff. Any dentist doing so is in violation of the code, and the ADA is assisting state boards in prosecuting these dentists, despite all the evidence of the toxicity of mercury.

The financial and legal implications of an admission by the ADA that mercury is toxic and harmful to health may be a possible motive behind this move. If the ADA was to admit that mercury amalgams are toxic health hazards, insurance companies or the government would possibly have to foot the bill for the removal of mercury amalgams from practically the entire population of the United States.

However, the growing number of research studies on biological dental techniques, the information coming out of Europe and Canada on mercury toxicity,[13] and increasing public awareness of some of the dangers of traditional dental practice are combining to build support for the small band of dentists risking their livelihood to practice safe dentistry in the United States. "Biological dentistry will, out of necessity, become the dental medicine of the 21st century," says Dr. Arana.

CHAPTER

5

Nutritional Supplements

HOW THEY CAN BENEFIT YOUR HEART

SINCE ATHEROSCLEROSIS and heart disease take many years to develop, a daily regimen of supplements may be helpful in preventing both. The amount of supplements needed varies from one individual to another depending on body weight and absorption levels, and it is best to consult with a nutritionally-skilled physician or naturopathic physician before embarking on a routine of supplements.

Matthias Rath, M.D., author of *Eradicating Heart Disease*, uses a program of supplements to reverse heart disease. "I firmly believe that America's number one killer can be prevented by an optimum intake of essential nutrients," he says. The supplements include vitamin C and other antioxidants, coenzyme Q10, amino acids, B vitamins, and minerals. Vitamin C is an important component because it helps prevent the formation of free radicals, which initiate artery obstruction by damaging arterial walls. It also helps to heal the damaged areas before they fill with cholesterol.

Reversing Heart Failure With Supplements

For example, George, a man in his fifties, came to Dr. Rath after experiencing sudden cardiac failure. This was a severe heart muscle weakness which resulted in decreased pumping function and enlargement of the heart chambers. George was no longer able to work full-time and had to give up

Dr. Rath's book, *Eradicating Heart Disease*, is available from Health Now, 387 Ivy Street, San Francisco, CA 94102; tel: 800-624-2442; fax: 800-582-8000. The nutrients are available as **Cardi-rite** from Carlson Laboratories, 15 College, Arlington Heights, IL 60004; tel: 847-255-1600 or 800-323-4141; fax: 847-255-1605.

most physical activities. Sometimes he felt so weak he had to hold an object with both hands to keep from dropping it and he was unable to climb stairs. His cardiologist recommended a heart transplant.

Dr. Rath put George on his supplement program for heart health. "Soon George could again fulfill his professional obligations on a regular basis and was able to undertake daily bicycle rides," says Dr. Rath. After two months on the program, his cardiologist reported that his heart enlargement had decreased. A month after that, George went on an overseas business trip and reported that physical limitations were no longer interfering with his work.

Vitamins

The following vitamins can help promote heart health:

Beta Carotene (vitamin A precursor)— Research done at Johns Hopkins University found that there were approximately 50% fewer heart disease cases among those study participants with the highest levels of beta carotene, compared to the group with the lowest levels.[1] A similar study at Harvard University found that of two groups with prior evidence of heart disease, the group given a beta carotene supplement had 40% fewer heart attacks than the group given a placebo.[2]

Vitamin B3 (niacin)—Niacin helps to lower cholesterol levels and lessen the risk of heart disease.[3] It has also

Dr. Rath's Nutrient Recommendations

The following are general supplement guidelines to promote heart health. Keep in mind that each person is unique and has different nutritional requirements. It is always best to consult a qualified health practitioner for assistance in designing a supplement program that meets your individual needs.

Vitamin C: 1,000 mg

Vitamin E: 600 IU

Beta carotene: 8,000 IU

L-proline: 500 mg

L-lysine: 500 mg

L-carnitine: 150 mg

Coenzyme Q10: 25 mg

Vitamin B1: 40 mg

Vitamin B2: 40 mg

Vitamin B3: (niacin) 50 mg

Vitamin B3: (niacinamide): 150 mg

Vitamin B5: (pantothenate): 200 mg

Vitamin B6: 50 mg

Vitamin B12: 0.1 mg

Folic acid: 0.4 mg

Vitamin D: 600 IU

Biotin: 0.3 mg

Calcium: 150 mg

Magnesium: 200 mg

Zinc: 30 mg

Manganese: 6 mg

Copper: 2 mg

Selenium: 0.1 mg

Chromium: 0.05 mg

Molybdenum: 0.02 mg

One of Dr. Abram Hoffer's patients came to him 20 years ago with angina pectoris. He was treated with niacin and has had no signs of angina since.

For more about **homocysteine**, see Chapter 1: What Causes Heart Disease?, pp. 33-37.

been shown to increase the longevity of patients who have suffered one heart attack. Over 8,000 middle-aged men who had suffered a heart attack were given supplements of either niacin, estrogen, thyroid hormone, or a placebo. The study results showed that only niacin was beneficial in lowering the death rate and increasing longevity.[4]

Abram Hoffer, M.D., Ph.D., of Victoria, British Columbia, treated a pilot who had not been able to fly for seven years because of heart problems. Dr. Hoffer put him on 3 g daily of niacin; after one-and-a-half years, he received a clean bill of health and was able to fly again. Another of Dr. Hoffer's patients came to him 20 years ago with angina pectoris. This patient was also treated with niacin and, according to Dr. Hoffer, has had no signs of angina since.

Vitamin B6—Researchers have found vitamin B6 to be a safe and inexpensive supplement which may be helpful in preventing heart attacks, strokes,[5] and atherosclerosis.[6] Recent studies have shown that vitamins B6, B12, and folic acid can dramatically lower homocysteine, a free-radical generator capable of oxidizing cholesterol, one of the major contributing factors in heart disease.[7]

Vitamin B6 is needed for the conversion of homocysteine to the harmless chemical cystathionine, thus preventing the homocysteine-induced oxidation of cholesterol.[8] It has also been suggested that vitamin B6 inhibits the platelet aggregation which occurs in atherosclerosis.[9] The typical American diet, however, leaves many people significantly deficient in this vital nutrient.

In 1949, Moses M. Suzman, M.D., a South African neurologist and internist, gathered a group of pre-cardiac patients who showed signs of arterial damage and had them take 100 mg of vitamin B6 per day, while patients who had already had heart attacks or angina were given 200 mg per day (half in a B complex including choline). In addition, the patients with the most serious conditions were given 5 mg of folic acid, 100-600 IU of vitamin E, magnesium, and zinc.[10]

Over the next 23 years, Dr. Suzman's patients recovered rapidly, as their angina and electrocardiographic irregularities diminished or disappeared. Those who dropped out of the vitamin and diet regimen, however, soon found their cardiac problems returning.[11]

Interest in vitamin B6 deficiency and its relationship to heart disease revived in 1969, when Kilmer S. McCully, M.D., a professor of pathology at Harvard Medical School, found that heart patients had nearly 80% less of the vitamin than healthy individuals did.[12] From this, Dr. McCully postulated that B6 may help the body resist the arterial damage that precipitates heart disease. He also found that patients who had already suffered a heart attack or angina, and were then given 200 mg of B6 daily (half in a B complex including choline) combined with a low-fat, mostly vegetarian diet, recovered rapidly.[13]

Vitamin B12—A deficiency in vitamin B12 is associated with elevated homocysteine levels.[14] When vitamin B12 is supplemented, homocysteine levels decrease.[15] This effect can be increased by also supplementing choline, folic acid, riboflavin, and B6.[16]

Folic Acid—Folic acid is essential for the proper metabolism of homocysteine.[17] Thus, folic acid supplementation can help prevent the arterial plaque buildup caused by an excess of homocysteine in the blood.

Antioxidants—Antioxidants such as vitamin E, vitamin C, selenium, and coenzyme Q10 have also proven in numerous studies to be effective in both the prevention and treatment of heart disease.[18]

Vitamin C—Vitamin C (ascorbic acid) is integral to heart health. It is believed to help prevent the formation of oxysterols.[19] By combining the amino acid lysine with vitamin C, it may be possible to dissolve clots in the bloodstream.[20]

Studies also reveal that vitamin C is required for collagen synthesis and is therefore necessary to maintain the integrity of the walls of arteries.[21] Nobel laureate Linus Pauling, Ph.D., believed that a deficiency of vitamin C may precipitate arteriosclerosis because it causes defects in the arterial walls due to reduced collagen synthesis.[22] Drs. Pauling and Rath have shown in preliminary studies that vitamin C supplementation can reverse arteriosclerosis in humans.[23]

In a study conducted on guinea pigs, it was found that the equivalent of the U.S. Recommended Daily Allowance (RDA) of vitamin C offered virtually no protection against arterial damage. When the amount of vitamin C was increased to a dose equivalent to 2,800 mg for a 154-pound human, the researchers were able to reverse the damage.[24]

"Vitamin C reverses oxidation and prevents free radical forma-

High doses of vitamin C can dramatically reduce your risk of heart attack or death from other degenerative diseases, according to research results from Tufts University. Those individuals who consumed more than 700 mg daily of vitamin C had a 62% reduced risk of dying from heart disease and a 50% reduced mortality rate overall.

High amounts of vitamin C taken over a prolonged period of time can leach calcium and other minerals out of the teeth, bones, and other tissues, according to Dr. Cowden. He recommends that high amounts of vitamin C (ascorbic acid) be balanced by mineral ascorbates containing magnesium, potassium, zinc, and manganese.

tion," states William Lee Cowden, M.D., of Richardson, Texas. "In a diet that involves reducing fats, vitamin C is an integral part of helping the body to repair itself." In patients with existing cardiovascular disease, Dr. Cowden recommends that vitamin C be taken to bowel tolerance (the maximum amount a person can take before causing loose stools or diarrhea). He suggests a minimum of three to four doses daily, increasing the amount until reaching bowel tolerance.

"For example," explains Dr. Cowden, "the first dose could be 1,000 mg, the second dose 2,000 mg, the third dose 3,000 mg, and the fourth dose 4,000 mg. Stay on bowel tolerance until cardiovascular disease is resolved, and then go on a 3,000-mg maintenance dose. For those who are well but want to prevent cardiovascular disease, 3,000 to 10,000 mg daily is sufficient." Higher doses of vitamin C should be taken with adequate amounts of water, magnesium, and vitamin B6, adds Dr. Cowden.

A study conducted by James E. Enstrom, M.D., an epidemiologist at the University of California at Los Angeles, suggests that men who consume vitamin C every day, at levels 500% to 666% of the U.S. RDA, live about six years longer than men who don't.[25]

High doses of vitamin C can dramatically reduce your risk of heart attack or death from other degenerative diseases, according to research results from Tufts University in Boston, Massachusetts. Scientists tracked the health outcomes of 725 volunteers, 60-101 years old (average age of 73), over a 12-year span. Those individuals who consumed more than 700 mg daily of vitamin C had a 62% reduced risk of dying from heart disease and a 50% reduced mortality rate overall, suggesting that adequate vitamin C intake actually increases lifespan. Concurrent blood analyses of the subjects confirmed that those with high levels of vitamin C in their plasma enjoyed these benefits. The scientists also demonstrated that the highest degree of protection was provided by combining vitamin C intake at this level and dietary foods, such as vegetables, high in natural vitamin C.[26]

Vitamin E—Vitamin E is a fat-soluble antioxidant which can help prevent abnormal blood clot formation. Richard Passwater, Ph.D., of Berlin, Maryland, believes that any nutrient that prevents the oxidation of cholesterol, such as vitamin E, beta carotene, and coenzyme Q10, offers a protective factor. Supplementation of vitamin E may also inhibit platelet aggregation[27] and help repair the lining of blood vessels.[28]

Studies published in the *New England Journal of Medicine* suggest that vitamin E can contribute greatly to the prevention of heart disease in both men and women.[29] In a study conducted by Harvard Medical School of 87,245 female nurses, it was found that those who took 100 IU of vitamin E daily for more than two years had a 46% lower risk of heart disease.[30] In another Harvard study, 39,910 male health professionals who took 100 IU of

> In a study conducted by Harvard Medical School of 87,245 female nurses, it was found that those who took 100 IU of vitamin E daily for more than two years had a 46% lower risk of heart disease.

vitamin E daily for an unspecified time period had a 37% lower risk of heart disease.[31] In groups who took higher doses of vitamin E for a longer time, the results were even greater.

In a study of 34,486 postmenopausal women with no tangible signs of heart trouble, those who consumed at least 100 IU of vitamin E daily from their foods were 62% less likely to die of coronary heart disease than those women consuming less vitamin E, according to the *New England Journal of Medicine* in May 1996.[32] An earlier study the same year showed that those with heart problems who took vitamin E experienced a 75% reduction in the rate of heart attacks.

A study funded by the World Health Organization found that among 16 European study populations, those with low serum levels of vitamin E were at greater risk for heart disease than those with high blood pressure and high cholesterol levels.[33] When 1,851 men and women with coronary heart disease, such as angina or atherosclerosis, took natural-source vitamin E at rates between 400 and 800 IU daily, researchers observed that this supplementation reduced the number of clinically significant coronary events. Specifically, the risk of non-

Remember, *oxidized* LDL cholesterol is the kind that leads to plaque formation on the artery walls. Research at the University of Minnesota discovered that subjects taking 800 IU of vitamin E daily for just two weeks had up to three times the resistance to oxidation of LDL cholesterol. Investigators at the University of Texas report that 800 IU of vitamin E is as good as a combination of vitamins E and C and beta carotene for the same purpose—that is, for reducing arterial damage.[36]

fatal heart attack was reduced by 77%. The effects were apparent after about 200 days of vitamin E supplementation.[34]

While it is generally recognized that vitamin E supplementation can reduce the risk of cardiovascular disease, there is some disagreement over what is the most effective dose. A recent study at the University of Texas has concluded that 400 IU daily provides the maximum protection and anything lower may not prevent LDL oxidation.[35]

High dosages of vitamin E are not recommended for people with hypertension, rheumatic heart disease, or ischemic heart disease, except under close medical supervision. However, in hypertensive or ischemic heart disease patients, if the dose of vitamin E is raised gradually, the blood pressure will usually not rise significantly and there will not be a greater workload placed on the heart, according to Dr. Cowden.

Minerals

The following minerals may be effective in the treatment and prevention of heart disease:

Calcium—Calcium supplementation may also decrease total cholesterol and inhibit platelet aggregation.[37] Researchers at the Malmö University Hospital in Malmö, Sweden, studied 33,346 individuals over a 10.8-year period and found direct correlations between calcium levels and heart disease, malignant disorders, and mortality.[38] Too much calcium, they said, can damage health and shorten lifespan. As blood levels of calcium rise, so does the risk of premature death.

According to the study, men under 50 years old who had blood levels of calcium greater than 2.45 mmol/L (the high end of "normal") showed a 20% increase in mortality compared to men with lower levels. Those with calcium levels greater than 2.60 mmol/L died at twice the rate of those with lower levels. Those with levels between 2.51 and 2.55 mmol/L

Lipoproteins are in two principal forms. *Low-density lipoproteins (LDLs)* are combination molecules of proteins and fats, particularly cholesterol. LDLs circulate in the blood and act as the primary carriers of cholesterol to the cells of the body. An elevated level of LDLs, the so-called "bad" cholesterol, is a contributing factor in causing atherosclerosis (plaque deposits on the inner walls of the arteries). A diet high in saturated fats can lead to an increase the level of LDLs in the blood. *High-density lipoproteins (HDLs)* are also fat-protein molecules in the blood, but contain a larger amount of protein and less fat than LDLs. HDLs are able to absorb cholesterol and related compounds in the blood and transport them to the liver for elimination. HDL, the so-called "good" cholesterol, may also be able to take cholesterol from plaque deposits on the artery walls, thus helping to reverse the process of atherosclerosis. A higher ratio of HDL to LDL cholesterol in the blood is associated with a reduced risk of cardiovascular disease.

While it is generally recognized that vitamin E supplementation can reduce the risk of cardiovascular disease, there is some disagreement over what is the most effective dose. A recent study at the University of Texas has concluded that 400 IU daily provides the maximum protection and anything lower may not prevent LDL oxidation.

had a 50% increased risk of premature death from all causes, compared to men with calcium levels at 2.31-2.45 mmol/L, the researchers said. Men with calcium levels exceeding 2.50 mmol/L had a 58% increased chance of dying from cardiovascular disease and a 28% increased risk of dying from malignant disorders, such as cancer.

Chromium—Several studies have linked chromium deficiency to coronary heart disease.[39] Supplementation with chromium has been shown to lower total cholesterol and triglycerides and raise HDL cholesterol.[40] It is even more effective in lowering cholesterol when combined with niacin (vitamin B3).[41]

Magnesium—It has been found that individuals who die suddenly of heart attacks have far lower levels of magnesium and potassium than do control groups.[42] Magnesium deficiency has been implicated in mitral valve prolapse (MVP, also called floppy valve syndrome, a malfunction in the valve between the left atrium and ventricle of the heart) and supplementation with magnesium may reverse symptoms.[43]

A recent study lends new support to these findings.[44] Of 141 people with "heavily symptomatic" MVP, 60% had low magnesium levels, compared to only 5% in the control group. After five weeks of magnesium supplementation, the percentage of those with chest pain dropped from 96% to 47%; with palpitations, from 93% to 51%; with anxiety, from 84% to 47%; low energy, from 74% to 34%; faintness, from 64% to 6%; and difficulty breathing, from 84% to 39%.

Magnesium helps to dilate arteries and ease the heart's pumping of blood, thus preventing arrhythmia (irregular heartbeat). Magnesium may also prevent calcification of the blood vessels, lower total cholesterol, raise HDL cholesterol, and inhibit platelet aggregation.[45] But simply taking oral magnesium supplements may not be sufficient. "Most doctors don't use the best form for optimum absorption," Dr. Cowden explains. "It's more effective to use magnesium

The amino acid L-arginine, when given intravenously at the rate of 20 grams over one hour, can produce significant increases in stroke volume and cardiac output in patients with congestive heart failure. Arginine therapy can also lower arterial blood pressure. Supplementation with the amino acid L-carnitine immediately after an acute heart attack can help damaged heart muscle expand again.

QUICK DEFINITION

The **Meyer's Cocktail** is an intravenous vitamin and mineral protocol developed by John Meyers, M.D., a physician in Baltimore, Maryland, in the 1970s. It contains magnesium chloride hexahydrate (5 cc given), calcium gluconate (2.5 cc), vitamin B2 (1,000 mcg/cc; 1 cc given), vitamin B5 (100 mg/cc; 1 cc given), vitamin B6 (250 mg/cc; 1 cc given) the entire vitamin B-complex (100 mg/cc; 1 cc given), and vitamin C (222 mg/cc; 6 cc given). The solution is slowly injected over a 5-15 minute period. The "Cocktail" is indicated for patients with chronic fatigue, depression, muscle spasm, asthma, hives, allergic rhinitis, congestive heart failure, angina, ischemic vascular disease, acute infections, and senile dementia.

glycinate, taurate, or aspartate, or even herbal magnesium such as red raspberry, but some patients need intravenous or intramuscular magnesium to quickly raise their magnesium to ideal levels."

Alan R. Gaby, M.D., of Kent, Washington, has found that cases of congestive heart failure respond well to an intravenous injection of a nutrient "cocktail" composed of magnesium chloride hexahydrate, hydroxocobalamin, pyridoxine hydrochloride, dexpanthenol, B-complex vitamins, and vitamin C. (This is a modification of the nutrient cocktail popularized by John Meyers, M.D.)

Potassium—High blood pressure is often present in heart disease. It has been found that supplements of potassium can help reduce a patient's reliance on blood pressure medication or diuretic drugs.[46] As calcium channel blockers, the most common form of medication for high blood pressure, can increase your risk of heart attack, heart failure, and stroke, lowering blood pressure through natural means is of obvious benefit to heart health.

Selenium—A positive relationship has been found between low serum selenium levels and cardiovascular disease, possibly related to selenium's antioxidant effects.[47] Selenium supplementation also reduces platelet aggregation,[48] and selenium is a cofactor for glutathione peroxidase, an important antioxidant enzyme.

Other Supplements for Heart Health

The following supplements have also proven useful in treating heart disease and maintaining heart health:

Amino Acids—The amino acid L-arginine, when given intravenously at the rate of 20 g over one hour, can produce significant increases in stroke volume and cardiac output in patients with congestive heart failure. Arginine therapy can also lower arterial blood pressure.[49]

Supplementation with the amino acid L-carnitine immediately after an acute heart attack can help damaged heart muscle expand again. In one study, L-carnitine, when given orally at the rate of 2 g daily for 28 days, improved the condition of 51 patients who had undergone heart attacks.[50] Specifically, the amount of damaged heart muscle after 28 days was significantly less, the incidence of angina pectoris and arrhythmia was reduced by 50%, and the number of cardiac events of any kind for those on L-carnitine was 15.6% compared to 26% for those taking a placebo.

In another study of 472 post–heart attack patients, taking 9 g daily of L-carnitine by intravenous infusion for five days, followed by an oral dosage of 6 g daily (in three divided doses) for the next 12 months, improved the ability of the heart muscle to widen to receive incoming blood.[51] A heart attack (myocardial infarction) otherwise leaves portions of the heart muscle (myocardium) dead (infarcted) and thus unable to expand.

Bioflavonoids—Lower than average dietary intake of bioflavonoids (antioxidants that enhance vitamin C activity), specifically those found in onions and apples, can increase the risk of coronary heart disease, according to a Finnish study of 5,133 men and women, 30-69 years old.[52] Bioflavonoids found in other fruits, black tea, and red wine were also helpful to the heart.

Coenzyme Q10—Coenzyme Q10 is a natural chemical substance essential to the generation of energy in the cells. It's called a "coenzyme" because it enhances the activity of other enzymes. Over 30 years ago, Karl Folkers, Ph.D., a biomedical scientist at the University of Texas in Austin, discovered that coQ10 helps to strengthen the heart muscle and energize the cardiovascular system in many heart patients. Since then, studies have revealed that coenzyme Q10 may protect

For more about the **dangers of conventional blood pressure medication**, see Chapter 8: What Causes High Blood Pressure?, pp. 152-160, and Chapter 9: Self-Care Options: How to Use Diet, Exercise, and Lifestyle Changes to Lower Your Blood Pressure, pp. 162-171.

Research is needed into the role of nutritional supplements in preventing and reversing heart disease.

For more on **red wine and heart benefits**, see "Here's to Your Health: Drinking and the Heart," Chapter 2: Caring for Yourself, p. 59.

Vitamin and Mineral Supplement Ranges

Vitamin	Adult US RDA	Adult Daily Supplement Range

FAT-SOLUBLE VITAMINS

Beta Carotene	Not Established	10,000-50,000 IU

(Pro-Vitamin A) Converted by the body to vitamin A as needed. Primary antioxidant which helps protect the lungs and other tissues.
Possible side effects: Prolonged ingestion of relatively high doses may cause a benign yellowing of the skin, especially palms and soles. Avoid beta carotene supplement while taking the prescription drug Accutane, especially during pregnancy.

Vitamin E	12-15 IU	200-800 IU

(Alpha Tocopherol) Primary antioxidant which protects red blood cells and is essential in cellular respiration.
Possible side effects: Prolonged ingestion of vitamin E may produce adverse skin reactions and upset stomach.

WATER-SOLUBLE VITAMINS

Vitamin C	60 mg	300-3,000 mg

(Ascorbic Acid) Primary antioxidant, essential for tissue growth, wound healing, absorption of calcium and iron, and utilization of the B vitamin folic acid. Involved in neurotransmitter biosynthesis, cholesterol regulation, and formation of collagen.
Possible side effects: Essentially nontoxic in oral doses. However, excessive ingestion may cause abdominal bloating, gas, flatulence, and diarrhea. Acid-sensitive individuals should take the buffered ascorbate form of vitamin C supplement.

Vitamin B3	16-20 mg	20-100 mg

(Niacin) Essential for food metabolism and release of energy for cellular function. Vital for oxygen transport in the blood, and fatty acid and nucleic acid formation. A major constituent of several important coenzymes.
Possible side effects: Essentially nontoxic in normal oral doses. High doses (100 mg+) may cause transient flushing and tingling in the upper body area as well as stomach upset. Prolonged ingestion of excess vitamin B3 (1,000-2,000 mg+/day) may elevate liver enzymes and cause liver damage.

Vitamin B6	2.0-2.5 mg	5-200 mg

(Pyroxidine) Involved in food metabolism and release of energy. Essential for amino acid metabolism and formation of blood proteins and antibodies. Helps regulate electrolytic balance.
Possible side effects: Prolonged high doses (500 mg+/day) may be toxic and cause neurological damage. Note: Prescription oral contraceptives may cause deficiency of vitamin B6.

Vitamin	Adult US RDA	Adult Daily Supplement
Vitamin B12	3.0-4.0 mg	10-500 mcg

(Cobalamin) Essential for normal formation of red blood cells. Involved in food metabolism, release of energy, and maintenance of epithelial cells (cells that form the skin's outer layer and the surface layer of mucous membranes) and the nervous system.
Possible side effects: Essentially nontoxic in oral doses.

Folate	400 mcg	200-800 mcg

(Folic Acid, Folacin) Essential for blood formation, especially red blood cells and white blood cells. Involved in the biosynthesis of nucleic acids, including RNA and DNA.
Possible side effects: Essentially nontoxic in oral doses. An excess intake of folate can mask a vitamin B12 deficiency. Note: B vitamins should be taken in a B-complex form because of their close interrelationship in metabolic processes.

MINERALS—The functions of minerals are highly interrelated to each other and to vitamins, hormones, and enzymes. No mineral can function in the body without affecting others.

Calcium	800-1,200 mg	200-1,200 mg

(CA ++) Essential for strong bones and teeth. Serves as a vital cofactor in cellular energy production, and nerve and heart function.
Possible side effects: Prolonged ingestion of excess calcium, along with excess vitamin D, may cause hypercalcemia of bone and soft tissue (such as joints and kidneys) and may also cause a mineral imbalance.

Chromium	50-200 mcg	200-500 mcg

(CR +++) Vital as a cofactor of GTF (glucose tolerance factor), which regulates the function of insulin. Involved in food metabolism, enzyme activation, and regulation of cholesterol.
Possible side effects: Essentially nontoxic in oral doses.

Magnesium	300-350 mg	150-600 mg

(MG ++) Essential catalyst for food metabolism and release of energy. A cofactor in the formation of RNA and DNA, and in enzyme activation and nerve function.
Possible side effects: Extremely high doses (30,000 mg+) may be toxic in certain individuals with kidney problems. Doses of 400 mg+ may produce a laxative effect, causing diarrhea.

continued on next page

Vitamin and Mineral Supplement Ranges (cont.)

Vitamin	Adult US RDA	Adult Daily Supplement Range
Potassium	Not established	1,875-5,625 mg*

(K+) A primary electrolyte, important in regulating pH (acidity/alkalinity) balance and water balance. Plays a role in nerve function and cellular integrity.
Possible side effects: Extremely high doses (25,000 mg+/day) of K chloride may be toxic in instances of kidney failure.
*A typical healthy diet contains adequate potassium. Very active individuals may require additional electrolytes.

Selenium	55-200 mcg	100-200 mcg

(SE) Important constituent of the antioxidant enzyme glutathione peroxidase, which is contained in white blood cells and blood platelets.
Possible side effects: Prolonged ingestion of excess selenium may be toxic.

against atherosclerosis and, through its antioxidant properties, may protect against the formation of oxysterols.[53] It can also protect your heart against the damaging effects of the cancer drug adriamycin.

In one study, 17 patients with mild congestive heart failure took 30 mg daily of coQ10; after four weeks, every patient had improved and 53% had become symptom-free. CoQ10 kept 38% of 641 patients from requiring hospitalization for the same condition; they took coQ10 at the rate of 150 mg daily for one year.

Patients with angina pectoris who took 150 mg per day for four weeks had a 53% reduction in chest pain episodes. After 12 weeks on coQ10, patients with cardiomyopathy (a disease of the heart muscle) enjoyed increased strength in their heartbeat and less shortness of breath. Patients undergoing heart surgery who took coQ10 for 14 days before and 30 days after surgery recovered faster and with fewer complications.

Garry F. Gordon, M.D., D.O., reports success in helping infants avoid risky and unnecessary surgery using supplements of coQ10, amino acids, and herbs. "In one case, I went to see a newborn diagnosed with myocardiopathy. I asked the attending doctor if he had tried coenzyme Q10 or carnitine [an amino acid]. He said that he had read about their effects, but would not use either. With the family's permission, I treated the baby with those supplements, as well as

In one study, 17 patients with mild congestive heart failure took 30 mg daily of coQ10; after four weeks, every patient had improved and 53% had become symptom-free.

with magnesium, vitamin C, a multiple vitamin/mineral product, liquid garlic, and the herbal extract of hawthorn berry. The baby recovered without the heart transplant surgery that was being recommended by the university medical center."

Although coenzyme Q10 is present in many foods (such as rice and wheat bran) and the body can make it from the raw materials in foods, many serious health conditions have now been linked to a shortage of coQ10 in the body's nutritional stocks. Some conventional medications can also deplete the supply. For example, Mevacor, taken to lower cholesterol, also dangerously lowers body levels of coQ10.

While coQ10 is not yet generally prescribed by physicians in the U.S., in Japan it is among the most widely used of drugs. Animal studies prove that even at high doses, coQ10 has no toxic side effects and is safe as a nutritional supplement. Generally it takes four to eight weeks for coQ10 to build up a peak concentration in the body and to produce noticeable effects. CoQ10 is best absorbed as a supplement when it's prepared dissolved in oil rather than as a powdered capsule; in fact, one of the leading authorities on the substance states that the body cannot absorb coQ10 unless it is made fat-soluble. Chewable wafers of coQ10 combined with fatty acids are available and work well.[54]

For more about **coenzyme Q10,** see Chapter 10: Preventing & Reversing High Blood Pressure: One Doctor's Approach, pp. 172-182.

CoQ10 is available as capsules from: Stan Jankowitz, 730 Galloping Hill Road, Franklin Lakes, NJ 07417; tel: 201-891-1104; fax: 201-848-1867.

Essential Fatty Acids (EFAs)—Omega-3 and omega-6 oils are the two principal types of essential fatty acids, which are unsaturated fats required in the diet. The digits "3" and "6" refer to differences in the oil's chemical structure with respect to its chain of carbon atoms and where they are bonded. A balance of these oils in the diet is required for good health. The primary omega-3 oil is called alpha-linolenic acid (ALA) and is found in flaxseed (58%), canola, pumpkin and walnut, and soybeans. Fish oils, such as salmon, cod, and mackerel, contain the other important omega-3 oils, DHA (docosahexaenoic acid) and EPA (eicosapentaenoic acid).

Omega-3 oils help reduce the risk of heart disease. Linoleic acid or cis-linoleic acid is the main omega-6 oil and is found in most plant

Is Fish Oil as Effective as Aspirin in Preventing Heart Attacks?

In the early 1980s, physicians began prescribing aspirin as a preventative to those patients at risk for heart attacks and strokes. Many cited aspirin's anticoagulant effects, noting that aspirin prevents the blood from clotting in plaque-occluded arteries. Dr. Cowden suggests that this approach may be misguided, since aspirin has been known to cause gastrointestinal bleeding and even perforated ulcers in some cases, whereas eicosapentaenoic acid (EPA), an omega-3 essential fatty acid from fish oils, has no such risks and has also been shown to significantly reduce death from coronary heart disease.[55]

In addition, EPA (especially when taken in conjunction with adequate antioxidant nutrients like vitamins E and C and beta carotene) works on reducing stickiness of clotting cells in the blood by affecting prostaglandin ratios (as aspirin does). However, EPA also favorably alters blood lipid ratios and helps to lower blood pressure (which aspirin does not).[56]

and vegetable oils, including safflower (73%), corn, peanut, and sesame. The most therapeutic form of omega-6 oil is gamma-linolenic acid (GLA), found in evening primrose, black currant, and borage oils. Once in the body, omega-6 is converted to prostaglandins, hormone-like substances that regulate many metabolic functions, particularly inflammatory processes.

Supplementing the diet with essential fatty acids may help to lower the level of homocysteine.[57] Omega-3 EFAs are useful in reducing high LDL cholesterol levels and may prevent heart attacks by eliminating clotting and arterial damage.[58] Omega-6 EFAs have been shown to decrease the aggregation or stickiness of platelets, allowing them to pass through the arteries without danger of clotting.[59] Evidence suggests that gamma-linolenic acid may help to regulate the cardiovascular system.[60] Dr. Cowden recommends taking at least equal amounts of omega-3 whenever taking omega-6 fatty acids.

FOS (Fructo-oligosaccharides)—A Japanese study found that when 23 hospital patients, 50-90 years old, took 8 g of fructo-oligosaccharides (FOS) daily for two weeks, the *Bifidobacteria* (beneficial bacteria) levels in their intestines increased by ten times. Benefits from increasing *Bifidobacteria* levels include cholesterol reduction, control of blood sugar levels, immune function enhancement, and a reduction of the detoxification load on the liver, among others. FOS also has been shown to lower blood pressure by 9% when taken at 11.5 g daily by people with high blood pressure.

Under the best of conditions, the estimated 100 trillion bacteria that live in the human intestines do so in a delicate balance. Certain bacteria such as *Lactobacillus* and *Bifidobacteria* are "friendly" bacteria that support numerous vital physiological processes. Other bacteria such as *E. coli*, *Staphylococcus*, and *Clostridrium* may be present in smaller numbers, but they are considered "unfriendly," even dangerous bacteria.

A healthy intestine maintains a balance of the various intestinal flora, but with current lifestyles and the use of antibiotics, drugs, and processed foods, this balance is often upset. For example, people who eat a high-fat, low-fiber diet have reduced *Bifidobacteria* populations in their intestines. Practitioners of alternative medicine often recommend using probiotics, which means deliberately introducing live "friendly" bacteria into the system through food products (yogurt or *Acidophilus* milk) or through special supplements.

A new approach, developed in Japan in the mid-1980s, is called *prebiotics*. Here you introduce nutrients that directly feed the beneficial bacteria already in place in a person's large intestine, most typically, *Bifidobacteria* and *Lactobacilli*. Japanese researchers determined that FOS, a naturally occurring form of carbohydrate found in certain foods in minute amounts, could be a perfect food for *Bifidobacteria*. FOS acts like an intestinal "fertilizer," selectively feeding the friendly microflora in the large intestine so that their numbers can usefully increase. *Bifidobacteria* work to lower the pH (acidity/alkalinity balance) in the large intestine to a slightly more acidic condition; this discourages the growth of unfriendly bacteria.

In recognition of the health benefits of FOS, in Japan today over 500 commercially prepared foods contain FOS (known there as "neosugar"), with the endorsement of Japan's Minister of Health. FOS, which is made by fermenting sucrose with a fungus called *Aspergillus niger* (*Aspergillus oryzae*, for example, is used to make miso and soy sauce), is about 30% as sweet as sucrose.[61]

QUICK DEFINITION

Friendly bacteria, or probiotics, refer to beneficial microbes inhabiting the human gastrointestinal tract where they are essential for proper nutrient assimilation. The human body contains an estimated several thousand billion beneficial bacteria comprising over 400 species, all necessary for health. Among the more well-known of these are *Lactobacillus acidophilus* and *Bifidobacterium bifidum*. Overly acidic bodily conditions, chronic constipation or diarrhea, dietary imbalances, overly processed foods, and the excessive use of antibiotics and hormonal drugs can interfere with probiotic function and even reduce their numbers, setting up conditions for illness.

For more information about **FOS,** contact: GTC Nutrition Company, 1400 W. 122nd Avenue, Suite 110, Westminster, CO 80234; tel: 303-254-8012; fax: 303-254-8201.

The standard American diet has been continually cited by numerous studies conducted since the 1960s as a contributing, causative factor in a variety of "killer" diseases, including coronary heart disease, atherosclerosis, strokes, and high blood pressure.

Why Do We Need Nutritional Supplements?

Ever since the term "vitamins" was coined almost 100 years ago to describe the discovery of the essential life substances in foods, scientists have debated the issue of nutritional adequacy. Medical science has long held that healthy adults do not need supplementation if they consume a healthful, varied diet. Until recently, it was widely believed that supplements were only considered necessary if a person had an outright, or "severe," nutrient deficiency, usually manifested by overt illness.

Today, research indicates that people can have "mild" or "moderate" nutrient deficiencies, and that nutritional supplements are necessary to maintain health, according to nutritionist D. Lindsey Berkson, M.A., D.C., of Santa Fe, New Mexico. These mild disorders may not cause tangible health disorders, making them difficult to diagnose, but can result in a variety of symptoms along with a general decrease in wellness. Unaddressed, these deficiencies can often put the body at risk for future health problems. Therefore, it is important for individuals to be sure they are receiving the proper amounts of nutrients for overall emotional and physical well-being.

The standard American diet has been continually cited by numerous studies conducted since the 1960s as a contributing, causative factor in a variety of "killer" diseases, including coronary heart disease, atherosclerosis, strokes, high blood pressure, diabetes, arthritis, and colitis. Additionally, other contributing factors such as environmental pollution and stressful life patterns are creating even greater nutrient requirements. As the typical American diet is resulting in dangerous deficiencies, people are requiring more nutrients to maintain good health, even though they may appear to be adequately fed.

The United States Department of Agriculture (USDA) has found that a significant percentage of the United States population receives well under 70% of the U.S. Recommended Daily Allowance (RDA) for vitamin A, vitamin C, B-complex vitamins, and the essential minerals calcium, magnesium, and iron.[62] A separate study found that most typical diets contained less than 80% of the RDA for calcium, magnesium, iron, zinc, copper, and manganese, and that the people most at risk were young children and women, adolescent to elderly.[63]

A new Healthy Eating Index study of 4,000 Americans, conducted by the USDA, reveals that 88% of the population does not get good grades for proper nutrition. More than 80% eat too much saturated fat and too little fruits, vegetables, and fiber-rich grains. The worst eaters are between 15 and 39 years old. In all, the American diet of the 1990s achieves only 63% of what the USDA considers good nutrition.

Recommended Daily Allowances

The generally accepted reference standard for nutritional adequacy in the United States is the RDA. Developed by a group of government-sponsored scientists, its function is to provide levels of essential nutrients that prevent classic deficiency diseases and to set marginal daily guidelines for average population groups. As it was difficult for the scientists to agree upon the RDAs, they built within the guidelines instructions to keep reviewing and changing the RDAs every four years as new information is discovered. Today, in the wake of overwhelming clinical evidence that shows a wide variance in each person's individual nutritional needs, a growing number of scientists have begun to dispute the validity of RDA standards.

While a diet adequate in RDAs may be appropriate to avoid severe nutritional deficiency diseases such as rickets, scurvy, or beriberi, it may not be appropriate to avoid more mild deficiency reactions such as nervousness, insomnia, mental exhaustion, improper immune function, or proneness to injury. Emmanuel Cheraskin, M.D., D.M.D., suggests that IDAs—Ideal Daily Allowances—should replace RDAs, to make up for the limiting nature inherent in the current method.

Scientists have increasingly begun to examine whether the standardized RDA guidelines are sufficient for individual nutritional needs. One of the first to question the guidelines was Roger Williams, Ph.D., a pioneering biochemist who discovered vitamin B5 (pantothenic acid) in the 1930s. In his book *Nutrition Against Disease*, Dr. Williams express-

Since the current U.S. RDAs are an inadequate guide to the therapeutic benefits of nutritional supplements, research should be conducted to determine accurate supplementation ranges.

The United States Department of Agriculture (USDA) has found that a significant percentage of the United States population receives well under 70% of the U.S. Recommended Daily Allowance (RDA) for vitamin A, vitamin C, B-complex vitamins, and the essential minerals calcium, magnesium, and iron.

es his belief that each person is genetically unique, and therefore requires slight variations in nutrient intake to function optimally. He calls this principle biochemical individuality. Dr. Williams also believes that all living creatures are greatly affected by the overall quality, balance, and quantity of food ingested.

The concept of biochemical individuality has brought about many changes, including the emergence of new preventive diagnostic procedures, such as nutrition assessment and risk factor analysis. These utilize physiological data, personal and family health history, dietary intake analysis, and scientifically advanced biochemical screenings to help nutritional practitioners determine individual biochemistry and nutritional status.

The current challenge for medicine and nutritional science is to look beyond statistical guidelines in order to gain a greater understanding of the role of nutrients and determine the levels appropriate for each individual to achieve and maintain a high level of wellness. Through education and involvement, people can develop an understanding of the proper diet and nutritional needs specifically suited to their individual chemistries, and make this knowledge an integral part of living well.

Essential Nutrients

"Essential nutrients are those nutrients derived from food that the body is unable to manufacture on its own," says Jeffrey Bland, Ph.D., of Gig Harbor, Washington. These are absolutely necessary for human life and include eight amino acids, at least 13 vitamins, and at least 15 minerals, plus essential fatty acids, water, and carbohydrates.

Amino acids are the building blocks of protein. The essential amino acids are L-isoleucine, L-leucine, L-valine, L-methionine, L-threonine, L-phenylalanine, and L-tryptophan.

Essential vitamins are broken up in two groups: fat-soluble and water-soluble. The essential vitamins classified as fat-soluble include A, D, E, and K. The water-soluble essential vitamins are C (ascorbic acid), B1 (thiamine), B2 (riboflavin), B3 (niacin), B5 (pantothenic acid), B6 (pyridoxine), B12, folic acid, and biotin.

The essential minerals include calcium, magnesium, phosphorus, iron, zinc, copper, manganese, iodine, chromium, potassium, sodium, and a number of trace elements. They make up part of the necessary elements of body tissues, fluids, and other nutrients and play an active role in the body's regulatory functions. Low levels of these nutrients have been linked to such conditions as heart disease, high blood pressure, cancer, osteoporosis, depression, schizophrenia, and problems relating to menopause.

Essential fatty acids (EFAs) required for proper metabolism include linoleic and linolenic acid, found in seafood and unrefined veg-

Today, an estimated 46% of adult Americans take nutritional supplements, many on a daily basis.

etable oils, plus oleic and arachidonic acids, found in peanuts and most organic fats and oils. As mentioned earlier, EFAs play an important role in reducing heart disease.

Accessory Nutrients

There are also many nonessential nutrients, called accessory nutrients or cofactors, that work in harmony with the essential nutrients to aid in the breakdown and conversion of food into cellular energy, and that also help support all of the body's physical and mental functions.

According to Dr. Bland, some of the accessory nutrients that help support metabolism include vitamin B-complex cofactors choline and inositol, as well as coenzyme Q10 (a close relative of the B vitamins) and lipoic acid.

Other accessory nutrients which have demonstrated preventative functions include B-complex cofactor PABA (para-aminobenzoic acid) and substance P, bioflavonoids which work with vitamin C. Certain amino acids found in protein are also considered nonessential because they can be synthesized by the body from the essential amino acids.

How Nutrients Work Together

Vitamins and minerals help regulate the conversion of food to energy in the body, according to Dr. Bland, and can be separated into two general categories: energy nutrients, which are principally involved in the conversion of food to energy, and protector nutrients, which help defend against damaging toxins derived from drugs, alcohol, radiation, environmental pollutants, or the body's own enzyme processes.

Nutritional supplements are not a panacea, however, and it is important to be aware of some potential risks. Prolonged intake of excessive doses of vitamins A, D, and B6, for example, may produce toxic effects. Other vitamins, minerals, and accessory nutrients can also sometimes cause side effects when they interact with medications, or due to health condition, or simply a person's biochemical individuality.

"The B complex vitamins and magnesium are examples of energy nutrients," says Dr. Bland, "for they activate specific metabolic facilitators called enzymes, which control digestion and the absorption and use of proteins, fats, and carbohydrates. These nutrients often work as a team, their mutual presence enhancing each other's function."

In the process of converting food to energy, oxygen–free radicals are produced that can damage the body and set the stage for degenerative diseases, including heart disease, arthritis, certain forms of cancer, and premature aging. Protector nutrients, such as vitamin E, beta carotene, vitamin C, and the minerals zinc, copper, manganese, and selenium, play a critical role in preventing or delaying these degenerative processes. Vitamins E, A, and C work together as a team, protecting against breakdown and helping each other maintain adequate tissue levels.

Dr. Berkson notes that vitamins and minerals are what make the chemical and electrical circuitry of the body work, and that the body's functioning is therefore profoundly affected by how nutrients either work together or against each other. Nutrients can help each other or inhibit each other when taken simultaneously. For example, iron is best absorbed when taken separately from pancreatic enzymes and also should not be taken with vitamin E, says Dr. Berkson. There are also certain nutrients that can help "potentiate" the other nutrients. For example, vitamin C taken with iron provides the maximum absorption of the iron.

Using Nutritional Supplements

Today, an estimated 46% of adult Americans take nutritional supplements, many on a daily basis.[64] It is no longer just a fad, but part of a growing trend as more and more people take a proactive approach to their own health care.

Although researchers are learning more every day about the connection between nutrients and health, there is still no definitive scientific "how-to guide" for the complexity of nutritional supplementation, especially since each individual's needs are different.

While it is always recommended that a person try to obtain as many nutrients as possible through the consumption of a variety of nutrient-dense foods, this can be unrealistic for many, due to: reduced calorie intake; the dislike of certain foods; loss of nutrients in cooking; the variable quality of food supply; lack of knowledge, motivation, or time to plan and prepare balanced meals; and nutrient depletion caused by stress, lifestyle, and certain medications. This is where nutritional supplements can play an important role in filling nutrient gaps.

Alternative practitioners may sometimes recommend dosages higher than those currently considered safe by conventional medicine. The scientific literature and numerous clinical trials support these elevated dosages for short periods of time and only under medical supervision. "For example," says Dr. Berkson, "many alternative practitioners use extremely elevated levels of vitamin A for several days to a week to act as a natural antibiotic for acute infection."

Nutritional supplements should also never take the place of appropriate medical care when warranted. If you are currently under medical care, taking any medications, or have a history of specific problems, it is important to consult with a physician before making any changes in diet or lifestyle, including the use of supplements.

It can take years of personal research and experimentation to put together a good dietary and supplement program. To eliminate a lot of guesswork and frustration, it is advisable to consult a qualified health professional trained in the intricacies of nutritional biochemistry for assistance in determining your individual needs and developing an effective dietary and nutritional supplement program tailored to those needs.

How to Take Nutritional Supplements

Before taking any nutritional supplement, you should ask what scientific data supports its safety and what are the safe intake levels. Drs. Bland and Berkson make the following recommendations:

■ Nutritional supplements should be taken with meals to promote increased absorption. Fat-soluble vitamins (such as vitamin A, beta carotene, and vitamin E) and the essential fatty acids linoleic and alpha linolenic acid should be taken during the day with the meal that contains the most fat.

Since nutritional supplements cannot be patented, there is little financial incentive for pharmaceutical companies to invest the millions of dollars needed to meet the government's stringent research requirements and thus receive FDA approval for their use in the treatment of specific conditions. Alternative sources of funding must be found in order to make nutritional supplements an accepted part of mainstream medicine.

■ Amino acid supplements should be taken on an empty stomach at least an hour before or after a meal, with fruit juice to help promote absorption. When taking an increased dosage of one particular amino acid, be sure to supplement with an amino acid blend.

■ If you become nauseated when you take tablet supplements, consider taking a liquid form, diluted in a beverage.

■ If you become nauseated or ill within an hour after taking nutritional supplements, consider the need for a bowel cleanse or rejuvenation program prior to beginning a course of nutritional supplementation.

■ If you are taking high doses, do not take the supplements all at one time, but divide them into smaller doses taken throughout the day.

■ Take digestive enzymes with meals to assist digestion. If you are taking pancreatic enzymes for other therapeutic reasons, be sure to take them on an empty stomach between meals.

■ Take mineral supplements separately from the highest fiber meals of the day as fiber can decrease mineral absorption.

■ When taking an increased dosage of a particular B vitamin, be sure to supplement with a B complex.

■ When taking nutrients, be sure to take adequate amounts of liquid to mix with digestive juices and to prevent side effects.

The standard American diet has been continually cited by numerous studies conducted since the 1960s as a contributing, causative factor in a variety of "killer" diseases, including coronary heart disease, atherosclerosis, strokes, high blood pressure, diabetes, arthritis, and colitis. As the typical American diet is resulting in dangerous deficiencies, people are requiring more nutrients to maintain good health, even though they may appear to be adequately fed.

How Herbs Can Aid Your Heart

THE WORD "HERB" as used in herbal medicine (also known as botanical medicine or, in Europe, as phytotherapy or phytomedicine) means a plant or plant part that is used to make medicine, food flavors (spices), or aromatic oils for soaps and fragrances. An herb can be a leaf, a flower, a stem, a seed, a root, a fruit, bark, or any other plant part used for its medicinal, food-flavoring, or fragrant property.[1]

Herbs for the Heart

According to David L. Hoffmann, B.Sc., M.N.I.M.H., of Sebastopol, California, past president of the American Herbalist Guild, "Some herbs have a potent and direct impact upon the heart itself, such as *Digitalis purpurea* (foxglove), and form the basis of drug therapy for heart failure."

While it's best to consult a skilled herbalist before taking herbs, the following is an example of a cardiac tonic that Hoffmann recommends: an equal combination of tinctures of hawthorn berries, *Ginkgo biloba*, and linden flowers (one-half teaspoon three times a day). He also suggests the addition of tincture of motherwort, to prevent palpitations, and garlic, to help manage cholesterol.

The following herbs can be beneficial to the heart and circulatory system:

Cayenne (*Capsicum annuum*)

Cayenne or red pepper is the most useful of the systemic stimulants. It stimulates blood flow, strengthening the heartbeat and metabolic rate.[2] A general tonic, it is helpful specifically for the circulatory and digestive systems. If there is insufficient peripheral circulation, leading to cold hands and feet and possibly chilblains (a form of cold injury characterized by redness and blistering), cayenne may be used. It is also useful for debility as well as for warding off colds.[3]

Chlorella

In Japan, *Chlorella pyrenoidosa*, a freshwater single-celled green algae, is more popular as a regular supplement than vitamin C. An estimated five million Japanese use this medicinal algae every day. Chlorella's broad spectrum health benefits, amply researched by Japanese scientists, include the impressive fact that it contains 60% protein, including all the essential amino acids, and high levels of beta carotene and chlorophyll.

For more information on **chlorella**, contact: Nature's Balance, Inc., 635A Southwest St., High Point, NC 27260; tel: 910-882-4102; fax: 910-882-4119; orders: 800-858-5198. Sun Wellness, Inc., 4025 Spencer Street, Unit 104, Torrance, CA 90503; tel: 800-829-2828 or 310-371-5515; fax: 310-371-0094.

It is to chlorella's high chlorophyll content (more chlorophyll per gram than any other plant) that many researchers (and enthusiastic users) attribute its multiple health benefits, but new research from Japan suggests that chlorella's secret might lie elsewhere—in its effect on albumin.

For more about **albumin** and **longevity**, see "A New Marker for Longevity: How's Your Albumin Level?" *Digest* #20, pp. 112-116.

Albumin, continually secreted by the liver, is the most abundant protein found in the blood. It acts as a major natural antioxidant, contributing an estimated 80% of all neutralizing activity against free radicals in the blood that would otherwise damage cells and tissues. Albumin transports key nutritional substances and detoxifies the fluid surrounding cells in the connective tissue. But most important, at least 38 recent scientific studies have demonstrated the strong relationship between high blood levels of albumin and the lifespan of cells.

This research, says Tim Sara, president of Nature's Balance, a major U.S. supplier of chlorella, "has confirmed that serum levels of albumin are extremely accurate indicators of overall health status and that low albumin levels exist at the onset and progression of virtually every nonhereditary, degenerative disease process, including cancers and cardiovascular heart disease." A series of studies with rats demonstrated that chlorella supplementation increases albumin levels by 16% to 21%.

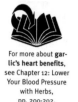

Garlic

Garlic has many properties that make it valuable in treating heart disease. It helps control cholesterol and contains sulfur compounds that work as antioxidants and aid in dissolving blood clots.[4]

For more about **garlic's heart benefits**, see Chapter 12: Lower Your Blood Pressure with Herbs, pp. 200-202.

Ginger (*Zingiber officinalis*)

In addition to its popular food flavoring qualities, ginger is well known for its cardiotonic properties.[5] It has been shown to lower cholesterol levels and make the blood platelets less sticky.[6]

Ginkgo (*Ginkgo biloba*)

Ginkgo is an excellent example of why protecting plants and animals from extinction can help create new medicine. Ginkgos are the oldest living trees on earth. They first appeared about 200 million years ago and, except for a small population in northern China, were almost completely destroyed in the last Ice Age. Ginkgo leaves contain several compounds called ginkgolides that have unique chemical structures. A standardized extract was developed in the past 20 years in Germany to treat a number of conditions associated with peripheral circulation.[7] It is currently licensed in Germany as a supportive treatment for peripheral arterial circulatory disturbances, such as intermittent claudication (a severe pain in the calf muscles resulting from inadequate blood supply).[8] Ginkgo leaf extracts are also used for heart diseases.[9]

One study found that a garlic-ginkgo combination lowered cholesterol rates in 35% of patients with levels ranging from 230 to 390—even during the Christmas holiday season when people tend to eat more high-fat foods. The supplement contained 150 mg of garlic and 40 mg of ginkgo (from a 50-to-1 extraction). Upon discontinuing the supplement, cholesterol levels rose again.[10]

Green Tea

Green tea (*Camellia sinensis*) is a highly popular beverage in China, Japan, and Korea, and may constitute 20% of the world's consumption of tea. In recent years, food scientists have identified health benefits connected to drinking tea. The primary chemical compounds found in green tea are called polyphenolic catechins and represent 17% to 30% of the dry weight of green tea leaves.

Catechins are many times stronger than vitamin E in defending the body against free radicals, thus supporting the immune system's responsiveness. They can reduce the risk of stroke and cardiovascular disease as well as stomach, pancreatic, and possibly lung cancers. A

No More Arrhythmia

John Sherman, N.D., of the Portland Naturopathic Clinic in Oregon, relates the case of Jolene, who came to his clinic complaining of heart palpitations. She was also concerned about the drugs she'd been prescribed for her heart arrhythmia. Jolene told Dr. Sherman that the drugs had been "sapping" her energy and only partially helping her heart problem. Dr. Sherman prescribed a combination herbal tincture of cactus, hawthorn, valerian, and lily of the valley, which is a standard combination naturopathic physicians use to combat arrhythmia and a "feeble" heart. He also analyzed her diet to determine her intake of specific minerals which affect the heart, including calcium, potassium, and sodium.

Jolene returned to Dr. Sherman's clinic two weeks later, still complaining of heart palpitations and feeling even more frustrated. Dr. Sherman decided to change the herbal formula slightly by adding Scotch broom. Within a few days, she happily reported the absence of any heart symptoms and was subsequently able to wean herself off the prescription drugs.

Japanese study showed that green tea can significantly lower blood pressure, reduce serum levels of LDL cholesterol, and keep blood sugar levels from rising inappropriately (as in diabetes and chronic weight-gain conditions).

To maximize the health benefits of catechins, Chemco Industries of Los Angeles, developed Polyphenon 60™ Green Tea Extract (under the Opti-Pure™ brand), a highly concentrated mixture obtained through organic nontoxic solvents, that contains 65.4% catechins. To put this in perspective, it takes about 909 pounds of green tea to extract 2.2 pounds of catechins. Optio™ Health Products, also in Los Angeles, uses Polyphenon 60 (a minimum of 20 mg in each tea bag) in its line of therapeutic green teas, which also contain *Ginkgo biloba*, bilberry, rose hips, and *Panax ginseng*.

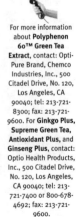

For more information about **Polyphenon 60™ Green Tea Extract**, contact: Opti-Pure Brand, Chemco Industries, Inc., 500 Citadel Drive, No. 120, Los Angeles, CA 90040; tel: 213-721-8300; fax: 213-721-9600. For **Ginkgo Plus, Supreme Green Tea, Antioxidant Plus,** and **Ginseng Plus,** contact: Optio Health Products, Inc., 500 Citadel Drive, No. 120, Los Angeles, CA 90040; tel: 213-721-7400 or 800-678-4692; fax: 213-721-9600.

Hawthorn

One of the most promising herbal remedies for the treatment of heart disease is the extract from the hawthorn berry, a commonly found shrub. Hawthorn berry has been found to help improve the circulation of blood to the heart by dilating the blood vessels and relieving spasms of the arterial walls.[11] According to Garry F. Gordon, M.D., D.O., "Hawthorn berry may render unnecessary medications that decrease the rate and force of heart contraction in

A Japanese study showed that green tea can significantly lower blood pressure, reduce serum levels of LDL cholesterol, and keep blood sugar levels from rising inappropriately as in diabetes and chronic weight-gain conditions.

For more on the **olive's heart benefits**, see Chapter 2: Caring for Yourself, pp. 52-54.

For a source of **olive leaf extract** , contact: Allergy Research Group (Prolive™ or Alive and Well™), 400 Preda Street, San Leandro, CA 94577; tel: 800-782-4274 or 510-639-4572; fax: 510-635-6730; e-mail: info@nutricology.com.

the treatment of heart disease as it performs a similar function to these drugs."

Olive Leaf Extract

Long a staple of Mediterranean cuisine, the olive and its oil have been linked to a lower incidence of heart disease in people of that region. Now evidence is mounting that an extract from olive leaves—oil comes from olive pulp—also has extensive therapeutic benefits, including lowering blood pressure, working against free-radical activity (which causes cell damage and leads to degeneration), repelling bacteria and viruses, and enhancing the immune systems of AIDS patients.

The active component of the olive leaf is oleuropein (the bitter element removed from olives when they are processed). The leaf also contains natural vitamin C helpers called bioflavonoids, such as rutin, luteolin, and hesperidin, which are needed for maintenance of the capillary walls and for protection against infection.[12] Analysis of oleuropein at the University of Messina in Italy demonstrated that olive leaf extract has distinct heart benefits. Researchers concluded that oleuropein increased blood flow to the heart and lowered blood pressure. Oleuropein found in olive leaf extracts had a stronger effect than oleuropein and the flavonoids in their isolated, purified form.[13]

Olive leaf extract may also have a heart-protecting effect due to its antioxidant ability, according to a study at the University of Milan in Italy. A high level of low-density lipoproteins (LDLs, the so-called bad cholesterol) in the blood—a result of a diet high in saturated fat—is considered a major risk factor for coronary heart disease. Oxidation of LDL (an undesirable chemical change produced by exposure to oxygen) is one of the factors that leads to the development of atherosclerotic lesions. Researchers found that oleuropein "interferes with biochemical events that are implicated in atherogenetic [heart] disease," such as blocking LDL oxidation by retarding the loss of vitamin E, a heart-protecting nutrient.[14]

The olive leaf's oleuropein may be effective against viruses. Some years ago, researchers at Upjohn, the pharmaceutical giant based in Kalamazoo, Michigan, reported that the main component in oleu-ropein, a salt extract called calcium elenolate, was "virucidal (virus-killing) for all viruses against which it has been tested." These include encephalomyocarditis, which attacks the brain and heart muscles. Upjohn researchers believed that calcium elenolate, interacting with the protein coat of the virus, managed to reduce the ability of these organisms to convey infections.

"The leaf and its extract may be of excellent nutritional value and will gain wide acclaim," says Stephen Levine, Ph.D., President and Director of Research at the Allergy Research Group in San Leandro, California. His company now markets an olive leaf extract in two forms: Alive and Well™ (for consumers) and Prolive™ (for medical professionals); both in 500-mg capsules. Dr. Levine suggests taking one capsule per day with meals for health maintenance, noting that it's advisable to con-sume extra amounts of pure **Olive leaf extract has distinct heart benefits. Researchers concluded that oleuropein increased blood flow to the heart and lowered blood pressure.** water while taking the extract, to help the body flush out toxins released under the influence of the olive leaf extract.

Herbs and Modern Medicine

Herbs have always been integral to the practice of medicine. The word drug comes from the old Dutch word *drogge* meaning "to dry," as pharmacists, physicians, and ancient healers often dried plants for use as medicines. Today, approximately 25% of all prescription drugs are still derived from trees, shrubs, or herbs.[15] Some are made from plant extracts; others are synthesized to mimic a natural plant com-pound. The World Health Organization notes that of 119 plant-derived pharmaceutical medicines, about 74% are used in modern medicine in ways that correlate directly with their traditional uses as plant medicines by native cultures.[16]

Yet, for the most part, modern medicine has veered from the use of pure herbs in its treatment of disease and other health disorders. One of the reasons for this is economic. Since herbs cannot be patent-ed and drug companies cannot hold the exclusive right to sell a par-ticular herb, they are not motivated to invest any money in that herb's

Of 119 plant-derived pharmaceutical medicines, about 74% are used in modern medicine in ways that correlated directly with their traditional uses as plant medicines by native cultures.

testing or promotion. The collection and preparation of herbs for medicine cannot be as easily controlled as the manufacture of synthetic drugs, making the profits less dependable.

In addition, many of these medicinal plants grow only in the Amazonian rain forest or politically and economically unstable places, which also affects the supply of the herb. Most importantly, the demand for herbal medicine has decreased in the United States because Americans have been conditioned to rely on synthetic, commercial drugs to provide quick relief, regardless of side effects.

However, the current viewpoint seems to be changing. "The revival of interest in herbal medicine is a worldwide phenomenon," says Mark Blumenthal, Executive Director of the American Botanical Council in Austin, Texas. This renaissance is due to the growing concern of the general public about the side effects of pharmaceutical drugs, the impersonal and often demeaning experience of modern health-care practices, as well as a renewed recognition of the unique medicinal value of herbal medicine.

Herbs Can Be Used in Many Forms

Herbs and herbal products are now available not only in natural food stores, but also grocery stores, drugstores, and gourmet food stores. Also, a number of multilevel marketing organizations sell a variety of herbal products, as do mail-order purveyors. Herbs come in many forms, including:

Whole Herbs: Whole herbs are plants or plant parts that are dried and then either cut or powdered. They can be used as teas or other products.

Teas: Teas come in either loose or tea-bag form. Because of the obvious convenience, most Americans today prefer to purchase their herbal teas in tea bags, which include one or a variety of finely cut herbs. When steeped in boiled water for a few minutes, the fragrant, aromatic flavor and the herbs' medicinal properties are released.

Capsules and Tablets: One of the fastest growing markets in herbal medicine in the past 15 to 20 years has been capsules and tablets. These offer consumers convenience and, in some cases, the bonus of not having to taste the herbs, many of which have undesirable flavor profiles, from intensely bitter (e.g., goldenseal root) due to the presence of certain alkaloids to highly astringent (e.g, oak bark) due to the presence of tannins.

Extracts and Tinctures: These offer the advantage of a high concentration in low weight and volume. They are also quickly assimilated by the body in comparison to tablets. Extracts and tinctures almost always contain alcohol. The alcohol is used for two reasons: as a solvent to extract the non-water-soluble compounds from an herb and as a preservative to maintain shelf life. Properly made extracts and tinctures have virtually an indefinite shelf life. Tinctures usually contain more alcohol than extracts (sometimes 70% to 80% alcohol, depending on the particular herb and manufacturer).

Essential Oils: Essential oils are usually distilled from various parts of medicinal and aromatic plants. Some oils, however, like those from lemon, orange, and other citrus fruits, are expressed directly from fruit peels. Essential oils are highly concentrated, with one or two drops often constituting adequate dosage. Thus, they are to be used carefully and sparingly when employed internally. Some oils may irritate the skin and should be diluted in fatty oils or water before topical application. Notable exceptions are eucalyptus and tea tree oils, which can be applied directly to the skin without concern of irritation.

Salves, Balms, and Ointments: For thousands of years, humans have used plants to treat skin irritations, wounds, and insect and snake bites. In prehistoric times, herbs were cooked in a vat of goose or bear fat, lard, or vegetable oils and then cooled in order to make salves, balms, and ointments. Today, a number of such products, made with vegetable oil or petroleum jelly, are sold in the United States and Europe to treat a variety of conditions. These products often contain aloe, marigold, chamomile, St. John's Wort, comfrey, or gotu kola.

How to Make an Herb Tea

Loose teas are usually steeped in hot water: three to ten minutes for leaves and flowers (this method is called infusion), or 15 to 20 minutes at a rolling boil for denser materials like root and bark (called a decoction).

Infusions: Infusions are the simplest method of preparing an herb tea and both fresh or dried herbs may be used, such as peppermint, chamomile, and rosehips. Due to the higher water content of the fresh herb, three parts fresh herb replace one part of the dried herb. To make an infusion:

■ Put about one teaspoonful of the dried herb or herb mixture for each cup into a teapot.

■ Add boiling water and cover. Let steep for five to ten minutes. Infusions may be taken hot, cold, or iced. They may also be sweetened.

■ Infusions are most appropriate for plant parts such as leaves, flowers, or green stems where the medicinal properties are easily accessible. To infuse bark, root, seeds, or resin, it is best to powder them first to break down some of their cell walls before adding them to the water. Seeds like fennel and aniseed should be slightly bruised to release the volatile oils from the cells. Any aromatic herb should be infused in a pot that has a well-sealing lid to reduce loss of the volatile oil through evaporation.

Decoctions: For hard and woody herbs, ginger root and cinnamon bark for example, it is best to make a decoction rather than an infusion, to ensure that the soluble contents of the herb actually reach the water. Roots, wood, bark, nuts, and certain seeds are hard and their cell walls are very strong, requiring more heat to release them than in an infusion. These herbs need to be boiled in the water. To make a decoction:

■ Put one teaspoonful of dried herb or three teaspoonfuls of fresh material for each cup of water into a pot or saucepan. Dried herbs should be powdered or broken into small pieces, while fresh material should be cut into small pieces.

■ Add the appropriate amount of water to the herbs.

■ Bring to a boil and simmer for 10 to 15 minutes.

When using a woody herb that contains a lot of volatile oil, it is best to make sure that it is powdered as finely as possible and then used in an infusion, to ensure that the oils do not boil away. Decoctions can be used in the same way as an infusion.

The Politics of Herbal Medicine

According to James Duke, Ph.D., a scientist and former USDA (United States Department of Agriculture) specialist in the area of herbal medicine, one of the reasons that research into the field of herbal medicine has been lacking is the enormous financial cost of the testing required to prove a new "drug" safe. Dr. Duke has seen that price tag rise from $91 million over ten years ago to the present figure of $231 million. Dr. Duke asks, "What commercial drug manufacturer is going to want to prove that

Additional research into the medicinal benefits of herbs will speed the integration of herbal medicine into the American health care system.

A 2,000-Year-Old Multi-Medicine from Deer Antlers

The cartilage of antlers from the velvet deer is poised to be one of the most versatile multipurpose natural remedies to arrive in the West. The Chinese have known about it for at least two millennia, according to an ancient medical scroll that recommends it for 52 health problems. Russians have used velvet deer antler for decades, especially as an endurance-building supplement for athletes, called Pantocrine. And for those living in Asia, Korea, and New Zealand, velvet deer antler is a medicinal food in high demand.

The medicinal claims for velvet deer antler are comprehensive and ambitious, and preliminary research tends to support most of them. Among the numerous claims, velvet deer antler can: improve blood circulation, reverse atherosclerosis, and possibly reduce the incidence of fatal heart attacks; increase the quality and quantity of blood production in treating kidney disorders and anemia; modulate the immune system, bringing it back to an even keel when it is depressed or overactive; increase muscular strength and nerve function; and generally boost energy.

What's in the antlers that can produce these effects? Cartilage, for one, which contains a substance called N-acetyl-glucosamine, which speeds up wound healing. The antlers also contain chondroitin sulfate, an anti-inflammatory substance that in concentrated form has been shown to reduce the incidence of fatal heart attacks reportedly by 400%, according to a six-year study. A natural growth hormone called IGF-1 is found in high levels in velvet deer antlers; this substance helps to keep the body lean and the muscles well-developed.[17]

Velvet deer antler is available as a powdered capsule (250 mg each) from the Prolongevity brand. The recommended dosage is one to four capsules a day for four weeks followed by one week off; users are advised that it may take 6 to 12 weeks to notice effects.

For information about **velvet deer antlers,** contact: Life Extension Foundation, P.O. Box 229120, Hollywood, FL 33022; tel: 1-800-544-4440.

saw palmetto is better than his multimillion dollar drug, when you and I can go to Florida and harvest our own saw palmetto?"

Other Alternatives for Heart Health

I N   C O N T R A S T   to conventional medicine, alternative medicine is providing exciting new options in treating heart disease. Instead of complicated, costly, and often dangerous surgery and drugs, many health-care professionals who practice alternative medicine work to correct the nutritional and biochemical imbalances that can affect the function of the heart and cause plaque deposits in the arteries.

In addition to the diet, exercise, and lifestyle recommendations and therapies covered in the preceding chapters, the following alternative medical techniques can be useful in restoring and maintaining heart health.

Ayurvedic Medicine

In treating heart disease, Ayurvedic physicians use several methods that can result in the reduction of the generation of free radicals, which, as we have discussed, can contribute to the disease process in the arteries and heart. "Meat, cigarette smoke, alcohol, and environmental pollutants all generate free radicals," explains Hari Sharma, M.D., president of Maharishi Ayurveda Medical Association. By using specific herbal food supplements and *pancha karma* (detoxification and purification techniques), says Dr. Sharma, "free radicals and lipid peroxides are reduced." As it is especially important for those with heart disease to lower their level of stress, Dr. Sharma also recommends a program of Transcendental Meditation.

Virender Sodhi, M.D. (Ayurveda), N.D., director of the American School of Ayurvedic Sciences in Bellevue, Washington, reports an interesting case of heart disease. Soram, a 55-year-old Asian male, had chest pain so severe that he could not walk more than ten steps before having to sit down. He came to Dr. Sodhi's office after receiving word from the local hospital that he needed immediate bypass surgery. The doctors told him that refusing the surgery would mean certain death.

Before beginning treatment, Soram underwent a battery of tests ordered by Dr. Sodhi. Angiographic studies showed that his coronary arteries were blocked—the left main coronary artery was 90% narrowed, the anterior descending was 80% narrowed, and the right coronary was 30% blocked. Blood tests indicated elevated cholesterol levels at 278 and decreased HDLs (high-density lipoproteins) at 38. Dr. Sodhi determined Soram's metabolic type according to Ayurvedic principles and started him on an appropriate cleansing program that included dietary changes and appropriate herbs.

After three months, Soram's cholesterol levels reportedly dropped more than 30% and his HDL level rose to 48. More importantly, though, his exercise tolerance had dramatically improved. "He was doing the treadmill exercise at the speed of five miles per hour for 45 minutes without any angina," reports Sodhi. More than two years later, Soram is doing fine. He now jogs up and down hills with no symptoms and his EKG has shown improvement. According to Dr. Sodhi, there is a hospital in Bombay, India, which has treated some 3,300 cases of coronary heart disease using this method with about 99% success.

Magnetic Field Therapy

The world is surrounded by magnetic fields: some are generated by the earth's magnetism, while others are generated by solar storms and changes in the weather. Magnetic fields are also created by everyday electrical devices: motors, televisions, office equipment, computers, microwave ovens, the electrical wiring in homes, and the power lines that supply them. Even the human body produces subtle magnetic

Ayurveda is the traditional medicine of India, based on many centuries of empirical use. Its name means "end of the Vedas" (which were India's sacred scripts), implying that a holistic medicine may be founded on spiritual principles. Ayurveda describes three metabolic, constitutional, and body types (doshas), in association with the basic elements of Nature in combination. These are *vata* (air and ether, rooted in intestines), *pitta* (fire and water/stomach), and *kapha* (water and earth/lungs). Ayurvedic physicians use these categories (which also have psychological aspects) as the basis for prescribing individualized formulas of herbs, diet, massage, breathing, meditation, exercise and yoga postures, and detoxification techniques.

For information about **Ayurvedic health products,** contact: Maharishi Ayur-Ved Products International Inc., P.O. Box 49667, Colorado Springs, CO 80949; tel: 719-260-5500; fax: 719-260-7400; e-mail: postmaster@mapi.com.

fields that are generated by the chemical reactions within the cells and the ionic currents of the nervous system.[1]

Recently, scientists have discovered that external magnetic fields can affect the body's functioning in both positive and negative ways, and this observation has led to the development of magnetic field therapy.

What is Magnetic Field Therapy?

The use of magnets and electrical devices to generate controlled magnetic fields has many medical applications and has proven to be one of the most effective means for diagnosing human illness and disease. For example, MRI (magnetic resonance imaging) is replacing X-ray diagnosis because it is safer and more accurate, and magnetoencephalography is now replacing electroencephalography as the preferred technique for recording the brain's electrical activity.

In 1974, researcher Albert Roy Davis, Ph.D., noted that positive and negative magnetic polarities have different effects upon the biological systems of animals and humans. He found that magnets could be used to arrest and kill cancer cells in animals, and could also be used in the treatment of arthritis, glaucoma, infertility, and diseases related to aging.[2] He concluded that negative magnetic fields have a

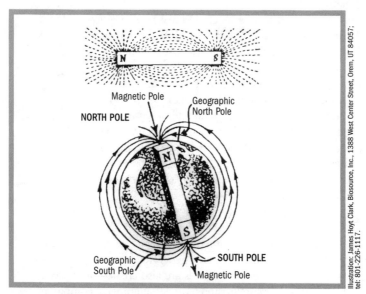

Negative *magnetic fields* have a beneficial effect on living organisms, whereas positive magnetic fields have a stressful effect.

"Symptoms of cardiac atherosclerosis and brain atherosclerosis have been observed to disappear after six to eight weeks of nightly exposure to a negative static magnetic field," reports Dr. Philpott.

beneficial effect on living organisms, whereas positive magnetic fields have a stressful effect.

"Scientifically designed, double-blind, placebo-controlled studies, however, have not been done to substantiate the claims of there being different effects between positive and negative magnetic poles," says John Zimmerman, Ph.D., president of the Bio-Electro-Magnetics Institute in Utah. "But numerous anecdotal, clinical observations suggest that such differences are real and do exist. Clearly, scientific research is needed to substantiate these claims."

Robert Becker, M.D., an orthopedic surgeon and author of numerous scientific articles and books, found that weak electric currents promote the healing of broken bones. Dr. Becker also brought national attention to the fact that electromagnetic interference from power lines and home appliances can pose a serious hazard to human health. "The scientific evidence," writes Dr. Becker, "leads only to one conclusion: the exposure of living organisms to abnormal electromagnetic fields results in significant abnormalities in physiology and function."[3]

According to Wolfgang Ludwig, Sc.D., Ph.D., director of the Institute for Biophysics in Horb, Germany, "Magnetic field therapy is a method that penetrates the whole human body and can treat every organ without chemical side effects." Magnetic field therapy has been used effectively in the treatment of atherosclerosis, circulatory problems, environmental stress, cancer, rheumatoid disease, infections and inflammations, headaches, sleep disorders, and fractures and pain. Dr. Ludwig notes that magnetic changes in the environment can affect the electromagnetic balance of the human organism and contribute to disease. Researchers suggest that magnetic therapy can be used to counter the effects caused by the electromagnetic pollution in the environment.

Kyoichi Nakagawa, M.D., director of the Isuzu Hospital in Tokyo, Japan, believes that the time people spend in buildings and cars reduces their exposure to the natural geomagnetic fields of the earth, and may also interfere with health. He calls this condition magnetic field deficiency syndrome, which can cause headaches, dizziness, muscle stiffness, chest pain, insomnia, constipation, and general fatigue.[4]

How Magnetic Field Therapy Works

"The healing potential of magnets is possible because the body's nervous system is governed, in part, by varying patterns of ionic currents and electromagnetic fields," reports Dr. Zimmerman. There are numerous forms of magnetic field therapy, including static magnetic fields produced by natural or artificial magnets, and pulsating magnetic fields generated by electrical devices. The magnetic fields produced by magnets or electromagnetic generating devices are able to penetrate the human body and can affect the functioning of the nervous system, organs, and cells. According to William H. Philpott, M.D., an author and biomagnetic researcher based in Choctaw, Oklahoma, magnetic fields can stimulate metabolism and increase the amount of oxygen available to cells. When used *properly*, magnetic field therapy has no known harmful side effects.

All magnets have two poles: one is called positive, and the other negative. However, as there are conflicting methods of naming the poles of a magnet, a magnetometer should be used as a standard method of determination (if one is using a compass to locate the poles, the arrowhead of the needle marked "N" or "North" will point to the magnet's negative pole). Dr. Philpott and other researchers claim that the negative pole generally has a calming effect and helps to normalize metabolic functioning. In contrast, the positive pole has a stressful effect, and with prolonged exposure interferes with metabolic functioning, produces acidity, reduces cellular oxygen supply, and encourages the replication of latent microorganisms.

The strength of a magnet is measured in units of gauss (a unit of the intensity of magnetic flux) or tesla (1 tesla=10,000 gauss), and every magnetic device has a manufacturer's gauss rating. However, the actual strength of the magnet at the skin surface is often much less than this number. For example, a 4,000-gauss magnet transmits about 1,200 gauss to the patient. Magnets placed in pillows or bed pads will render even lower amounts of field strength at the skin surface because a magnet's strength quickly decreases with the distance from the subject.

QUICK DEFINITION

Metabolism is the biological process by which energy is extracted from the foods consumed, producing carbon dioxide and water as by-products for elimination. Biochemically, metabolism involves hundreds of different chemical reactions, necessitating the involvement of hundreds of different enzymes, each of which handles a specific reaction. There are two kinds of metabolism constantly underway in the cells: anabolic and catabolic. In anabolic metabolism, the upbuilding phase, larger molecules are constructed by joining smaller ones together; in catabolic metabolism, the deconstructing phase, larger molecules are broken down into smaller ones. The anabolic function produces substances for cell growth and repair, while the catabolic function controls digestion (called hydrolysis), disassembling food into forms the body can use for energy.

> **"A negative magnetic field can function like an antibiotic in helping to destroy bacterial, fungal, and viral infections,"** says Dr. Philpott, **"by promoting oxygenation and lowering the body's acidity."**

How Magnets are Used Therapeutically

Magnetic therapy can be applied in many ways, and devices range from small, simple magnets to large machines capable of generating high magnitudes of field strength (used for treating fractures and pseudoarthrosis, a false joint forming after a fracture). Magnetic blankets and beds have also been manufactured for the purposes of promoting sleep and reducing stress. Specially designed ceramic, plastiform, and neodymium (a rare earth chemical element) magnets can be placed either individually or in clusters over the various organs of the body, on lymph nodes, or on various points of the head.

Research into the therapeutic benefits of magnetic field therapy is needed. This type of therapy could provide a safe and effective way to curb rising health care costs.

In Japan, small *tai-ki* magnets have been designed to stimulate acupuncture points, but no clinical studies have yet explored this procedure. Magnetic devices are popular in Germany, where the use of certain devices is covered by medical insurance. After simple instruction is given to the patient, these devices can be used at home.

Magnetic Field Therapy Treatment

Treatment can last from just a few minutes to overnight and, depending upon the situation and severity, may be applied several times a day or for days or weeks at a time. The following cases illustrate both the potential for success and wide range of application of magnetic field therapy. Sometimes the results can be dramatic, as in this case of heart flutter cited by Dr. Ludwig:

Heart Flutter–A 46-year-old man had suffered for years from severe heart flutter, diarrhea, and nausea. No treatment seemed to help, but when a magnetic applicator with less than one gauss of energy was placed upon his solar plexus for only three minutes, his symptoms immediately ceased. Two years later, he had experienced no relapse.

Atherosclerosis–According to Dr. Philpott, "Symptoms of cardiac atherosclerosis and brain atherosclerosis have been observed to disappear after six to eight weeks of nightly exposure to a negative static magnetic field." A man, 70, with atherosclerotic heart disease, underwent a multiple bypass operation. Two years later his heart pain returned, leaving him unsteady on his feet and subject to disorientation in familiar surroundings; his speech grew thick and he became chronically depressed.

Dr. Philpott had him sleep with the negative pole of several magnets (ferrous ceramic, 2,000-4,000 gauss in strength) placed at the crown of his head. During the day, the man also wore a magnet strapped to the skin over his heart. Within a week, his symptoms improved and after one month of this treatment, he had no heart pain, his balance returned, his speech became distinct, and his depression was gone. Through this method, "the mental confusion, disorientation, and depression of cerebral atherosclerosis is remarkably reduced or even completely relieved," reports Dr. Philpott.[5]

Stress—A negative magnetic field applied to the top of the head has a calming and sleep-inducing effect on brain and body functions, due to the stimulation of the production of the hormone melatonin, according to Dr. Philpott. Melatonin has been shown to be antistressful, anti-

As there are literally hundreds of diseases that are related to stress, infections, and aging, magnetic field therapy could be considered an important adjunct in their treatment and researchers are currently studying its contributions.

For more information about **magnetic therapy**, contact: William Philpott, M.D., P.O. Box 50655, Midwest City, OK 73140; tel: 405-390-1444.

aging, anti-infectious, and anticancerous, and to have control over respiration and the production of free radicals.[6] A free radical is a highly destructive molecule that is missing an electron and readily reacts with other molecules. Free radicals contribute to the aging of cells, hardening of muscle tissue, wrinkling of skin, and, in general, decreased efficiency of protein synthesis.

Bacterial, Fungal, and Viral Infections—"A negative magnetic field can function like an antibiotic in helping to destroy bacterial, fungal, and viral infections," says Dr. Philpott, "by promoting oxygenation and lowering the body's acidity." Both these factors are beneficial to normal bodily functions but harmful to pathogenic (disease-causing) microorganisms, which do not survive in a well-oxygenated, alkaline environment.

Dr. Philpott theorizes that the biological value of oxygen is increased by the influence of a negative electromagnetic field, and that the field causes negatively charged DNA (deoxyribonucleic acid) to "pull" oxygen out of the bloodstream and into the cell. The negative electromagnetic field keeps the cellular buffer system (pH or acid-alkaline balance) intact so that the cells remain alkaline. The low acid balance also helps maintain the presence of oxygen in the body, which is essential to the health of the cells, blood and circulation, and all organs including the heart.

Pain Relief—A negative magnetic field normalizes the disturbed metabolic functions that cause painful conditions such as cellular edema (swelling of the cells), cellular acidosis (excessive acidity of the cells), lack of oxygen to the cells, and infection.

Dr. Philpott cites the case of a woman in her seventies who for 33 years had experienced pain and weakness in her left leg stemming from a blood clot in the groin area. She could not climb stairs without stopping several times due to pain. After a year of sleeping on a negative magneto-electric pad, the woman found that she could walk up a long flight of stairs without any pain or weakness in her leg.

While a negative magnetic field may relieve pain, a positive magnetic field can increase pain due to its interference with normal metabolic function. However, magnetic therapy should not be considered a replacement for local anesthetics or pain relievers.

Oxygen Therapy

Studies at Baylor University in the 1970s found that an intravenous drip of hydrogen peroxide into leg arteries of atherosclerotic patients cleared arterial plaque.[7] In cardiopulmonary resuscitations, hydrogen peroxide infusions often stopped ventricular fibrillation (rapid, ineffective contractions by ventricles of the heart), the heart's response to insufficient oxygen.[8] Charles Farr, M.D., reports success alternating treatments of intravenous diluted hydrogen peroxide and chelation therapy to bring patients out of high-output heart failure (where the heart fails even though it is pumping a high amount of blood).

CAUTION The body's subtle electromagnetic fields can be affected by even the weakest of magnets. Since even minor alterations in the fields can cause mild to serious symptoms, magnetic therapy should be practiced only under the supervision of a qualified professional.

Dr. Philpott adds the following precautions:

■ Industrial magnets often have different positive and negative pole identifications than the magnets used in medicine and therapy. Use a magnetometer or compass to confirm proper identification.

■ Don't use magnets on the abdomen during pregnancy.

■ Don't use a magnetic bed for more than eight to ten hours.

■ Wait 60 to 90 minutes after meals before applying magnetic therapy to the abdomen, to prevent interference with peristalsis (wavelike contractions of the smooth muscles of the digestive tract).

■ Do not apply the positive magnetic pole unless under medical supervision. It can produce seizures, hallucinations, insomnia, and hyperactivity; stimulate the growth of tumors and microorganisms; and promote addictive behavior.

Traditional Chinese Medicine

For more on **oxygen therapy**, see Chapter 16: Oxygen Therapy, pp. 244-256; for **traditional Chinese medicine**, see Chapter 11: Chinese Medicine, pp. 184-199.

Traditional Chinese medicine (TCM) views heart disease as a problem stemming from poor digestion, which causes the buildup of plaque in the arteries. Harvey Kaltsas, Ac. Phys. (FL), D. Ac. (RI), Dipl. Ac. (NCCA), president of the American Association of Acupuncture and Oriental Medicine, recommends herbs to strengthen digestive functioning. "It has been understood in China for thousands of years that the circulation needs to flow unimpeded," states Dr. Kaltsas.

An herbal extract made from a plant known as *mao-tung-ching* (*Ilex puibeceus*) is often used to dilate the blocked vessels. According to Dr. Kaltsas, a study was conducted in China in which *mao-tung-ching* was administered daily (4 ounces orally, 20 mg intravenously) to 103 patients suffering from coronary heart disease. In 101 out of the 103 cases, there was significant improvement.[9]

Maoshing Ni, D.O.M., Ph.D., L.Ac., vice president of the Yo San University of Traditional Chinese Medicine in Santa Monica, California, views heart disease as either a weakness or block in the body's energy system. He generally refers patients with acute heart problems to a Western physician, stating that TCM is more suited to the treatment of chronic heart problems. For these, Dr. Ni uses a combination of acupuncture and herbs to dissolve plaque, lower cholesterol levels, raise blood flow rates, and relieve angina.

One patient came to Dr. Ni after having an angioplasty because of 70% blockage of the coronary arteries. After the angioplasty, he still had 55% blockage. Dr. Ni treated him with herbs and acupuncture and, within four months, the blockage was reduced to 35%.

Additional Alternative Therapies

Self-Care

The following therapies for the treatment and prevention of heart disease can be undertaken at home under appropriate professional supervision:

- Fasting
- Yoga
- Aromatherapy: To strengthen heart muscle—garlic, lavender, peppermint, marjoram, rose, rosemary. For palpitations—lavender, melissa, neroli, ylang-ylang.
- Juice Therapy: Carrot, celery, cucumber, beet (add a little

garlic or hawthorn berries); Blueberries, blackberries, black currant, red grapes.

■ Hydrotherapy: Constitutional hydrotherapy two to five times weekly.

Professional Care
The following therapies can only be provided by a qualified health professional:
- ■ Alexander Technique
- ■ Biofeedback Training
- ■ Cell Therapy
- ■ Environmental Medicine
- ■ Guided Imagery
- ■ Hypnotherapy
- ■ Meditation
- ■ Osteopathy
- ■ Body Therapy: Acupressure, reflexology, *shiatsu*, massage.
- ■ Chiropractic: To improve mid-back mobility and breathing.

■ Hydrotherapy: Leon Chaitow, N.D., D.O., reports that the neutral bath (patient immersed in water 35°C for two hours) has been effective in treating mild heart failure problems that result in fluid retention.

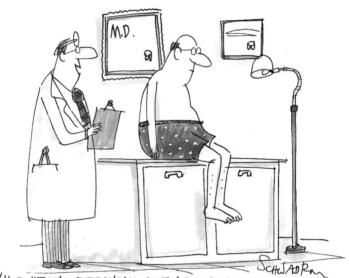

"YOUR HEART'S GREAT. IT'S ALL THOSE ASPIRIN COMMERCIALS THAT ARE MAKING YOU SICK."

PART TWO

High
Blood
Pressure

(Hypertension)

What Causes High Blood Pressure?

HIGH BLOOD PRESSURE (clinically known as hypertension) is the most common cardiovascular disease in industrialized nations and is a major cause of heart attack, stroke, and congestive heart failure. In 1994 alone, high blood pressure killed 38,130 Americans and was a factor in 180,000 additional deaths.[1] Hypertension accounts for an estimated 28.3 million annual office visits to conventional physicians, or about 7.2% of all doctors' appointments in a year. This amount is twice that for acute upper respiratory infection, the next most prevalent health condition on a list of the top ten, according to data compiled by *Scott-Levin's Physician Drug and Diagnosis Audit* in 1996.

Approximately 50 million Americans (nearly one out of five) currently suffer from high blood pressure and two-thirds of them are under 65 years of age, which indicates that hypertension is not an inevitable result of aging but rather a condition affected by a number of risk factors, including smoking, obesity,[2] stress,[3] excessive alcohol consumption, and a diet high in fats and sodium chloride (table salt).[4] According to William Lee Cowden, M.D., of Richardson, Texas, "Individuals with diabetes are especially susceptible, as are those with a family history of hypertension. Stress and a sedentary lifestyle are other factors to consider when diagnosing and treating this condition."

The Heart Under Pressure

To understand high blood pressure, you need to know a few facts about the heart. The human heart beats on average 70 times per minute, 100,000 times a day, and 2.5 billion times in a lifetime. With each heartbeat, about 2.5 ounces of blood are pumped through the heart—that is 1,980 gallons every day.

The term blood pressure refers to the force of the blood against the walls of arteries, veins, and the chambers of the heart as it is pumped through the body. Greater than normal force

Approximately 50 million Americans (nearly one out of five) currently suffer from high blood pressure and two-thirds of them are under 65 years of age.

exerted by the blood against the arteries (when high blood pressure is present) begins to weaken the cellular walls and makes it easier for harmful substances, such as toxins and oxidized cholesterol, to form dangerous deposits on the arterial walls.

Hypertension takes two forms: essential hypertension, when the cause is unknown; and secondary hypertension, when damage to the kidneys or endocrine dysfunction causes blood pressure to rise. Of

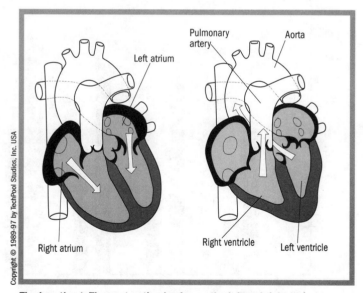

Copyright © 1989-97 by TechPool Studios, Inc. USA

The heartbeat. The contraction begins as the left and right atria squeeze blood downward into the ventricles and then continues as both ventricles squeeze upward. The right ventricle pumps blood into the pulmonary artery, then to the lungs to be re-oxygenated. The left ventricle pumps oxygenated blood into the aorta, then out to all parts of the body.

The symptoms of hypertension are far-reaching and include dizziness, headache, fatigue, restlessness, difficulty breathing, insomnia, intestinal complaints, and emotional instability.

the diagnosed cases of hypertension in the United States, over 90% are essential hypertension.[5] The symptoms of hypertension are far-reaching and include dizziness, headache, fatigue, restlessness, difficulty breathing, insomnia, intestinal complaints, and emotional instability. In advanced stages, the hypertensive patient often suffers from other forms of cardiovascular disease as well as damage to the heart, kidneys, and brain.

Diagnosing High Blood Pressure

Blood pressure is measured by placing an inflatable cuff around the

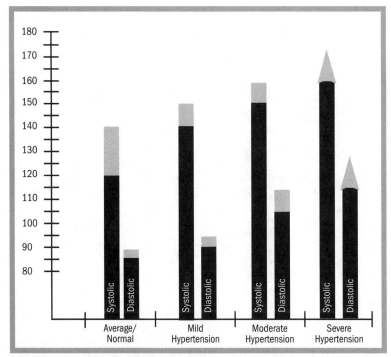

High blood pressure (hypertension) is usually measured as a range of the systolic (when the heart contracts) and diastolic (when the heart rests, filling with more blood) values.

upper arm. As the cuff is inflated, the arm is squeezed tight. At this point the pulse cannot be heard through the stethoscope. As the cuff is slowly deflated, the pulse is heard again. This is the high number and measures the systolic pressure, when the heart is contracting to pump blood into the body. A second reading is taken as the cuff is deflated even further.

The pulse sound disappears again and when it returns, that reading is the low number and measures the diastolic pressure, when the heart is relaxing to refill with blood. The ratio of the two numbers represents blood pressure, as in 120/85, an "average" or healthy reading. A patient has hypertension if the high reading is above 140 and the low reading is above 90, when tested on two separate occasions.

Causes of High Blood Pressure

"High blood pressure often occurs due to a strain on the heart, which can arise from a variety of conditions, including diet, atherosclerosis [narrowing and hardening of the arteries], high cholesterol, diabetes, environmental factors, as well as lifestyle choices," according to Dr. William Lee Cowden. When these factors combine with a genetic predisposition, hypertension can occur in two out of three individuals.[6]

Hypertension is closely associated with the Western diet and is found almost exclusively in developed countries.

Dietary Factors

Hypertension is closely associated with the Western diet and is found almost exclusively in developed countries.[7] Recent studies of residents in remote areas of China, New Guinea, Panama, Brazil, and Africa show virtually no evidence of hypertension, even with advanced age. But when individuals within these groups moved to more industrialized areas, the incidence of hypertension among them rose. The studies concluded that changes in lifestyle, including dietary changes and increased body mass and fat, significantly contributed to the higher levels of blood pressure.[8]

"Although a combination of genetic and environmental factors such as behavior patterns and stress are believed to contribute to hypertension, the main cause appears to be a diet high in animal fat and sodium chloride, especially if high in relation to potassium and magnesium organic salts," says Dr. Cowden.

Research concurs that a diet high in sodium chloride and deficient in potassium has been associated with hypertension. Lack of potassium and other nutritional deficiencies play a significant role in the development of hypertension. Magnesium levels have also been found to be consistently low in patients with high blood pressure.[9] High blood pressure can also develop as a symptom of adult-onset diabetes (see Chapter 11: Chinese Medicine: How It Can Help Reverse High Blood Pressure).

Lifestyle Factors

Lifestyle choices, including smoking and consumption of coffee and alcohol, have been shown to cause hypertension. A recent study conducted in Paris, France, showed higher systolic and diastolic levels in coffee drinkers compared to nondrinkers, with levels rising in direct correlation to the amount of coffee consumed each day.[10] Even moderate amounts of alcohol can produce hypertension in certain individuals, and chronic alcohol intake is one of the strongest predictors of high blood pressure.[11] In the face of this evidence, restricting alcohol and avoiding caffeine are recommended.

Smoking is a contributing factor to hypertension, due in part to the fact that smokers are more prone to increased sugar, alcohol, and caffeine consumption.[12] However, even smokeless tobacco (chewing tobacco, snuff, etc.) causes hypertension through its nicotine and sodium content.[13]

Atherosclerosis and High Blood Pressure

Atherosclerosis involves the accumulation of plaque in the blood vessels, which restricts blood flow and increases blood pressure. Consequently it is a common cause of hypertension as well as the main cause of coronary heart disease and strokes.

According to Leon Chaitow, N.D., D.O., of London, England, "Blood pres-

---

Blood Pressure Drug May Cause Cancer

According to a study involving 5,000 patients over 70 years old, conducted by scientists at the University of Tennessee in Memphis, the regular use of calcium channel blockers, the most widely prescribed group of high blood pressure drugs, is associated with a 72% higher rate of cancer. In research published in *The Lancet* (August 1996), this percentage increase is equal to eight new cancers per 100 people using the drugs for five years.

sure rises when the blood leaving the heart has to be pumped more vigorously due to a thicker consistency of the blood or to a greater resistance from the blood vessels themselves. The vessels may have become narrower, less elastic, or the muscles which surround them may be exerting more tension. The function of the muscles and breathing apparatus may also be inefficient in helping the heart to function properly. The relative health of the kidneys and liver (which filter the blood) also influences blood pressure."

Environmental Factors

Environmental factors such as lead contamination from drinking water, as well as residues of heavy metals such as cadmium, have also been shown to promote hypertension.[14] People whose hypertension has been left untreated have been shown to have blood cadmium levels three to four times higher than those with normal blood pressure.[15] It is important to check for both lead and cadmium toxicity when treating hypertension.

Lead Contamination and High Blood Pressure

A low level of lead exposure and accumulation in tissues in adults is now linked to both hypertension and impaired kidney function, according to the *Journal of the American Medical Association* (April 1996). In two studies involving over 1,000 men, the exposure to lead was at levels previously considered safe. Those with the highest levels of bone lead were 50% more likely to have hypertension than those with the lowest.

Researchers at the Harvard School of Public Health found that high levels of childhood exposure to lead are linked to adult obesity, according to their 1995 study of 79 overweight adults.[16] Adults who had absorbed high lead levels as children gained the most weight between the ages of 7 and 20. Both excess weight and high lead concentrations are associated with high blood pressure in adults.

Reversing High Blood Pressure Caused by Heavy Metal Toxicity

Jonathan Wright, M.D., of Kent, Washington, treated Jonas, who had unexplained high blood pressure (156/100). His blood, urine, and kidney examinations were all normal and his lifestyle habits were exemplary. He avoided sugar, refined flour, caffeine, and excess salt; his diet was high in vegetables and fruits; and he took vitamin C and E supplements. He also exercised regularly and did not smoke.

However, Jonas was an industrial painter and Dr. Wright suspected that heavy metals in the paints were the problem. Pubic hair analysis confirmed his suspicions, showing higher than usual amounts of lead, cobalt, and cadmium. Dr. Wright started Jonas on a zinc supplement, to force the cadmium out of his system, and increased his vitamin C intake to bowel tolerance. He also recommended extra vitamin B6 to prevent the increased vitamin C from causing kidney stones, and added selenium, which is known to protect against cadmium toxicity.

Dr. Wright further suggested linseed oil, which contains essential fatty acids noted for reducing hypertension. After six months, Jonas' blood pressure had dropped to 154/96; after 12 months to 142/90; and after 18 months to 134/80. At that point, Dr. Wright cut the supplement dosages, but zinc and vitamin C were continued to prevent recurrence since Jonas continued in his profession.

The Hypothyroidism Connection

For more about the thyroid, see "The Reason Behind Weight Gain, Fatigue, Muscle Pain, Depression, Food Allergies, Infections...." Digest #16, pp. 52-56.

According to Broda O. Barnes, M.D., low thyroid function (hypothyroidism) is correlated with a tendency to develop high blood pressure.[17] "I have seen many patients

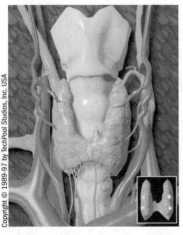

The thyroid gland, one of the body's seven endocrine glands, is located just below the larynx in the throat with interconnecting lobes on either side of the trachea. The thyroid is the body's metabolic thermostat, controlling body temperature, energy use, and, for children, the body's growth rate. The thyroid controls the rate at which organs function and the speed with which the body uses food; it affects the operation of all body processes and organs. Of the hormones synthesized in and released by the thyroid, T3 (triiodothyronine), represents 7%, and T4 (thyroxine), accounts for almost 93% of the thyroid's hormones active in all of the body's processes. Iodine is essential to forming normal amounts of thyroxine. The secretion of both these hormones is regulated by thyroid-stimulating hormone, or TSH, secreted by the pituitary gland in the brain. The thyroid also secretes calcitonin, a hormone required for calcium metabolism.

Copyright © 1989-97 by TechPool Studios, Inc. USA

Drugs Associated with a Higher Incidence of High Blood Pressure (Hypertension)

According to the *Physicians' Desk Reference*, the following drugs are associated with hypertension. (Statistics refer to the percentage of individuals affected.)

- Alfenta Injection (18%)
- Aredia for Injection (up to 6%)
- Clozaril Tablets (4%)
- Dobutrex Solution Vials (most patients)
- Epogen for Injection (0.75% to approximately 25%)
- Habitrol Nicotine Transdermal System (3%-9%)
- Lupron Depot 3.75 mg (among most frequent); Injection (5% or more)
- Methergine Injection, Tablets (most common)
- Orthoclone OKT3 Sterile Solution (8%)
- Polygam, Immune Globulin Intravenous (Human) (3-6%)
- Procrit for Injection (0.75%-24%)
- Sandimmune IV Ampules for Infusion, Oral Solution (13%-53%)
- Sandimmune Soft Gelatin Capsules (13%-53%)
- Sufenta Injection (3%)
- Tolectin (200, 400, and 600 mg) (3%-9%)
- Velban Vials (among most common)
- Ventolin Inhalation Aerosol and Refill (less than 5%)
- Wellbutrin Tablets (4.3%)

with hypertension—mild, moderate, and even severe—respond to thyroid therapy," Dr. Barnes said.

Hypothyroidism is a condition of low or underactive thyroid gland function that can produce numerous symptoms. Among the 47 clinically recognized symptoms: fatigue, depression, lethargy, weakness, weight gain, low body temperature, chills, cold extremities, general inappropriate sensation of cold, infertility, rheumatic pain, menstrual disorders (excessive flow or cramps), repeated infections, colds, upper respiratory infections, skin problems (itching, eczema, psoriasis, acne, skin pallor, dry, coarse, and scaly skin), memory disturbances, concentration difficulties, paranoia, migraines, oversleep, "laziness," muscle aches and weakness, hearing disturbances, burning/prickling sensations, anemia, slow reaction time and mental slug-

See "Hyperthyroidism," p. 934; "Hypothyroidism," pp. 936-937.

Based on a long-term study of 1,500 of his own patients, Dr. Barnes concluded that thyroid treatment (supplementation with an oral thyroid extract) yielded considerably fewer cases of high blood pressure than would be expected in a population of that age and health status.

gishness, swelling of the eyelids, constipation, labored and difficult breathing, hoarseness, brittle nails, and poor vision. A resting body temperature (measured in the armpit), below 97.8°F, indicates hypothyroidism; menstruating women should take the underarm temperature only on the second and third days of menstruation.

Based on a long-term study of 1,500 of his own patients, Dr. Barnes concluded that thyroid treatment (supplementation with an oral thyroid extract) yielded considerably fewer cases of high blood pressure than would be expected in a population of that age and health status. Patients on thyroid therapy had "marked protection against the development of elevated blood pressure" despite their age, and those who were initially hypertensive experienced a reduction in their high blood pressure from thyroid therapy alone (without antihypertensive medications).

"High blood pressure often occurs due to a strain on the heart, which can arise from a variety of conditions, including diet, atherosclerosis [narrowing and hardening of the arteries], high cholesterol, diabetes, environmental factors, as well as lifestyle choices," according to William Lee Cowden, M.D., of Richardson, Texas. When these factors combine with a genetic predisposition, hypertension can occur in two out of three individuals.

Self-Care Options

HOW TO USE DIET, EXERCISE, AND LIFESTYLE CHANGES TO LOWER YOUR BLOOD PRESSURE

ONVENTIONAL HIGH BLOOD pressure medications treat hypertension by reducing the heart output, lowering the blood pressure, or reducing fluid retention through the use of diuretics. These medications may relieve the symptoms of hypertension but do little to address the cause. As many of these drugs have unwanted side effects and can actually increase the risk of life-threatening heart disease, an alternative for reducing blood pressure is warranted.

Alternative medical approaches inevitably begin with a careful evaluation of the factors[1] contributing to the patient's illness. Such an evaluation often reveals a need for dietary changes and lifestyle changes such as increased exercise, weight loss, and stress management.

Diet

A diet low in fat, sugar, and salt, and rich in foods containing potassium, calcium, magnesium, and fiber is highly recommended for hypertensives. Also, garlic and other members of the onion family should be included in any diet that aims to lower high blood pressure, as they significantly reduce both systolic and diastolic pressure.[2]

Making relatively simple changes in diet, such as eating less fat and more fruits and vegetables, can lower blood pressure as effectively as conventional hypertension drugs. This conclusion comes from a

There was a significant reduction in both systolic and diastolic blood pressures in the subjects eating fish and/or taking fish-oil supplements, particularly those on a low-fat diet.

study directed by the Kaiser Permanente Center for Health Research in Portland, Oregon, in cooperation with researchers at Johns Hopkins, Harvard, and Duke Universities.[3]

The study enrolled 459 adults (50% women, 60% African American) with a starting blood pressure of less than 160/80-95 (high blood pressure was considered 140/90 or higher). The participants were divided into three groups, each of which followed a different diet. The first group ate a conventional American diet (typically high in fats, sugar, meat, and processed foods); the second group ate the same diet complemented with a high level of fruits and vegetables. The third group practiced a diet low in fats, fat comprising only 31% of the total calories compared to 37% in a typical American diet. This group kept their consumption of fats and cholesterol low and their consumption of fruits, vegetables, and low-fat dairy products high.

Changes in blood pressure were noticeable within two weeks. For those in the third group, blood pressure values dropped by an average of 5.5/3, while for those in the second group, the readings declined an average of 2.8/1.1. In the view of the researchers, both changes were significant. Even more impressive, those in the third group who started with high blood pressure experienced drops of 11.4/5.5.

Another study compared the effects of omega-3 fatty acids in fish or fish-oil supplements on 125 men with moderately high blood pressure consuming high-fat or low-fat diets. The subjects ate fish, took fish-oil supplements, or had a combination providing an average total of 3.65 g per day of omega-3 fatty acids. There was a significant reduction in both systolic and diastolic blood pressures in the subjects eating fish and/or taking fish-oil supplements, particularly those on a low-fat diet, compared with control subjects.[4]

A third study of 2,300 middle-aged people, all moderately overweight and with blood pressure in the high

QUICK DEFINITION

Omega-3 and omega-6 oils are the two principal types of essential fatty acids, which are unsaturated fats required in the diet. The digits "3" and "6" refer to differences in the oil's chemical structure with respect to its chain of carbon atoms and where they are bonded. A balance of these oils in the diet is required for good health. The primary omega-3 oil is called alpha-linolenic acid (ALA) and is found in flaxseed (58%), canola, pumpkin and walnut, and soybeans. Fish oils, such as salmon, cod, and mackerel, contain the other important omega-3 oils, DHA (docosahexaenoic acid) and EPA (eicosapentaenoic acid). Omega-3 oils help reduce the risk of heart disease. Linoleic acid or cis-linoleic acid is the main omega-6 oil and is found in most plant and vegetable oils, including safflower (73%), corn, peanut, and sesame. The most therapeutic form of omega-6 oil is gamma-linolenic acid (GLA), found in evening primrose, black currant, and borage oils. Once in the body, omega-6 is converted to prostaglandins, hormone-like substances that regulate many metabolic functions, particularly inflammatory processes.

ᴡɪᴛʜɪn two weeks of starting a nutritional supplement program, Dr. Braverman's patient was off medication and his blood pressure had dropped from 150/90 to 128/82.

normal range, found that those who lost around ten pounds within six months and cut the sodium in their diet experienced a 60% lowering of their blood pressure.[5]

Lowering Hypertension with Diet and Supplements

Eric R. Braverman, M.D., director of Place for Achieving Total Health (PATH) in New York City, treats hypertension with a program centered around diet and nutritional supplementation.

To contact **Eric Braverman, M.D.**, or order his book, *How to Lower Your Blood Pressure and Reverse Heart Disease Naturally* (1995), contact: PATH, 274 Madison Ave., 4th Floor, Room 402, New York, NY 10016; tel: 212-213-6155; fax: 212-213-6188.

Dr. Braverman's diet is low in sodium, low in saturated fat, high in vegetables from the starch group, and high in protein (particularly fish). In addition, the diet features large amounts of fresh salad. Simple sugar, alcohol, caffeine, nicotine, and refined carbohydrates are reduced dramatically or eliminated altogether. His nutritional supplement program for a typical hypertensive patient includes fish oil (containing omega-3 fatty acids), garlic, evening primrose oil, magnesium, potassium, selenium, zinc, vitamin B6, niacin, vitamin C, tryptophan, taurine, cysteine, and coenzyme Q10.

One of Dr. Braverman's patients had been treated with medication for hypertension for two years and his blood pressure was still 150/90. Dr. Braverman started him on multivitamins and supplements of B6, folic acid, B12, magnesium, taurine, garlic, and evening primrose oil. Within two weeks, he was off medication and his blood pressure had dropped to 128/82.

When John, 62, first came to Dr. Braverman, he had suffered from high blood pressure for ten years. His levels for total cholesterol, triglycerides, and high-density lipoproteins (HDLs), which are key indicators of heart health, were highly imbalanced. He was taking strong daily doses of three conventional medications. When John began Dr. Braverman's program, his blood pressure was 140/90.

First, Dr. Braverman put John on a low-carbohydrate, high-protein diet to help him lose weight. Next, he started John on daily supplementation with evening primrose and fish oils, a niacin-garlic formula, safflower oil, and a hypertension nutrient formula Dr. Braverman had specially developed for his blood pressure–lowering program. The formula consisted of:

High Blood Pressure Drugs—
Another Heart Disease Risk Factor

For adults with borderline to mild high blood pressure, the use of conventional antihypertensive drugs is not only often unneeded, but also can increase the risk of heart attack by nearly four times, according to physicians at Malmö University Hospital in Malmö, Sweden. Lead researcher Juan Merlo noted that despite mounting doubt about the effectiveness of high blood pressure drugs in preventing heart attacks, the trend of physicians routinely prescribing them continues to grow. In the Malmö University Hospital study, 484 men, born in 1914, were tracked between 1969 and 1992, and their use of antihypertensive drugs recorded.

Out of this group, 13% who had a diastolic blood pressure below 90 mm Hg (mild high blood pressure) and were taking antihypertensive drugs experienced a rate of heart attacks 3.9 times greater than men with similar blood pressures not taking any heart drugs. For men with blood pressures exceeding 90 mm Hg (high blood pressure) and who were taking antihypertensive drugs, the risk of having a serious heart attack was doubled.[6]

Calcium channel blockers also pose threats to heart health. A study of 900 elderly people with high blood pressure found that taking one kind of calcium channel blocker (the short-acting form of nifedipine, marketed as Procardia and Adalat) doubled the likelihood of dying within five years after using the drug, typically from heart attacks, heart failure, and strokes. American doctors wrote two million prescriptions for this drug in 1994, despite the lack of rigorous scientific trials by either the FDA or drug companies to prove its safety.[7]

- garlic powder (200 mg)
- magnesium (oxide, 50 mg)
- zinc (chelate, 4 mg)
- niacinamide (50 mg)
- molybdenum (40 mg)
- beta carotene (1222.33 IU)
- amino acid taurine (200 mg)
- potassium (chloride, 6.7 mg)
- chromium (chloride, 26.7 mcg)
- vitamin C (40 mg)
- vitamin B6 (50 mg)
- selenium (sodium selenite, 20 mcg)

John took six pills daily of this formula along with a magnesium formula, containing vitamin B6 (65 mg), magnesium (oxide, 470 mg), and zinc (chelate, 15 mg).

Two weeks into the program, John's cholesterol had dropped from 264 to 131, his triglycerides had decreased from 161 to 100, his blood pressure was 120/80, and his HDLs increased positively from 59 to 64. John was able to stop taking his conventional medications. After another week on the nutrients, his blood pressure was a healthier 110/80. Over the following months, Dr. Braverman reduced John's nutrient program and adjusted his diet. John continued to be

Researchers at Johns Hopkins University in Baltimore stated that "the higher the oats intake, the lower the blood pressure," regardless of other factors such as age and weight, or alcohol, sodium, or potassium intake, which are known to affect blood pressure.

medication-free, his energy level and sexual drive had increased, and he was "doing fantastically well," reports Dr. Braverman.

What a Bowl of Oatmeal Can Do for Your Heart

While people living in the British Isles may take it for granted, making oatmeal a mainstay of the diet makes smart nutritional sense. In recent years, at least 37 clinical studies have affirmed the ability of oatmeal and oat bran to reduce blood cholesterol levels, lower blood pressure, and generally reduce the long-term risk of heart disease.

In recognition of these now well-established benefits, in 1996, the U.S. FDA granted manufacturers or packagers of oatmeal (as a food category) the right to make specific health claims about this food. It was the first such permissible health claim ever accorded to a food by the FDA, an agency that generally has favored drugs over natural substances. The FDA's proposed health claim (now in the process of public review) states that diets high in oatmeal or oat bran may reduce the risk of heart disease.

Among the numerous studies that have demonstrated the health benefits of oatmeal, at least four put the food's health advantages in clear focus. In 1995, researchers at Johns Hopkins University in Baltimore, Maryland, reported that people who regularly consumed even a modest portion of oatmeal (one ounce, cooked, daily) had lower blood pressure and cholesterol readings than those who never ate oatmeal.[8] The study was based on evaluation of 850 men, 17-77 years old, living in China; their oatmeal consumption ranged from 25-90 g daily.

The researchers stated that "the higher the oats intake, the lower the blood pressure," regardless of other factors such as age and weight, or alcohol, sodium, or potassium intake, which are known to affect blood pressure.

According to chief researcher Michael Klag, M.D., it is oatmeal's high content of water-soluble fiber (called beta glucan) that produces the heart benefits. A six-year study involving 22,000 middle-aged Finnish males showed that consuming as little as three g daily of soluble fiber (from the beta-glucan fiber component of oats, barley, or rye) reduced the risk of death from heart disease by 27%.[9]

Another study of oatmeal's heart benefits was conducted by scientists at the Chicago Center for Clinical Research in Illinois. The researchers enlisted 156 adults, all of whom had a diagnosis of high cholesterol or multiple heart risk factors, and had them consume differing amounts of oatmeal or oat bran. In this case, more was not necessarily better. Those who ate 56 g (two ounces, dry weight) of oat bran daily for six weeks achieved the best results (15.9% reduction of low-density lipoprotein cholesterol), followed by those who consumed 84 g (three ounces) daily of oatmeal (11.5% reduction).[10]

A related study involved 206 adults, 30-65 years old, who consumed 60 g daily of oatmeal or oat bran, in addition to reducing their fat intake, for 12 weeks. The results also showed that eating oats at a "moderate and practical level" produced important decreases (at least 5.2%) in blood cholesterol levels.[11]

Studies have also certified the widely circulated folk saying that a bowl of oatmeal "sticks to your ribs" throughout the morning. William Evans, Ph.D., director of the Noll Physiological Research Center at Pennsylvania State University at State

Lifestyle plays a major role in the development of hypertension, and any program to reduce blood pressure must take this into consideration.

College, tested oatmeal's ability to sustain athletic performance in 18 college students.

The study participants were divided into three groups, each consuming equal-calorie portions of oats in three different forms: oatmeal; oat rings, a snack food; and dry oat cereal. Then they exercised on stationary bicycles as long as they could, stopping just short of exhaustion. Students who had oatmeal were able to exercise for five hours compared to four hours for the other two groups, according to Dr. Evans. The results confirm that oatmeal at breakfast can help keep you feeling "energized" throughout the morning.

This same advantage translates into benefits for diabetics, too. A recent study enrolled eight men, with an average age of 45, who had diabetes but did not require insulin injections.[12] Over a 12-week period, those eating oat bread (34 g of oat fiber intake) daily had more stability in their blood sugar (glucose) levels. Large fluctuations in glucose often lead to serious problems in diabetics. The men reported a "longer delay in the return of hunger" after eating oatmeal than

Meditation is so effective in reducing stress that in 1984 the National Institutes of Health recommended meditation over prescription drugs for mild hypertension.

with other foods, particularly white bread, indicating oatmeal helped them achieve more control of their daily blood sugar levels.

Lifestyle and Exercise

Lifestyle plays a major role in the development of hypertension, and any program to reduce blood pressure must take this into consideration. Dr. Cowden notes that any changes that are implemented must be maintained if blood pressure is to be controlled on a long-term basis. Smoking should be moderated or, preferably, totally avoided, and alcohol intake should be kept to a minimum. Weight loss reduces blood pressure in those with and without hypertension, and should be a primary goal for hypertensives who are obese or moderately overweight. Other lifestyle factors important in reducing and controlling hypertension are stress management and increased exercise.

For more about **biofeedback,** see Chapter 13: Alternative Medicine Options for Lowering High Blood Pressure, pp. 217-221.

QUICK DEFINITION

Biofeedback training is a method of learning how to consciously regulate normally unconscious bodily functions (such as heart rate, blood pressure, and breathing). It uses a monitoring device to measure and report back immediate information about the heart rate, for example, transmitting one blinking light or beep per heartbeat. The person being monitored learns techniques such as meditation, relaxation, and visualization to slow their heart rate and then uses the flashes or beeps to check their progress and make adjustments accordingly.

Stress Management

Stress-reduction techniques from the various disciplines of mind/body medicine such as biofeedback, yoga, meditation, *qigong*, relaxation exercises, and hypnotherapy have all proven successful in lowering blood pressure.[13] In fact, meditation is so effective in reducing stress that in 1984 the National Institutes of Health recommended meditation over prescription drugs for mild hypertension.[14]

To reduce stress and improve digestion and thus improve absorption of nutrients from food and supplements, Dr. Cowden has his patients perform stress-reduction techniques before meals and at bedtime. Says Dr. Cowden, "The nutrients we recommend have to be absorbed out of the gastrointestinal tract. But if the gut is in a stressed state, it will not absorb those nutrients nearly as well as if it is in a relaxed state."

Biofeedback has proven particularly valuable in working to lower hypertension. Patients in one study were able to sustain lower blood pressure readings than those registered prior to treatment after three years of using biofeedback.[15] Combining biofeedback with other stress-reduction techniques can also help patients achieve optimum results. A study of mildly hypertensive males treated with either biofeedback, autogenic training, or breathing relaxation training showed a significant reduction in both systolic and diastolic blood pressure. The higher the pretreatment blood pressure, the greater the effects of relaxation training.[16]

Self-guided relaxation techniques can be a quick and effective way to lower blood pressure, according to researchers at the National Taiwan University in Taiwan.[17] Hypertension is widespread there with 27% of men and 13% of women having readings of at least 140/90.

Based on a study group of 590 individuals with high blood pressure, Taiwanese researchers found that practicing progressive relaxation techniques (from a taped cassette) coupled with home study of healthful practices led to an average drop of blood pressure to 130/85 after two months. No drugs or other treatments were involved other than the power of self-directed relaxation.

Exercise

Regular exercise reduces stress and blood pressure, so it is highly recommended that it be an integral part of your life. Consistent aerobic exercise can both prevent and lower hypertension.[18] In a study of 902 people, 45 to 69 years old, with hypertension, positive long-term effects on blood pressure and all cholesterol levels were achieved with increased exercise along with a lower-fat diet.[19]

Swimming, which is frequently prescribed as a non-impact exercise to lower high blood pressure, can produce a significant decrease in resting heart rate (a sign of cardiovascular health) and resting systolic blood pressure in previously sedentary people with elevated blood pressure.[20]

> ## Exercise Lowers High Blood Pressure in Black Men
>
> Seventy-one percent of black men over age 60 have high blood pressure. In a study conducted by the Veterans Affairs Medical Center in Washington, D.C., 46 black men with hypertension rode an exercise bicycle strenuously for 45 minutes daily for 32 weeks, after which time, their blood pressure had dropped and the men were able to reduce their medications by 30%-40%.

CAUTION
Before undertaking any exercise program, an individual with hypertension should consult a physician.

Rebounding and the Benefits of Aerobic Exercise

For more about **herbal medicine,** see Chapter 12: Lower Your Blood Pressure With Herbs, pp. 200-206; for **nutritional supplements,** see Chapter 13: Alternative Medicine Options for Lowering High Blood Pressure, pp. 208-226.

Aerobic training of any kind, including rebounding, improves your cardiovascular fitness in a variety of ways, according to John A. Friedrich, M.D., of Duke University, who first reported on the effects of aerobic exercise on the body in the *Journal of Physical Education* (May/June 1970).

Aerobics can strengthen heart muscles and produce other cardiovascular changes so that the heart can pump more blood with fewer beats. This means your resting (normal) heart rate will be lower, which is good. By regularly working your heart harder during exercise, you improve its overall function so that it doesn't have to work as hard during your normal activities, Dr. Friedrich wrote.

"A conditioned person may have a resting heart rate 20 beats per minute slower than a deconditioned person," says Dr. Morton Walker. "He saves 10,000 beats in one night's sleep." Reducing the day-to-day workload of your heart can lessen your chances of developing heart disease, Dr. Walker adds.

Aerobic exercises such as rebounding increase red blood cell count, allowing faster oxygen transport through the body, and can help lower elevated blood pressure. According to Dr. Friedrich's research, aerobic exercise helps dissolve blood clots and increases the amount of high-density lipoproteins (HDLs, the so-called good cholesterol and a major factor in the prevention of atherosclerosis) in the blood.

The capacity of the lungs also increases, enabling them to process more air and replenish oxygen in the cells of the body's tissues and organs more quickly. Metabolism (conversion of food into energy) is enhanced and you tend to absorb nutrients from your food more efficiently. Any tendency towards constipation, kidney stones, or diabetes is reduced by this form of exercise.

Lower Your High Blood Pressure Naturally

Here are easy alternatives to blood-pressure-lowering drugs for mild to moderate hypertension, according to naturopath Michael T. Murray, N.D.

If you have mild hypertension (140-160/90-104):

■ Reduce your weight.

■ Eliminate your salt intake and avoid alcohol, caffeine, and smoking.

■ Exercise more and practice stress-reduction techniques (such as biofeedback, self-hypnosis, yoga, meditation, and muscle relaxation).

■ Change your diet to include more potassium-rich foods (such as potatoes, avocado, cooked lima beans, bananas, flounder), fiber, and complex carbohydrates.

■ Eat more celery, garlic, onions, and vegetable oils high in omega-3 fatty acids, but eat less animal fats.

■ Take supplements, including calcium (1,000-1,500 mg/day), magnesium (500 mg/day), vitamin C (1-3 g/day), zinc (in picolinate form, 15-30 mg/day), and flaxseed oil (1 tablespoon/day).

■ Maintain this program for at least three months, and preferably for six months; if your blood pressure isn't normal after this period, see a doctor.

If you have moderate hypertension (140-180/105-114):

■ Do all of the above.

■ Take hawthorn herbal extract (100-250 mg, 3 times daily, provided the extract contains 10% procyanidins).

■ Take coenzyme Q10 (20 mg, 3 times daily).

■ Follow this program for three months; if there is no change in your blood pressure, see a physician.[21]

Preventing & Reversing High Blood Pressure

ONE DOCTOR'S APPROACH

WHEN IT COMES to heart disease, prevention is easier than cure, says cardiologist Stephen T. Sinatra, M.D., executive director of the New England Heart Center in Manchester, Connecticut. Based on 20 years of experience as a board-certified cardiologist, Dr. Sinatra strongly believes that "if you do have heart disease, you can slow its progression and even reverse it." One of the best places to start is to reduce high blood pressure, a major risk factor for cardiovascular illness, says Dr. Sinatra. It may be major, but it's also *controllable*, using natural nondrug approaches, he adds.

To accomplish this, Dr. Sinatra offers a comprehensive alternative program of dietary change, nutritional supplements, exercise, and psychological counseling, in addition to some conventional prescription of beta blockers and other "antihypertensive" drugs. Dr. Sinatra's approach addresses the mind and body, the physiology and emotions, of the individual with high blood pressure. "There is definitely a heart/brain 'hotline,'" he notes in his book *Heartbreak & Heart Disease*. "The identification of people at risk for sudden death depends not only on the hidden possibilities of heart disease, but also on the psychological and emotional status of the one afflicted."

Coenzyme Q10:
An Energy Nutrient for the Heart

Pamela, 47, came to Dr. Sinatra with a seriously high blood pressure of 205/105. About two years earlier, physicians had placed her on standard antihypertensive drugs, including beta blockers, calcium channel blockers, and ACE inhibitors. These had left her excessively fatigued, coughing, and dissatisfied with the results.

For more on **coenzyme Q10**, see Chapter 5: Nutritional Supplements, pp. 115-119.

Dr. Sinatra immediately started Pamela on coenzyme Q10, at a dosage of 30 mg, three times daily; at the same time he reduced her intake of high blood pressure drugs by half. CoQ10, a substance found naturally in sardines, salmon, mackerel, and beef heart (but not made by the human body) is an essential feature of Dr. Sinatra's program because it helps prevent the depletion of substances that recharge the cellular energy system in the body.

"As the heart muscle continually uses oxygen and consumes huge amounts of energy, heart muscle cells can greatly benefit from the energy boost of coenzyme Q10," says Dr. Sinatra. In fact, levels of coQ10 are usually ten times higher in the healthy heart than in any other organ. This is why a coQ10 deficiency is most likely to primarily affect the heart and contribute to heart failure. It is estimated that 39% of patients with high blood pressure have a coQ10 deficiency.

The heart requires a constant supply of coQ10 to meet its energy needs. It is both "extremely vulnerable to nutritional deficiencies" and highly receptive to the

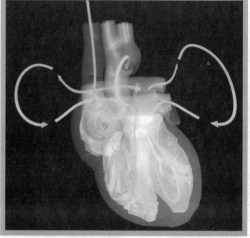

Copyright © 1989-97 by TechPool Studios, Inc. USA

"As the heart muscle continually uses oxygen and consumes huge amounts of energy, heart muscle cells can greatly benefit from the energy boost of coenzyme Q10," says Dr. Sinatra.

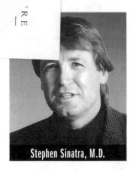

Stephen Sinatra, M.D.

"The identification of people at risk for sudden death depends not only on the hidden possibilities of heart disease, but also on the psychological and emotional status of the one afflicted," says Dr. Sinatra.

benefits of "targeted nutrition," Dr. Sinatra says. Clinical research indicates it usually takes 4 to 12 weeks for coQ10 to have a noticeable effect on blood pressure.

"I regard coQ10 as one of the best medical discoveries of the 20th century," he states. "I've been using it for ten years and have probably thousands of patients on it now. It is absolutely essential for strengthening the biochemistry of the heart cells." CoQ10 functions like a vitamin, "rescuing" body tissues that have been damaged by free radicals. "CoQ10 taken for cardiovascular conditions may enable some patients to reduce the dosage of their medications by up to 50%," notes Dr. Sinatra.

For these reasons, Dr. Sinatra starts almost all his cardiovascular patients on coQ10 at the initial low dose of 90 mg daily, then gradually increases it. "Extremely few people are oversensitive to it and may experience nausea—very rarely do I see side effects," says Dr. Sinatra. After one week, he increased Pamela's coQ10 dosage to 60 mg, three times daily. The standard dose for coQ10, as commonly prescribed by physicians, is "sub-therapeutic" and probably too low to be effective, says Dr. Sinatra. If you take 90-120 mg daily, you're likely to have a blood level of 1.5 ug/ml of usable coQ10, while what the body requires for a strong therapeutic response is 2.5 to 3.5 ug/ml.

As a general heart-protective dose, Dr. Sinatra himself takes 180 mg daily, but for high blood pressure, he usually builds toward a daily dose of 180 to 360 mg, and for serious congestive heart failure, 360-400 mg daily. For preventive maintenance for someone without a specific heart problem, Dr. Sinatra recommends a dosage of 30 to 90 mg daily.

The Value of a Mediterranean Diet

Dr. Sinatra also recommended that Pamela institute major changes in her diet. Specifically, he said her diet should consist of 30% fats, 20%-

A coenzyme Q10 deficiency is most likely to primarily affect the heart and contribute to heart failure. It is estimated that 39% of patients with high blood pressure have a coQ10 deficiency.

25% protein, and 45%-50% carbohydrates. The fats should come from fish such as salmon, mackerel, Greenland halibut, cod, and bluefish, but not tuna because of possible mercury contamination. Large amounts of red meat should be avoided while fresh fruits and vegetables are emphasized. Dr. Sinatra calls this the traditional Mediterranean diet.

For more about **olive oil**, see Chapter 2: Caring for Yourself, pp. 52-54.

A now classic study conducted in the 1980s investigating the rate of heart attacks over a ten-year period for individuals in European nations revealed that the island of Crete reported zero heart attacks as a cause of death, even though many of the residents had dangerously high cholesterol levels, a presumed risk factor for heart disease.

According to Dr. Sinatra, "the Mediterranean diet, rich in monounsaturated fat (olive oil) and antioxidants, has proved to be crucial in cardiovascular protection." Dr. Sinatra says this diet is low in saturated fats (such as dairy products and meats), high in fiber and antioxidants (from fresh fruits and vegetables) such as vitamin C, beta carotene, and vitamin E, and high in essential fatty acids, found in flax and other omega-3 oils. Avocados and asparagus, commonly eaten in this diet, are rich in L-glutathione, an amino acid that can scavenge harmful free radicals, while garlic and onions have ingredients that help protect the heart, and olive oil is "the healthiest of oils, no doubt."

Underlying the success of the Mediterranean diet is a biochemical principle, Dr. Sinatra says. It is called insulin resistance or hyperinsulinism. Insulin is a key digestive hormone, secreted by the pancreas for regulating the absorption of glucose (blood sugar) and the metabolism of carbohydrates and fats. In general, most Americans are eating too many carbohydrates, which in turn leads to excess insulin secretion (hyperinsulinism) and to insulin resistance, says Dr. Sinatra.

"When you've had too much insulin circulating in your bloodstream for too long—as is often the case when people doggedly stick to high-carbohydrate, low-fat diets—specialized receptor cells lose their ability to respond to insulin." The resulting insulin resistance can lead to higher blood pressure, thickened, less elastic arterial walls, increased cravings for carbohydrates, and higher blood sugar

QUICK DEFINITION

Omega-3 and omega-6 oils are the two principal types of essential fatty acids, which are unsaturated fats required in the diet. The digits "3" and "6" refer to differences in the oil's chemical structure with respect to its chain of carbon atoms and where they are bonded. A balance of these oils in the diet is required for good health. The primary omega-3 oil is called alpha-linolenic acid (ALA) and is found in flaxseed (58%), canola, pumpkin and walnut, and soybeans. Fish oils, such as salmon, cod, and mackerel, contain the other important omega-3 oils, DHA (docosahexaenoic acid) and EPA (eicosapentaenoic acid). Omega-3 oils help reduce the risk of heart disease. Linoleic acid or cis-linoleic acid is the main omega-6 oil and is found in most plant and vegetable oils, including safflower (73%), corn, peanut, and sesame. The most therapeutic form of omega-6 oil is gamma-linolenic acid (GLA), found in evening primrose, black currant, and borage oils. Once in the body, omega-6 is converted to prostaglandins, hormone-like substances that regulate many metabolic functions, particularly inflammatory processes.

levels, says Dr. Sinatra.

This factor contributes to heart disease in two ways. First, as insulin secretion increases, so does the level of arachidonic acid. (This is a fatty-acid precursor to prostaglandins and is found almost entirely in animal foods.) Further biochemical changes resulting from this cause blood vessels to constrict and blood to clot, and this sets up a risk factor for both higher blood pressure and serious heart problems.

The second problem with too much insulin is that it is antagonistic to the cells (called endothelial) that line the blood vessels and keep them free of obstructions, Dr. Sinatra says. As insulin levels rise, the structural integrity of the endothelial cells suffers and the type of muscles in the blood vessels changes. The result can be blood vessels that are prone to developing plaque deposits, which again can lead to high blood pressure, he adds.

"The benefit of the Mediterranean diet is that everything in it helps prevent excess insulin release," says Dr. Sinatra. The diet, through saltwater fish, shellfish, and flaxseed, contains high levels of alpha-linolenic and omega-3 fatty acids, which are "the most important essential fatty acids for the protection of cardiovascular health."

Dr. Sinatra also generally recommends minimizing the consumption of "high glycemic carbohydrates." This means foods such as flour pastas, white potatoes, and white rice, whose carbohydrate portion enters the bloodstream quickly, leading to higher levels of insulin to handle the sudden glucose load. Examples of fruits with a low-glycemic index (slow absorption by the blood) include grapefruit, cherries, peaches, plums, kiwi, and rhubarb. Pamela was also instructed to avoid preservatives, processed foods and meats, canned vegetables, diet soft drinks, and chemical ingredients.

Under Dr. Sinatra's supervision, Pamela added tofu, navy beans, and seaweeds to her diet for their magnesium content. She also started taking an antioxidant vitamin-mineral formula (containing no copper or iron) developed by Dr. Sinatra under the brand name Optimum Health. Pamela started taking a daily formula containing 1,000 mg of calcium and 500 mg of magnesium. These amounts were in addition to the vitamin-mineral supplement which contained lower amounts of both (280 mg of magnesium, 250 mg of calcium). "Magnesium prevents spasming of blood vessels which is why it's one of the most important mineral treatments for high blood pressure," says Dr. Sinatra.

Dr. Sinatra also encouraged Pamela to begin a regular exercise program, preferably vigorous walking. "I don't recommend jogging. If you can do a brisk walk lasting 15 minutes twice a day, that's all the exercise you really need," says Dr. Sinatra. As an alternative, he advises dancing (and practices it himself) as a "heart nurturing" form of daily rhythmic exercise. Regularity, not intensity, of exercise is paramount, he says.

At Pamela's next appointment two weeks later, her blood pressure had dropped to 170/90, "a big improvement," says Dr. Sinatra. He kept her on the diet and supplement program, including coQ10 at 180 mg daily; he took her off calcium channel blocker but kept her on a low dose of beta blocker. She maintained a daily walking program of one to two miles. After about three months on the Sinatra program, Pamela's blood pressure had come down to a safe 140-145/80-85. "I was satisfied with that," Dr. Sinatra says.

Hawthorn Helps Colin's Heart Relax

Dr. Sinatra offers another case involving Colin, 65, who came to him with a history of heart attacks and progressive heart failure. His problem was that his heart's pumping ability was severely reduced. Colin's blood pressure was 180/90, he was unable to tolerate most conventional heart drugs, and his mitral valve (one of the heart's four valves) was leaking blood as a result of his high blood pressure. Colin had chronic shortness of breath and was unable to walk much without getting winded.

Dr. Sinatra started Colin on the Mediterranean diet; coQ10, magnesium, calcium, and potassium supplements; and hawthorn herbal extract (from hawthorn berries) beginning at 500 mg daily, then increasing to 1,000 mg. Clinical studies have shown that hawthorn can help reduce blood pressure by reducing or blocking the constriction of blood vessels directly serving the heart. This is crucial because when blood vessels constrict, blood pressure rises. "I gave Colin hawthorn to reduce his blood pressure, strengthen his heart, and give him a good quality

EDITOR'S NOTE

Dr. Sinatra is board certified in Internal Medicine and Cardiology and is a certified bioenergetic therapist in the tradition of Alexander Lowen, M.D. Dr. Sinatra has served as chief of cardiology at the Manchester Memorial Hospital in Connecticut and as assistant clinical professor at the University of Connecticut. He is the editor of the monthly newsletter, *HeartSense*, and the author of *Heartbreak & Heart Disease* (1996), Keats Publishing, Inc., 27 Pine Street, New Canaan, CT 06840; tel: 203-966-8721; fax: 203-972-3991; and *Optimum Health* (1997), Bantam Doubleday, New York, NY.

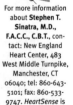

For more information about **Stephen T. Sinatra, M.D., F.A.C.C., C.B.T.**, contact: New England Heart Center, 483 West Middle Turnpike, Manchester, CT 06040; tel: 860-643-5101; fax: 860-533-9747. *HeartSense* is available from Philips Publishing, Inc., P.O. Box 60042, 7811 Montrose Road, Potomac, MD 20859; tel: 800-211-7643; 12 issues/$100. For information about the Optimum Health line of heart supplements, contact Dr. Sinatra's office.

"Magnesium prevents spasming of blood vessels which is why it's one of the most important mineral treatments for high blood pressure," says Dr. Sinatra.

For more on **homocysteine**, see Chapter 1: What Causes Heart Disease?, pp. 34-37.

of life," which means improved health without the unpleasant side effects of drugs.

Colin also began taking B vitamins, specifically 40 mg each of B1, B2, and B6, 40 mcg of B12, and 800 mcg of folic acid. "I recommend B vitamins for anybody with heart disease because they are the antidote to a condition we call hyperhomocysteinemia," says Dr. Sinatra.

Here is how it works: Red meat contains methionine, an essential amino acid and protein building block. But if your system is deficient in B vitamins, methionine does not get broken down into simpler substances and instead forms homocysteine. Too much homocysteine contributes to premature heart disease and aging, explains Dr. Sinatra.

After about six weeks on the program, Colin's blood pressure dropped to 140-145/90-95. There was less leakage at his mitral valve; he was not taking any conventional drugs; he was able to walk, play golf, and exercise more freely; and "he felt he was in terrific control of his life," says Dr. Sinatra.

Often an individual with high blood pressure or heart disease suffers from depression and sexual dysfunction, including impotence, Dr. Sinatra notes. Sometimes these conditions are caused by conventional drugs; other times, they result from diminished nutrition and unresolved emotional issues. To help shift the depression that can accompany heart problems, Dr. Sinatra prescribes the amino acid L-tyrosine. Getting a person off conventional heart drugs and onto a solid nutritional support program often completes the turnaround, he adds.

"When you empower patients with nutritional support, diet, and exercise, they have control over their destiny and develop a much greater optimism. When you have this optimism about participating in your health, you become alive sexually. I've seen this many times. I tell them I am not their doctor but their nurse. In other words, I will nurse them along and nurture their healing, but *they* have the power to get well."

Uncovering the Anger in Ray's Blood Pressure

It's important not to overlook the crucial role that emotions can play in the development of high blood pressure, notes Dr. Sinatra. "The psychological risk factors can be just as lethal as the more accepted

Clinical studies have shown that hawthorn can help reduce blood pressure by reducing or blocking the constriction of blood vessels directly serving the heart.

physical risk factors," he says. Unresolved emotions, such as anger, hostility, and rage, and the way one reacts to stress, are hidden risk factors in heart disease that many cardiologists fail to acknowledge.

To many, both physicians and patients, these emotions represent the "dark side" or shadow portion of the personality that tends to get denied or suppressed. "But I think that getting in touch with these powerful hidden emotions and becoming aware of their contribution to heart disease is critical to healing and protecting the heart," Dr. Sinatra says. Ray's case perfectly demonstrates this point.

Ray, 44, was a corporate executive in a position of high responsibility and stress. His blood pressure was "horrendous" at 220/115 and was not responding at all to conventional antihypertensive drugs when he first came for treatment. Dr. Sinatra performed an emotional stress test on Ray, using a computerized device called a Cardiac Performance Laboratory (CPL) that in effect measures anger by evaluating the degree to which the blood vessels are constricted from hypertension. The CPL measures 17 dynamic circulatory changes inside the heart and blood vessels.

Dr. Sinatra asked Ray to perform mental arithmetic, put his hands in ice-cold water, and answer stressful questions. The test registers the changes in blood pressure, literally with each heartbeat, in accordance with these requests. If you are a reasonably calm person, putting your hands in ice water will elevate your blood pressure five to ten points, says Dr. Sinatra, but if you are what is called a "hot reactor" or physiological overreactor, the jump may be 30-40 points.

"With Ray, I was dealing with a man who was very calm on the outside, but on the inside, he was a hot reactor. When I asked him questions about his mother or his personal life, he virtually went off the walls with his blood pressure." He saw it rise dangerously to 240/125 under stress. "Ray was a young man but in tough shape—a risk for sudden death."

During his interview with Ray, Dr. Sinatra observed how much anger Ray held in his body, as evidenced by his clenched jaw and shallow breathing. Dr. Sinatra then understood why the antihypertensive drugs were having no useful effect on Ray: his anger was the prime cause of his high blood pressure.

"Are you aware of how much anger you have?" Dr. Sinatra asked

How Well is Your Heart Working?
The Cardiac Performance Lab Can Tell You

The Cardiac Performance Lab (CPL) from SoftQue Inc. of Mesa, Arizona, is a noninvasive diagnostic system that measures heart and circulatory performance. CPL, which looks at heart stroke volume, cardiac output, total systemic resistance, and 14 other heart functions, provides more information than the standard electrocardiogram (EKG) yet is not as expensive or invasive as heart catheterization.

Impedance cardiography (as this process is called) originated in the 1930s and was used by NASA during the Apollo space program. It uses elec-

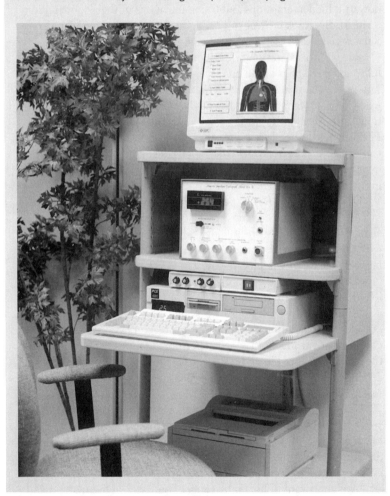

trical resistance (impedance) to measure cardiac performance. All substances, including body tissues, have a higher or lower opposition (resistance) when an electrical current passes through them. Copper, the most common conductor, has a low resistance to electricity; that is to say, it has a low electrical impedance. In body tissues, electrical resistance is lower in wet tissue than in dry, and blood is a particularly good electrical conductor because it has low resistance compared to other tissues.

CPL in effect turns the chest cavity into an electrical conductor and then measures changes in resistance which reflect changes in blood flow. A high-frequency, low-intensity alternating current is conducted through the chest of the subject (with no discomfort) from electrodes attached to the forehead and abdomen. EKG leads attached to the body monitor resistance levels throughout the area and send this information to the CPL computer. As blood is pumped through the heart and into the body, resistance in the chest cavity fluctuates because of the changing concentration of blood. These changes are recorded by the CPL computer, which displays heart and circulatory performance along with blood pressure fluctuations in wave patterns on a continuous graph giving an accurate picture of cardiac activity.

The CPL test is adjusted for each individual to accommodate for demographic information, such as age, sex, height, and weight. These values help establish normal ranges for the individual. Changes in cardiac performance under stress are induced using five standard tests: the subject goes through a series of different postures and movements and performs mental tests to simulate "real world" stress. The results are then compared to normal ranges for the individual to evaluate heart function under these conditions.

Some of the heart and circulatory factors measured by CPL include blood pressure (systolic, diastolic, and mean); cardiac output (stroke volume times heart rate); left ventricular ejection time (time for blood to be pumped from the left ventricle); stroke volume index (stroke volume divided by body surface area); vascular rigidity index (pulse pressure per change in stroke volume per body surface area); and total systemic resistance (mean arterial pressure times 80 then divided by cardiac output).

For more information about **Cardiac Performance Laboratory**, contact: SoftQue Inc., 2427 East Huber, Mesa, AZ 85213; tel: 602-834-1318; fax: 602-835-6559.

him. Ray responded: "Yes, but I can't get it out or show it." He then admitted he had never shared this secret with anybody nor had he ever allowed himself to show his anger. "Then Ray started to cry because he was seeing this side of himself for the first time. Crying is very healthy for the heart. I try to reframe a patient's anger and make it a healing rather than a destructive energy."

After this meeting, Ray started psychotherapy with a practitioner trained in the way emotions can be lodged in the body. Soon after,

Ray's corporation transferred him to another city, but when Dr. Sinatra heard from him about six months later, Ray reported that his blood pressure was completely normal.

Ray's case underscores another important insight gained from the heart study of the Cretans, particularly the men, says Dr. Sinatra. Equally as important as their Mediterranean diet is the fact that men in that region tend to talk more openly with other men about their feelings, families, dreams, and spiritual beliefs.

Men in this Mediterranean culture tend not to wear social masks, but feel comfortable arguing, crying, supporting, even holding one another, says Dr. Sinatra. This quality of comradery and the respect for the "healing powers of nurturing relationships" is a major factor accounting for the low level of coronary heart disease among that population, he says.

Best of all—for his patients—Dr. Sinatra tries to be a good example of what is required to keep one's heart healthy and unpressured. He works hard but he listens to his body so he does not become highly stressed. He takes coQ10, practices the Mediterranean diet, and loves to dance. "I cry when I want to and have my anger—I experience my dark-side, shadow emotions."

He never forgets that becoming ill, whether with high blood pressure or other heart ailments, "is really a form of disease that emerges from the chaotic imbalance of mind, body, and spirit." For a cardiovascular therapy to be completely successful, says Dr. Sinatra, it must heal this "disturbed relationship," addressing heart stress at the metabolic, physiological, psychological, and even spiritual levels.

It's important not to overlook the
crucial role that emotions
can play in the development of high
blood pressure, notes Dr. Sinatra.
"The psychological risk factors
can be just as lethal as the more accepted
physical risk factors," he says.
Unresolved emotions, such as anger,
hostility, and rage, and the way one reacts
to stress, are hidden risk factors
in heart disease that many
cardiologists fail to acknowledge.

Chinese Medicine

HOW IT CAN HELP REVERSE HIGH BLOOD PRESSURE

TRADITIONAL CHINESE medicine (TCM) is a well-established method of health care that combines the use of medicinal herbs, acupuncture, food therapy, massage, and therapeutic exercise. It has proven effective for many conditions, including high blood pressure.

As a result of imbalance in the body, high blood pressure can begin to creep up even in an otherwise seemingly healthy person. If left untreated, it can lead to more serious heart disease. High blood pressure can also develop as a symptom of other conditions, such as adult-onset diabetes and a liver imbalance. In the following section, acupuncturist **Ira J. Golchehreh, Lic.Ac., O.M.D.**, of San Rafael, California, explains how this can happen and how traditional Chinese medicine can reverse it and prevent the development of more serious conditions.

High Blood Pressure on the Way to Diabetes

Many people in the West develop serious health problems, such as heart disease, diabetes, cancer, or arthritis, when they reach middle age. Although these may seem to arise out of nowhere, almost always there is a medical history of many chronic conditions that were never treated correctly.

Based on my experience with acupuncture and Chinese herbs, I can say confidently that serious illness at midlife does not have to happen. With the strategic use of Chinese medicine, for example, you can successfully *prevent* a series of chronic problems from becoming one big acute problem later. The case of Ronald shows this perfectly.

When I first met Ronald, 44, he presented the classic symptoms of a lifelong liver imbalance. Technically, in Chinese medicine we call this "hyperactivity of liver yang." It represents a liver whose energy, or "fire," is so overactive, or "yang," and, therefore, so imbalanced, that it creates problems throughout the mind and body.

When I first treated Ronald, I made an emergency house call, as he didn't feel well enough to come to my office. His acute symptom was painful, bright red, and terribly itchy skin lesions on his inner thighs and groin. I knew at once this was a flare-up along his liver meridian. When I learned that he had a job with much pressure and responsibility, I understood that these factors might have precipitated this crisis from the basis of a liver energy imbalance. I also noted that as it was spring and the liver is the organ of this season in Chinese medical thinking, the timing of the flare-up was appropriate.

I applied needles to acupuncture points on the front of Ronald's body to redirect healing energy (or *qi*) to the area of inflammation. I also gave him *Gypsum fibrosum* powder (calcium sulfate) to apply topically (moistened with water) to the lesions and to take internally to "cool down" his system because there was too much "heat" in his liver.

One week later, Ronald came to my office, where I took his complete health history. As a child, he suffered from colitis and constipation, angry outbursts, and nearsightedness. As an adult, Ronald had been bothered with chronic indigestion, bloating, gas, heartburn, multiple food allergies, a recurrent dry cough, night sweats, periodic irritability, and fluctuating body temperature. His complexion was pale, he was overweight, his abdomen was tight and distended, and his breathing was shallow. Ronald's pulse, as we "read" it in Chinese medicine, was fast and taut, especially for his liver.

Ronald's blood sugar level at 150 was high, as normal is 80-120. His body temperature was two degrees below normal; his blood pressure was elevated at 130/89; and the oxygen saturation of his blood was a dangerously low 87% (normal is 95%-97%). In his immediate family, there was a history of diabetes, gallbladder dysfunction, and bloating.

What an Unbalanced Liver Can Do

It was clear to me that Ronald was well on the way towards developing adult-onset diabetes with possible prostate and heart complica-

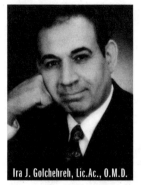

Ira J. Golchehreh, Lic.Ac., O.M.D.

"Many people in the West develop serious health problems, such as heart disease, diabetes, cancer, or arthritis, when they reach middle age. Based on my experience with acupuncture and Chinese herbs, I can say confidently that serious illness at midlife does not have to happen," says Ira J. Golchehreh, Lic.Ac., O.M.D.

tions. One never knows for sure, but he could have been as close as five years from these problems. With Ronald, a single organ—the liver—was clearly the cause of many symptoms. Chinese medicine has a name for the quality of Ronald's liver energy. We call it "rebellious *qi*." The energy of his liver was excessive and too strong. It rose up through his system like a volcano and was subject to periodic eruptions, which he might experience as angry outbursts. His liver was in rebellion, energetically speaking, against his other organs.

The healthy liver is the source of an estimated 13,000 different enzymes and biochemicals which it produces every day. The enzymes in Ronald's liver were wild and hyperactive, exploding throughout the body like sparks from a volcano. Even though he had too many enzymes, his system could not use them to digest his food; hence, he had many digestive problems.

The liver heat dried up his lungs, making them contract and stiffen. That's why his blood-oxygen level was so dangerously low. This, in turn, meant his heart and other organs were becoming oxygen-deprived. The cough was an attempt by his lungs to suck more air into them. Although he exercised regularly and ate a low-fat diet, Ronald was both overweight and undernourished, conditions caused by faulty metabolism, thanks to the liver.

The liver imbalance also upset Ronald's pancreas, which produces insulin to regulate blood-sugar levels, hence, his blood sugar was high. Finally, the overactive liver was depleting Ronald's basic life force, which Chinese medicine says is stored in the kidneys. Three years earlier he had been sick for a month with a bladder infection; this of course is a sign of an underlying kidney imbalance.

When you understand the *root* cause that produces many health

When you understand the *root* cause that produces many health problems in a person, you see that all the signs and symptoms of illness actually make perfect sense. In Ronald's case, they all resulted from a liver imbalance.

problems in a person, you see that all the signs and symptoms of illness actually make perfect sense. In Ronald's case, they all resulted from a liver imbalance that he was probably born with. With this in mind, I developed my treatment plan.

Taming the Volcano

As he arrived for his second treatment, Ronald told me that his cough had become constant. He could not speak without coughing. To help this, I applied six vacuum glass cups to the surface of his back. These would open his lungs, draw toxins out of them and towards the skin surface, and enable him to breathe better. Next, I applied two hydro hot packs to the

To contact **Dr. Ira J. Golchehreh, Lic.Ac., O.M.D.:** Bay Park Business Center, 2175 Francisco Blvd., Suite D, San Rafael, CA 94901; tel: 415-485-4411; fax: 415-485-0857.

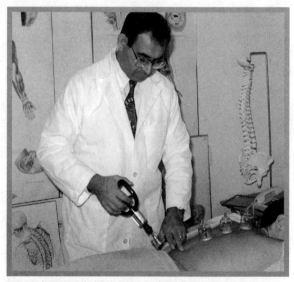

Chinese medicine uses a practice called *cupping* in which vacuum glass cups are applied to the skin's surface, in this case, on the back, to "open" the lungs, draw toxins out of them and towards the skin surface, and to facilitate better breathing.

QUICK DEFINITION

Acupuncture meridians are specific pathways in the human body for the flow of life force or subtle energy, known as *qi* (pronounced *CHEE*). In most cases, these energy pathways run up and down both sides of the body, and correspond to individual organs or organ systems, designated as Lung, Small Intestine, Heart, and others. There are 12 principal meridians and eight secondary channels. Numerous points of heightened energy, or *qi*, exist on the body's surface along the meridians and are called acupoints. There are more than 1,000 acupoints, each of which is potentially a place for acupuncture treatment.

Eriobotrya and *Ophiopogon* **Combination** contains Prince Ginseng root (*Radix Ophiopogonis*), white mulberry leaves (*Morus alba*), calcium sulfate (*Gypsum fibrosum*), licorice, sesame seed, apricot kernel, and ginseng. **CO-197** contains honeysuckle flower, forsythia fruit, reed grass root, bamboo, mint, false perilla leaves, soybean, platycodon root, burdock, and licorice. This product is available as part of the ProBotanixx line from: Sun Ten Labs, Irvine, CA 92718. *Ma Huang Coix Combination* contains Coix lachryma (dried seeds), ephedra, apricot seed, and licorice. **Resplex** is available from: PhysioLogics, 6565 Odell Place, Boulder, CO 80301.

same points on his back. These are thick hot tubes containing minerals that release heat through the skin to the lungs.

Then I focused two mineral infrared lamps onto the lung and liver areas of his back. These lamps project heat through a filter containing 33 different minerals and nutrients; the skin absorbs the energy of these elements and conducts it inwards. I gave Ronald several capsules of the herb *Ephedra* to ease his cough and further open his lungs. Finally, I applied about 50 needles to points on the Liver, Lung, Spleen, and Stomach acupuncture meridians. Normally I do not use this many needles, but it was important to treat many organs and energy systems at once to start bringing his entire system into harmony.

I told Ronald to take two capsules of *Ephedra* three times daily, for a daily total of 1,800 mg, to help open his lungs so he could breathe more fully and saturate his blood with more oxygen. I gave him another Chinese herb called *Bupleurum* to help disperse excess liver heat, to keep the liver from "exploding" with too much energy, to regulate blood pressure, and to destroy pathogens in his system. He would take one teaspoon of this mixed in water, twice daily.

Next, I gave Ronald CO-197 containing ten Chinese herbs, to be taken three times daily. In addition, I asked him to drink at least $\frac{1}{2}$ gallon of pure water every day; this would promote the excretion of toxins from the system through frequent urination.

Finally, I asked him to radically change his diet to one that was high-protein, low-fat and low-carbohydrate, and completely yeast-free. I asked Ronald to eat vegetable soups, whole grains (excepting wheat), lots of protein (preferably chicken and fish as he was allergic to beans), and no fruit, no fresh raw vegetables, nothing yeasted, no coffee, alcohol, salt, sugar, spices, or dairy products of any kind. The purpose of the diet was to give Ronald's liver some breathing space to clean itself out thoroughly after many years of having to deal with foods that upset it. To my relief, Ronald said he realized he needed to completely overhaul his diet and welcomed my guidance.

One week later, Ronald returned for his third treatment. He had kept a journal of all his daily symptoms. This was quite instructive because it showed me how the energy was starting to move around in his body, temporarily producing both physical and emotional symptoms. When I checked his vital signs, I was pleased with the results. His blood sugar had dropped to 120, his oxygen saturation had climbed to 97, and his blood pressure was better at 120/78. He was less bloated and his coughing was about 50% reduced.

This time I treated acupoints on Ronald's front, focusing on the Liver, Spleen, and Pancreas meridians. As before, I used a lot of needles and let him lie on the table for about an hour as they helped to harmonize his organs. This time, I sent Ronald home with a new herbal formula called *Eriobotrya* and *Ophiopogon* Combination, one teaspoon mixed in water, to be taken twice daily.

This blend would help remove the "heat" from the lungs so that they could expand more fully; it would also help to harmonize the energies of the spleen and stomach. I also put Ronald on Resplex, a respiratory formula containing beta carotene, vitamin E, wild cherry bark, horehound, lobelia, pleurisy root, hyssop, and mullein, to be taken three times daily, two capsules each time.

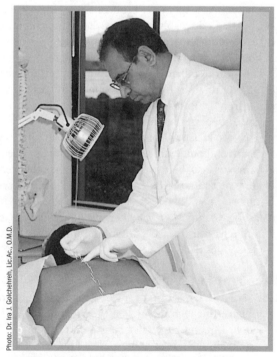

Photo: Dr. Ira J. Golchehreh, Lic.Ac., O.M.D.

Mineral infrared lamps (pictured here) **project heat through a filter containing 33 different minerals and nutrients; the skin absorbs the energy of these elements and conducts it inwards.**

Out of the Woods After a Month

By the time of the fourth treatment, one month after beginning with Ronald, he was out of the woods as far as his acute problems were concerned. By the way, he had taken only one day off from work during this period, although he slept heavily on the weekends.

When you reset the energy patterns of a major organ, especially the liver, which influences so much else in the body, and after a lifetime of imbalance, it takes many weeks for one's full supply of energy to return. It's like trying to irrigate a parched field for the first time; the water reserves are stretched at first because the ground is so dry. That's why Ronald was exhausted every Saturday. Had he taken two weeks off from work, his total healing time would have been reduced to about five weeks instead of what ended up taking ten weeks.

At this point, Ronald's vital signs were the best yet. His blood sugar was 78, his pulse was much calmer, oxygen saturation was 97%, and blood pressure was a much more balanced 119/88. His cough was only sporadic, probably 80% improved. Ronald's complexion was noticeably rosier, as the higher blood-oxygen content had brought more life, literally, to his face. This time I again treated acupoints that would harmonize the interactions of all his organs. For his fifth treatment, I worked on harmonizing the energies flowing among the liver, lungs, and kidneys by placing needles at points on the front of Ronald's body. Following this treatment, he reported that he felt energized and vibrant.

Two weeks later, Ronald returned for another treatment but his vital signs and pulse indicated he actually did not need one. His blood pressure was even better at 116/81, while the other readings remained stable. I kept him on the *Ephedra*, Resplex, *Eriobotrya* and *Ophiopogon* Combination, and the restricted diet, and added two more herbal formulas. I gave him *Ma Huang Coix* including *Ephedra*, taken at the rate of nine pills daily. I also started him on another *Bupleurum* powder, two teaspoons daily in water.

Excellent in Four Months

One month later, Ronald returned for a checkup and maintenance treatment. After two months on the program, he had lost 20 pounds and looked fit and rosy. His energy had returned to normal, his liver was calm, and he was in good spirits. This time I used the needles to fine-tune the energies of his liver, lungs, and other organ systems.

I was gratified to see how well he had responded to the treatment. There was no doubt the body was healing itself after a lifetime of imbalance. I asked Ronald to remain on the diet for another month to complete the liver's total detoxification. All of his original symptoms were gone. Four months after beginning treatment, Ronald's blood pressure was a healthy 112/78, his oxygen level was 98%, and his liver pulse was calm. Provided he continues with a moderate diet and periodic acupuncture checkups, it is quite likely the symptoms will not return for the rest of his life.

In retrospect, I can see now that Ronald's initial health crisis of inflammation on his thighs and groin was sufficiently acute to get him into treatment for what proved to be a lifetime disorder seated in his liver. This is a good example of how an acute problem today can also be an opportunity to *prevent* something far more serious just around the corner in a person's life. ■

Fundamentals of Traditional Chinese Medicine

TCM has been practiced for over 3,000 years and, at present, one-quarter of the world's population makes use of one or more of its therapies. A complete system of medicine, it has been selected by the World Health Organization for worldwide propagation to meet the health care needs of the twenty-first century.[1]

TCM's approach to health and healing is very different from modern Western medicine. TCM looks for the underlying causes of imbalances and patterns of disharmony in the body, and views each patient as unique. Western medicine generally provides treatment for a specific illness, whereas traditional Chinese medicine addresses how the illness manifests in a particular patient and treats the patient, not just the disease. As Roger Hirsh, O.M.D., L.Ac., Dipl. NCCA, of Beverly Hills, California, explains, "The conventional Western physician focuses predominantly on the pathogenic factor (the disease), rather than the response of the patient to the factor."

The philosophy of traditional Chinese medicine is preventive in nature and views the practice of waiting to treat a disease until the symptoms are full-blown as being similar to "digging a well after one has become thirsty."[2] In line with this, TCM makes a point of educating patients with regard to lifestyle so that they can assist in their own therapeutic process. The TCM practitioner educates the patient about diet, exercise, stress management, rest, and relaxation.

The terms yin and yang are used by the TCM practitioner to describe the opposing physical conditions of the body. These terms

The philosophy of traditional Chinese medicine is preventive in nature and views the practice of waiting to treat a disease until the symptoms are full-blown as being similar to "digging a well after one has become thirsty."

stem from a basic Chinese concept describing the interdependence and relationship of opposites. Much as hot cannot be understood or defined without having experienced cold, yin cannot exist without its opposite yang, and yang cannot exist without yin.

Roger Jahnke, O.M.D., an acupuncturist based in Santa Barbara, California, explains that when applying these concepts to the human body, "Yin refers to the tissue of the organ, while yang refers to its activity. In yin deficiency, the organ does not have enough raw materials to function. In yang deficiency, the organ does not react adequately when needed."

These two conditions are forever connected, though, "in a system of interdependence and interrelatedness," adds Maoshing Ni, D.O.M., Ph.D., L.Ac., president of Yo San University of Traditional Chinese Medicine in Santa Monica, California. For example, says Dr. Ni, a yin deficiency in thyroid hormone levels, the raw material of the thyroid gland, would eventually cause a yang deficiency in the thyroid, as its function becomes impaired by the lack of hormones. Likewise, poor thyroid function, a yang deficiency, would eventually result in a yin deficiency, as the gland's output of hormones decreased.

Traditional Chinese medicine also introduces a major component of the body, *qi* (also referred to as chi), that Western medicine does not even acknowledge. *Qi*, according to Dr. Ni, is difficult to define. "We call it life force. It is all-inclusive of the many types of energy within the body and is essential for life itself," he says. This vital life energy flows through the body following pathways called meridians.

These meridians flow along the surface of the body, and through the internal organs, with each meridian being given the name of the organ through which it flows, such as "Liver," or "Large Intestine." Organs can be accessed for treatment through their specific meridians, and illness can occur when there is a blockage of *qi* in these channels. Therefore it is essential in traditional Chinese medicine to keep the *qi* flowing in order to maintain health. The healthy individual has an abundance of *qi* moving smoothly through the meridians and organs. With this flow, the organs are able to harmoniously support each other's functions.

Five Phase Theory

The interrelationship of the body's organs is another important concept in traditional Chinese medicine. Ten organs are arranged into a system that places each in one of five categories: fire, earth, metal, water, and wood. This system, called the Five Phase Theory, is based on the premise that each organ either nourishes or inhibits the proper functioning of another organ, just as the basic elements act either adversely or beneficially on each other. "The Chinese have, for thousands of years, watched how things worked around them in order to understand why things happen, why things transform from one thing to another," says Dr. Ni. "They've taken this same conceptual model and applied it to the human body and found it really works well."

For example, as fire melts metal, the heart, which is associated with fire, controls the lungs, which are associated with metal. Likewise, as metal cuts wood, the lungs control the liver; as wood penetrates the earth, the liver controls the spleen; as the earth dams water, the spleen controls the kidneys; and as water quenches fire, the kidneys control the heart.

Under traditional Chinese medical treatment, the patient's blood pressure dropped from 180/130 to 130/90 in less than two weeks.

The organs are also divided up into two groups of yin and yang organs. "The heart, spleen, lungs, kidney, and liver belong to the yin group, because they are what we call more substantial organs, more solid," explains Dr. Ni, "whereas, the yang organs are hollow organs like the small intestine, stomach, large intestine, and bladder, where things just pass through. They're more functional—remember, yang is function, action, and yin is more passive, solid, substantial—that's why they're categorized that way."

ELEMENT	YIN ORGAN	YANG ORGAN
Fire	Heart	Small intestine
Earth	Spleen	Stomach
Metal	Lungs	Large intestine
Water	Kidney	Bladder
Wood	Liver	Gallbladder

According to TCM, essential hypertension is usually due to a problem in the circulation of energy *(qi)* in the body. Treatment is aimed at bringing the energy flow of the body back into balance through a combination of acupuncture and herbs.

The Practice of Traditional Chinese Medicine

In treating a patient, a TCM practitioner first looks for patterns in the details of his or her clinical observations of that patient. This allows the practitioner to discover the disharmony in the system of that individual. Familiar with symptoms that are standard to each disease, the doctor also considers what symptoms or behaviors would be especially telling to the individual patient. For example, some people are very active and constantly moving, even red in the face, yet these appearances may not indicate any malady. On the other hand, it is perfectly normal for others to exhibit slowness and inactivity. It is against this individual landscape that the TCM practitioner attempts to correctly assess the pattern of disharmony when an individual becomes ill.

A pattern may be so commonly associated with a certain treatment that the pattern and treatment carry the same name. But often the doctor must develop a strategy by carefully balancing many details. Stomach ulcers, for instance, may originate in very different patterns of disharmony, although the resulting ulcers may appear identical. Therefore, each type of ulcer may require a very different type of treatment, and the wrong treatment could worsen the condition.

"Yet in Western medicine, ulcers are generally treated with whatever anti-ulcer medication there may be, without differentiating," says Dr. Ni. "What Chinese medicine does is decipher the response of the patient. How is the patient's body reacting to the illness, to the cause of the illness? It's these patterns that we seek to determine and then treat accordingly." Alternatively, people with different symptoms, but the same pattern of disharmony, can often be treated by the same medicines or therapies.

Methods of Diagnosis

A first-time patient, accustomed to Western medicine, may be surprised that TCM diagnosis does not require procedures such as blood tests, X rays, endoscopy (the inspection of the inside of a body cavity by an endoscope), or exploratory surgery. Instead, the TCM practitioner performs the five following, noninvasive methods of investigation:

■ Inspection of the complexion, general demeanor, body language, and tongue

■ Questioning the patient about symptoms, medical history, diet, lifestyle, history of the present complaint, and any previous or concurrent therapies received

■ Listening to the tone and strength of the voice

■ Smelling any body excretions, the breath, or the body odor

■ Palpation (feeling with the fingers) of the pulse at the radial arteries of both wrists (pulse diagnosis), the abdomen, and the meridians and/or acupuncture points

Through pulse diagnosis, a skilled practitioner can examine the strength or weakness of the *qi* and "blood," which includes lymph and other bodily fluids, and assess how these affect each of the organs, tissues, and layers of the body. The practitioner will also look at the impact of a wide range of personal and environmental factors. Mood influences, activity, sex, food, drugs, weather, and seasons of the year can each affect health and the healing process. "All these factors need to be weighed when making a diagnosis," states Dr. Hirsh, "but the presence of one factor doesn't always warrant a disease outcome."

Dr. Ni explains that what TCM practitioners try to do with all

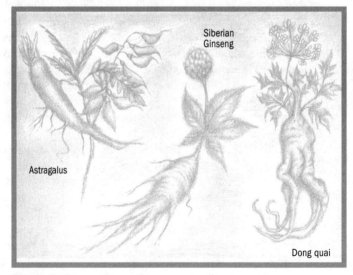

Chinese herbs

forms of diagnosis is look at illness in the body from the point of view of function. "Too much function or too little function—illness can really be simplified in this way," says Dr. Ni.

Treatments in Traditional Chinese Medicine

Herbs are a primary part of a TCM treatment. A prescription consists of generous piles of ingredients, distributed in paper packets containing one-day or two-day doses. The visually intriguing ingredients—perhaps bark, roots, or oyster shell—come from the vegetable, animal, and mineral kingdoms. The formulas may contain from 6 to 19 different substances and are assembled with great care. These are prescribed to treat the root of the disease and its manifestation, and the formula must also be balanced within itself.

Although the herbs are taken internally as decoctions (herbs boiled in water), TCM doctors also prescribe pills, powders, syrups, tinctures, inhalants, suppositories, enemas, douches, soaks, plasters, poultices, and salves. Specific foods may also be part of the protocol.

Acupuncture is also extensively used in traditional Chinese medicine. Using the meridian system and its thousands of corresponding surface points, acupuncture uses special needles placed strategically into these "acupoints" to help correct and rebalance the flow of energy within the specific meridian, consequently relieving pain and restoring health. Moxibustion, the burning of special "moxa" herbs on or above a specific acupoint, is another technique TCM employs.

Massage and manipulation are integral parts of the modern practice of TCM, including professional remedial massage therapies such as osteopathic and chiropractic adjustments. "There are many different massages in Chinese medicine," says Dr. Ni. "We have one massage called *Tui Na*, which is a combination of acupressure, massage, and manipulation.

"The purpose of massage is not dissimilar to acupuncture, in that the whole goal is to promote the flow of *qi* and to remove blockages, thereby alleviating any imbalances." Dr. Ni adds that massage is most often used in conjunction with other treatment therapies, such as acupuncture. "They are often used together for musculoskeletal problems such as a sprain."

Qigong and other therapeutic exercises are another aspect of TCM, particularly as a means of stress reduction and preventative therapy. Meditative relaxation, calisthenics, internal energy exercises, and the laying on of hands are all incorporated into the overall Chinese medicine approach, along with an emphasis on spiritual meditation.

With early diagnosis and TCM treatment, not only can hypertension be alleviated, but complications including damage to the heart, brain, kidneys, and liver can be prevented.

Conditions Treated by
Traditional Chinese Medicine

Traditional Chinese medicine addresses the full range of human illness. While best known for treating chronic illnesses such as high blood pressure, asthma, allergies, headaches, gallbladder disease, lupus, diabetes, and gynecological disorders, TCM also treats acute, infectious illness. Extensive research is continuously being pursued in a wide range of TCM applications and reported on in scores of medical journals published around the world.[3] Research has shown that TCM can effectively complement modern Western medicine when the two systems are used in concert for acute, chronic, or life-threatening diseases.[4]

According to TCM, high blood pressure is usually due to a problem in the circulation of energy (*qi*) in the body. Diet and long-term emotional distress such as chronic nervousness, anger, and depression can lead to this condition. "Treatment is aimed at bringing the energy flow of the body back into balance through a combination of acupuncture and herbs," says Harvey Kaltsas, Ac. Phys. (FL), D.Ac. (RI), Dipl. Ac. (NCCA), of Sarasota, Florida, former president of the American Association of Acupuncture and Oriental Medicine.

"Secondary hypertension often occurs when the energy reserves become exhausted (called 'kidney yin deficiency' in traditional Chinese medicine), and can also be treated with a combination of acupuncture and herbs to build up and restore one's energy."

With early diagnosis and treatment, not only can hypertension be alleviated, but complications including damage to the heart, brain, kidneys, and liver can be prevented. In addition to acupuncture and herbs, other important elements of treatment include exercises such as qigong, meditation, and a diet high in vegetables and low in fat, sugar, and alcohol.

Mark T. Holmes, O.M.D., L.Ac., director of the Center for Regeneration in Beverly Hills, California, relates two cases in which TCM successfully controlled hypertension. The first case involved a 46-year-old white male attorney with essential hypertension, whose

High Blood Pressure Reversed with Chinese Herbs

Dr. Wu, a famous Chinese physician, was visited by a 42-year-old man who had been diagnosed with hypertension and the early stages of coronary heart disease. He complained of throbbing temples and soreness at the top of his head. An examination identified the following elements: red (not pink) tongue, dark yellow urine, constipation, poor appetite, painful teeth and eyes, insomnia, pain on the right side of the body, and excessive dreaming. His pulse was "wiry and sinking." The man was diagnosed with "constrained liver *qi* accompanied by liver fire ascending to disturb the head."

The treatment called for harmonizing the liver, cooling the liver fire, and transforming mucus. Twelve herbs were given as a tea for three days and another combination for nine additional days. With this treatment, the patient's blood pressure dropped from 180/130 to 130/90, well within normal range, and soon all his symptoms disappeared. A final herbal prescription was then given. The patient then took this for a longer period of time to ensure that his blood pressure remained normal.

blood pressure was 160/90. Additional symptoms included impotence, insomnia, red eyes, nervousness, and a decreased desire to exercise.

An inability to relax after work, combined with a nightly habit of drinking two bottles of wine were determined to be causative factors. Laboratory tests revealed elevated liver enzymes. In TCM this is referred to as a "flaring up of liver fire." After seven months of daily herbal intake combined with regular acupuncture treatments, the patient's hypertension was reversed, his incidence of impotency was significantly reduced, and all the other symptoms abated.

Dr. Holmes also successfully treated an 80-year-old woman suffering from secondary hypertension. Her blood pressure was unusually high, around 210/90. With conventional drugs, it dropped moderately to 180/90. Using Chinese herbs combined with bimonthly acupuncture and homeopathic remedies, Dr. Holmes was able to stabilize her blood pressure at 130-140/85. A subsequent Western clinical examination revealed a 20% increase of carotid artery circulation.

Traditional Chinese medicine also introduces a major component of the body, *qi* (also referred to as chi), that Western medicine does not even acknowledge. *Qi*, according to Dr. Ni, is difficult to define. "We call it life force. It is all-inclusive of the many types of energy within the body and is essential for life itself," he says. This vital life energy flows through the body following pathways called meridians.

CHAPTER 12

Lower Your Blood Pressure With Herbs

MANY BOTANICALS and herbs have hypotensive (blood pressure–lowering) properties. These include garlic, ginseng, hawthorn, valerian, maitake and other medicinal mushrooms, and noni, discussed in this chapter. In many cases, the correct use of simple herbs can make a clinically important difference in the status of your blood pressure and make the use of harsh conventional drugs entirely unnecessary.

Garlic (*Allium sativum*)

Garlic is probably the most well-recognized medicinal herb. According to David Hoffmann, B.Sc., M.N.I.M.H., of Sebastopol, California, eating a clove of raw garlic daily will help considerably in preventing or reversing the effects of high blood pressure. While garlic has been used for centuries in traditional cultures throughout the world as a multipurpose medicinal food, in recent decades more than 2,000 clinical studies have validated many of the folk-healing claims for "the stinking rose," as garlic was once called.

Prominent among these substantiated claims is garlic's ability to lower blood pressure, inhibit cholesterol production, promote blood circulation, and discourage clot formation. Yu-Yan Yeh, Ph.D., of the Department of Nutrition at Pennsylvania State University, reviewed extensive multi-laboratory studies on garlic's ability to reduce cardiovascular disease and concluded, "Collectively, the results suggest that garlic may lower the risk for this disease by reducing plasma lipids, lowering blood pressure, and depressing platelet adhesion and aggregation [clotting]."

A scientific panel of the European community has endorsed garlic for its cardiovascular benefits.[1] In Germany, garlic extracts are approved over-the-counter drugs to supplement dietary measures in patients with elevated blood lipid (fat) levels and to avert age-associated vascular changes."[2]

In a Chinese study, 70 patients with clinically diagnosed high blood pressure took garlic oil for several weeks. At the end of the study, 35 registered a "marked" lowering of their blood pressure, while another 14 subjects experienced "moderate" drops. Garlic can not only lower high blood pressure, but apparently elevate low blood pressure as well, leading researchers to propose that its true effect is in *normalizing* blood pressure.

Prominent among the substantiated healing claims of garlic is its ability to lower blood pressure, inhibit cholesterol production, promote blood circulation, and discourage clot formation.

In a study published in *Atherosclerosis*, 20 patients with elevated levels of lipoproteins took garlic for four weeks. At the end of the period, all subjects showed a 10% drop in blood pressure and blood cholesterol levels. Researchers studying a vegetarian community in India found that those who consumed "liberal" amounts of garlic (and onions) had an average of 25% lower cholesterol levels than those who did not.

A study directed by Benjamin H.S. Lau, M.D., Ph.D., of the School of Medicine at Loma Linda University in Loma Linda, California, studied the effect of garlic supplementation on 32 subjects with high cholesterol.[3] During the six-month study, subjects took four capsules daily of liquid garlic extract, after which time cholesterol levels had returned to normal in 65% of the participants. More specifically, levels of HDL cholesterol (believed to protect the heart) rose steadily, while levels of LDL cholesterol (believed to harm the heart) dropped. Garlic appears to produce its cholesterol-lowering effect by slowing down the synthesis of cholesterol by the liver in the first place.

Garlic has also been shown to promote blood circulation, both peripheral (to the hands and feet) and "microcirculation" (into the tiniest capillaries). It can also interrupt the harmful tendency of the

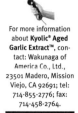

For more information about **Kyolic® Aged Garlic Extract™**, contact: Wakunaga of America Co., Ltd., 23501 Madero, Mission Viejo, CA 92691; tel: 714-855-2776; fax: 714-458-2764.

platelets and fibrin in the blood to form clots, a condition associated with heart attacks and stroke. Researchers reported in the *Journal of the American College of Nutrition* (October 1994) the results of a clinical study involving 45 men, 30-70 years old, with high cholesterol levels. Of this group, 66% received "beneficial effects" in these levels and in platelet activity after taking garlic extract (at 700 mg, nine times daily for six months). The result was "cardiovascular risk reduction."

According to Brenda Lynn Petesch, nutritionist with Wakunaga of America Co., Ltd., manufacturers of Kyolic® Aged Garlic Extract™, garlic can prevent the spread of smooth muscle cells in blood vessels that would otherwise further the progression of heart disease. Petesch also notes that a recent Australian study showed that garlic extract "may afford protection against the onset of atherosclerosis [hardening of the arteries]."

Finally, with respect to existing heart conditions, dietary garlic may reduce the risk of having a second heart attack as well as the general risk of dying from heart disease. Over a study period of three years, based on a group of 432 subjects, regular use of garlic reduced the rate of repeat heart attack by 30% in the second year and by 60% in the third year . Researchers proposed that garlic's benefit is cumulative, building with continuous use.[4]

Studies indicate general benefits from almost any type of garlic, be it raw garlic, dried garlic, garlic oil, or a prepared commercial product, such as the odorless or odor-controlled garlic preparations which enable the user to avoid the bad breath associated with garlic consumption.[5] However, garlic liquid extract that has been aged for at least one year appears to produce better results than fresh raw garlic. A Bulgarian study on cats showed that fresh garlic juice produced only a "slight and temporary" decrease, while aged garlic extract produced more significant and sustained drops in blood pressure.

Ginseng (*Panax ginseng*, Oriental ginseng; *Panax quinquefolius*, American ginseng)

Ginseng has an ancient history and has accumulated much folklore about its actions and uses. The genus name *Panax* is derived from the Latin word panacea, meaning "cure-all." Many of the claims that surround ginseng are exaggerated but it is clearly an important remedy, receiving attention from researchers around the world.[6] It is a powerful adaptogen (supporter of the adrenal glands),[7] aiding the body to cope with stress.[8] In addition, ginseng may lower blood cholesterol.[9] If

After eight weeks on hawthorn, the blood pressure of 40 heart patients dropped from an average of 171/115 to 164/110 and their ability to tolerate the heart stress of physical work increased.

ginseng is abused, however, side effects can occur, including headaches, skin problems, and other reactions. For this reason, the proper dosage for the individual should be determined and respected.

Hawthorn (*Crataegus oxyacantha*)

Hawthorn has been used in folk medicine in Europe and China for centuries. Europeans have employed both the edible fruit as well as the leaves and flowers, primarily for their beneficial effects on the cardiovascular system. Hawthorn is one of the primary heart tonics in traditional medicine. Fruit and leaf extracts are known for their cardiotonic, sedative, and hypotensive (blood pressure–lowering) activities.

Hawthorn has been extensively tested on animals and humans and is known to cause: a decrease in blood pressure with exertion; increase in heart muscle contractility (the ability to contract or shorten); increase in blood flow to the heart muscle; decrease in heart rate; and decrease in oxygen use by the myocardium (the middle layer of the walls of the heart).[10] In Germany, hawthorn extracts are used clinically for a number of heart-related conditions, often in conjunction with digoxin, the primary conventional pharmaceutical drug. Hawthorn extracts are approved by the German Ministry of Health for declining heart performance, sensations of pressure or restrictions in the heart area, senile heart in cases where digitalis is not yet required, and mild forms of bradyarrhythmia (slow heartbeat).[11]

"An infusion of hawthorn berries drunk twice daily is a gentle and effective way of helping the body to normalize blood pressure," says David Hoffmann. "The infusion can be strengthened by combining linden flowers or by adding chamomile or valerian, if tension or headaches are present."

In a study conducted by A. Schmidt, M.D., of Cologne, Germany, 40 patients (average age, 60) with high blood pressure and "stable coronary insufficiency" took doses of hawthorn extract at the rate of 200 mg, three times daily, for eight weeks. Before taking the hawthorn, they tired easily and had diminished physical ability, but after eight weeks on hawthorn, these symptoms occurred 42% fewer times. Blood pressure dropped from 171/115 to 164/110 and the patients' ability to tolerate the heart stress of physical work increased.

QUICK DEFINITION

Adaptogens are substances that provide a nonspecific effect on the entire body by increasing resistance to stress and toxins (physical, chemical, or biological) and promoting a balancing or normalizing condition. The key function of adaptogens is support for the adrenal glands, which are located near the kidneys and are activated in response to stress. Chronic stress can overwhelm the adrenals, leading to symptoms including fatigue, reduced immune function, and poor blood sugar metabolism. Adaptogens help reinvigorate and support the adrenals, enabling the body to deal more effectively with stress. In addition to adrenal support, adaptogens enhance central nervous system activity, provide protection for the liver, act as antioxidants, and increase stamina. Herbs that are considered adaptogenic include Asian and Siberian ginseng, *Ashwagandha*, *Astragalus*, *Codonopsis* ("*Dangshen*"), and *Schizandra*.

In a related study by German physicians K. Bödigheimer, M.D., and D. Chase, M.D., 36 patients (average age, 61) who had angina, a history of heart attacks and arrhythmia, and who were 20% overweight, took 300 mg daily of hawthorn extract for 28 days. As a result, their cardiovascular health and performance improved, both during the stress of exercise and the rest period.[12]

Siberian Ginseng or Eleuthero (*Eleutherococcus senticosus*)

Siberian ginseng is one of the best adaptogen herbs, increasing the body's ability to resist and endure stress. This herb has a very low toxicity. A wealth of clinical and laboratory research has been conducted on Siberian ginseng in the former Soviet Union. Initial findings from controlled experiments indicate a dramatic reduction of total disease occurrence, especially in diseases related to environmental stress.[13] There is a long list of illnesses that improve with the use of this herb, including chronic gastritis, diabetes, and atherosclerosis (hardening of the arteries).

Valerian (*Valeriana officinalis*)

The odorous root of valerian has been used in European traditional medicine as a stimulant for centuries. In Germany, valerian root and its teas and extracts are approved as over-the-counter medicines for "states of excitation" and "difficulty in falling asleep owing to nervousness."[14] A scientific team representing the European community has reviewed the scientific research on valerian and concluded that it is a safe nighttime sleep aid.

These scientists also found that there are no major adverse reactions associated with the use of valerian and, unlike barbiturates and other conventional drugs used for insomnia, valerian does not have a synergy with alcohol,[15] meaning it is safe to have a drink while taking valerian. Herbalist Christopher Hobbs, L.Ac., founder of the American School of Herbalism, notes that other uses for valerian include application for nervous heart conditions. He recommends a valerian-hops preparation as a daytime sedative, as it will not interfere with or slow one's reflexive responses.[16]

A 73-year-old man saw his blood pressure drop from 170 to ⌐⌐ after taking four grams of maitake daily for only three weeks. A heavy drinker, 48, dropped his blood pressure from 180 to 130 in only two weeks at the rate of three grams daily of maitake.

Other Useful Botanicals

Maitake Mushroom

Prized for centuries by Japanese herbalists for its ability to strengthen health, Maitake mushroom (which means "dancing mushroom") is now being investigated in Japan and America for its healing abilities in a number of diseases, including hypertension.

Maitake is available in tablet form as Grifron® from: Maitake Products, P.O. Box 1354, Paramus, NJ 07653; tel: 800-747-7418.

In over 30 cases, maitake mushrooms gradually decreased high blood pressure to normal levels.[17] A woman, 61, had taken hypotensive drugs for 20 years but could never get her systolic blood pressure lower than 150; it was usually 190. After taking maitake at five grams daily for 30 days, it went down to 130. A 73-year-old man saw his blood pressure drop from 170 to 128 after taking four grams daily for only three weeks. A diabetic man, 45, reduced his blood glucose from 139 to 80 and his blood pressure from 165 to 132 after only three weeks, taking four grams daily. A heavy drinker, 48, dropped his blood pressure from 180 to 130 in only two weeks of taking three grams daily of maitake.

Reishi Mushroom

Chinese herbal medicine physicians regard the reishi mushroom as an "elixir of immortality." Research confirms that reishi is an effective cardiotonic. In a study of 54 people (average age, 58.6) whose blood pressure was over 140/90 and who were unresponsive to hypertension medication, those taking reishi mushroom extract in tablet form three times a day for four weeks experienced a significant drop in their blood pressure compared to the control group.[18] The blood pressure of all the test subjects fell below 140/90.

Tahitian Noni

Among the lay healers of Tahiti, the reputation of the noni fruit (*Morinda citrifolia*) as a medicinal food ranks high. The plant itself is found throughout French Polynesia and can grow as high as 20 feet,

For more information about **Morinda Tahitian Noni**, contact: Pascal Sureau, 5020 Lee Street, Torrance, CA 90503; tel/fax: 310-792-7275.

bearing noni fruits the size of potatoes. In Malaysia, it is known as *Mengkudu* and is used for urinary problems, coughs, and painful menstruation, while in the Caribbean, people know it as the Pain Killer Tree. People throughout the region have long used the noni fruit as a dietary staple.

Anecdotal reports suggest that juice from this fruit can be significantly helpful in numerous health conditions, such as hypertension, wounds and infections, ulcers, skin rashes, digestive disorders, colds, influenza, arthritis, and cancer. Mitchell Tate, director of the Center for Lifestyle Disease in St. George, Utah, reports that while researching noni at the University of Honolulu in Hawaii (noni also grows in Hawaii), he found that "a significant amount of research had been done on the plant and that most of it substantiated claims by the Tahitians." One study confirmed the belief that noni helps lower blood pressure.

Research by R.M. Heinicke, Ph.D., at the University of Hawaii, suggests that the active ingredient in noni is xeronine, a digestive enzyme similar to bromelain in pineapple. Dr. Heinicke emphasizes that noni must be consumed on an empty stomach, preferably upon rising in the morning, for the enzyme to become activated by the intestines. Dr. Heinicke believes that, once activated, xeronine helps to repair damaged cells by regulating the rigidity and shape of particular proteins comprising those cells. "Since these proteins have different functions within the cells, this explains how the administration of noni juice causes a wide range of physiological responses," states Dr. Heinicke.

According to Morinda, the product's manufacturer, about 25% of the users of noni experience a noticeable difference after using the drink for three weeks, while 50% notice benefits after three to eight weeks of daily use. Mitchell Tate suggests a daily dosage of two tablespoons for general health maintenance, but three to four tablespoons daily for an existing health condition.

In a study published in *Atherosclerosis*, 20 patients with elevated levels of lipoproteins took garlic for four weeks. At the end of the period, all subjects showed a 10% drop in blood pressure and blood cholesterol levels. Researchers studying a vegetarian community in India found that those who consumed "liberal" amounts of garlic (and onions) had an average of 25% lower cholesterol levels than those who did not.

Alternative Medicine Options

FOR LOWERING HIGH BLOOD PRESSURE

I N   A D D I T I O N to the therapies for high blood pressure covered in the preceding chapters and those for general heart health and heart disease discussed in Part One, the following alternative treatment methods can be effective for preventing and reversing high blood pressure.

Aromatherapy

Victor Marcial-Vega, M.D., of Miami, Florida, relates a case of successfully lowering blood pressure using aromatherapy. Martin had dangerously high blood pressure, topping 182/130. After taking his blood pressure and recording this level, Dr. Marcial-Vega asked Martin to gently inhale the aroma of ylang-ylang essential oil after rubbing it on his palms. After breathing its vapor for only five minutes, Martin's blood pressure dropped to 135/80. Dr. Marcial-Vega recommends applying the oil onto the palms, rather than on a cloth, because whatever is not inhaled as aroma is absorbed directly through the skin.

As often as five times a day, Dr. Marcial-Vega himself daubs a few drops of an essential oil on his palms, rubs it in, cups his palms around his nose, and gently inhales.

Before and after patients occupy his office, he mists the air with a blend of various aromas such as lavender, tea tree, eucalyptus, or myrrh (dispersed in water), all of which have strong actions against ambient bacteria, viruses, or fungi. Equal parts of ylang-ylang, orange, or patchouli oils also impart a cleansing atmosphere. When patients arrive and inhale the aromas, they are likely to relax, facilitating their recovery.

Dr. Marcial-Vega also recommends a foot bath or full-body soak as an antidote to stress. Take a large Pyrex glass tray, fill it with warm water, dribble in a few drops of lavender oil, and immerse your feet for 20 minutes. Similarly, you can fill a bath and disperse five drops of a single oil or a blend into the water, and soak yourself until you feel relaxed.

Aromatherapy is More than Aroma

Aromatherapy is a unique branch of herbal medicine that utilizes the medicinal properties found in the essential oils of various plants. Through a process of steam distillation or cold-pressing, the volatile constituents of the plant's oil (its essence) are extracted from its flowers, leaves, branches, or roots. According to Dr. (rer. nat.) Kurt Schnaubelt, director of the Pacific Institute of Aromatherapy, the term "aromatherapy" is somewhat misleading, as it can suggest an exclusive role for the aroma in the healing process. "In actuality," says Dr. Schnaubelt, "the oils exert much of their therapeutic effect through their pharmacological properties and their small molecular size, making them one of the few therapeutic agents to easily penetrate bodily tissues."

Aromatherapy has been used to lower blood pressure and is highly effective for bacterial infections of the respiratory system,[1] immune deficiencies such as Epstein-Barr virus (a form of herpes virus believed to be the causative agent in infectious mononucleosis), and numerous skin disorders.[2] The immediate and often profound effect that essential oils have on the central nervous system also makes aromatherapy an excellent method for stress management[3] and therefore of additional benefit in the treatment of hypertension.

History of Aromatherapy

Plants and their essential oils have been used therapeutically from ancient times in countries as diverse as Egypt, Italy, India, and China.[4] In most of the world, plant essences remain popular as therapeutic

CAUTION

Dr. Marcial-Vega cautions however that not every version of ylang-ylang oil will produce this remarkable result in five minutes. You need to use oils that are pure and of the highest quality to achieve these effects. People with low blood pressure should not use ylang-ylang oil in this way because it could further lower their blood pressure. Dr. Marcial-Vega reports using this oil with many people with normal to high blood pressure, without side effects.

For more about **aromatherapy applications,** contact: Victor Marcial-Vega, M.D., 4037 Poinciana Avenue, Miami, FL 33133; tel: 305-442-1233; fax: 305-445-4504. For information about the **aromatherapy oils,** contact: Phyto Medicine Company, 6701 Sunset Drive, Suite 100, Miami, FL 33143; tel: 305-662-6396; fax: 305-667-5619.

Research shows that oils such as orange, jasmine, and rose have a tranquilizing effect and work by altering the brain waves into a rhythm that produces calmness and a sense of well-being. In the same way, the so-called stimulating oils—basil, black pepper, rosemary, and cardamom—work by producing a heightened energy response.

agents and are utilized in everything from antiseptic creams and skin ointments to liniments for arthritic pain.

The term aromatherapy was coined in 1937 by the French chemist René-Maurice Gattefossé. While working in his family's perfume laboratory, Dr. Gattefossé burned his hand. He knew lavender was used in medicine for burns and inflammation, and immediately immersed his hand in a container of pure lavender oil he had on his workbench. When the burn quickly lost its redness and began to heal, he was impressed enough by the oil's regenerative ability to begin researching the curative powers of other essential oils. This marked the beginning of the modern-day science of aromatherapy for the treatment of common ailments. In the United States, the popularity of aromatherapy

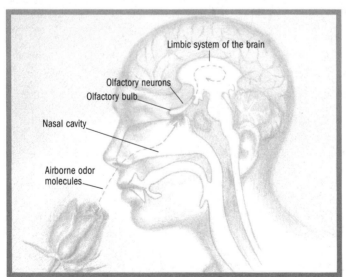

Aromas affect the *limbic system*, which is connected to the part of the brain that controls heart rate, blood pressure, and stress levels.

has grown rapidly over the last ten years, fueled by the increasing demand for nontoxic restorative therapies.

How Aromatherapy Works

According to Dr. Schnaubelt, "The chemical makeup of essential oils gives them a host of desirable pharmacological properties ranging from antibacterial, antiviral, and antispasmodic to use as diuretics (promoting production and excretion of urine), vasodilators (widening blood vessels), and vasoconstrictors (narrowing blood vessels). Essential oils act on the adrenal glands, ovaries, and the thyroid and can energize or pacify, detoxify, and facilitate the digestive process." The oils' therapeutic properties also make them effective for treating infection, interacting with the various branches of the nervous system, modifying immune response, and harmonizing moods and emotions.

Aromatic molecules that interact with the top of the nasal cavity give off signals that are modified by various biological processes before traveling to the limbic system, the emotional switchboard of the brain.[5] There they create impressions associated with previous experiences and emotions. The limbic system is directly connected to those parts of the brain that control heart rate, blood pressure, breathing, memory, stress levels, and hormone balance. As scientists have learned, oil fragrances may be one of the fastest ways to achieve physiological or psychological effects.

> After breathing ylang-ylang oil vapor for only five minutes, Martin's blood pressure dropped from 182/130 to 135/80.

John Steele, Ph.D., of Sherman Oaks, California, and Robert Tisserand, of London, England, leading researchers in the field of aromatherapy, have studied the effects on brain-wave patterns when essential oils are inhaled or smelled. Their findings show that oils such as orange, jasmine, and rose have a tranquilizing effect and work by altering the brain waves into a rhythm that produces calmness and a sense of well-being. In the same way, the so-called stimulating oils—basil, black pepper, rosemary, and cardamom—work by producing a heightened energy response.[6]

Inhaling the fragrance of certain essential oils can help clear sinuses or free congestion in the chest, as well as alter the neurochemistry of the brain to produce changes in mental and emotional behavior. Even aromas too subtle to be consciously detected can have significant effects on central nervous system activity, sometimes to the point of cutting in half the amount of time needed to perform a visual search task.[7]

Conditions Benefited by Aromatherapy

The value of aromatherapy in the treatment of infectious diseases has gained increased attention in recent years. Its use for this purpose is widespread in France, where a system of aromatherapeutic medicine has been developed.[8] French physicians routinely prescribe aromatherapy preparations, and French pharmacies stock essential oils alongside the more conventional drugs. In England, aromatherapy is used mainly for stress-related health issues. Hospital nursing staffs administer essential-oil massage to relieve stress and pain and to induce sleep.[9] English hospitals also use a variety of vaporized essential oils (including lemon, lavender, and lemongrass) to help combat the transmission of airborne infectious diseases.[10] Essential oils are also used topically on wound sites to counter infection.

Essential oils like citronella and *Eucalyptus citriodora* can be diffused in the air or rubbed on the wrists, solar plexus, and temples for quick and effective relaxation. Mandarin is a fragrance favored by children, and its calming qualities can slow hyperactivity. Lavender oil added to the bath or sprayed on the bed sheets reduces tension and enhances relaxation.[11] Roman chamomile (*Anthemis nobilis*) is also recommended to calm an upset mind or body. A drop rubbed on the solar plexus can bring rapid relief of mental or physical stress.

In their pure state, certain oils, such as clove and cinnamon, can cause irritation or skinburn. These oils call for careful and expert application. It is recommended that they be diluted with a less irritating essential oil before being applied to the skin. Essential oils can cause a toxic reaction if ingested. Consult a physician before taking any oils internally.

For more information about **aromaSpa™** aromatic steam capsule, contact: Variel Health International, 9618 Variel Avenue, Chatsworth, CA 91311; tel: 818-407-4717; fax: 818-407-0738. The single-seater "Serene" unit sells for about $1500; the two-seater "Gemini" model sells for about $2300.

Aromatherapy Spa: Detoxify, Relax Muscles, and Enhance Immunity

Physicians have long known of the many therapeutic benefits of steam heat, also known as hyperthermia or heat stress detoxification. Similarly, the benefits of aromatherapy—the inhalation of the vapors of essential plant oils—are widely recognized among alternative practitioners. Now, Variel Health International has combined both modalities in the form of the aromaSpa™ aromatic steam capsule, suitable for home use as a portable health spa.

The unit stands 5'6", weighs about 68 pounds, may be easily disassembled, and plugs into any standard 115-volt socket. Its walls and sliding door are made of transparent polycarbonate, used to make airplane windows. The steam generator and aroma diffuser are located on the floor of the unit. Any of at least 250 aromatherapy oils may be used, singly or in combination, to support muscle relaxation, detoxification, and immune system stimulation, or for eliminating fatigue, lifting mood, revitalizing skin, or general rejuvenation.

Other self-care benefits include general mind and body relaxation, stress reduction, energizing, emotional cleansing, and "customized personal pampering," depending on the aromatherapy formula used, says Variel's Cathy Dammann.

In the self-contained aromatherapy and steam heat diffuser, soothing mists carrying aromatic molecules envelop the entire body surface for maximum absorption and benefit.

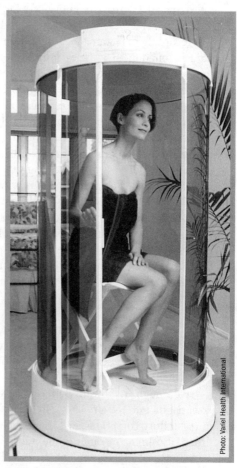

The aromaSpa uses one quart of distilled water (preferable to chlorinated and fluoridated tap water) for a 40-minute steam heat session, and inside temperatures can reach 115°-120° within about 10 minutes. These temperatures are necessary, as hyperthermia provides its benefits by temporarily raising the body temperature to between 101° and 103° and inducing perspiration. Clinical information suggests that steam heat may have therapeutic advantages over the dry heat associated with most saunas, says Dammann.

The aromaSpa was tested in 1994 by Jerry Schindler, Ph.D., director

Photo: Variel Health International

Steam heat therapy using aromatherapy essences may increase blood circulation and heighten immune response by stimulating white blood cell production.

of the Sports Health Science Human Performance Lab at Life College School of Chiropractic in Marietta, Georgia. Dr. Schindler reported that the unit was effective in decreasing the risk of everyday and athletic injuries, primarily by increasing muscle flexibility, blood flow, and oxygen delivery to the muscles.

Dr. Schindler demonstrated these benefits by way of thermographic studies (which register nerve sense pathways) comparing the left and right sides of a test subject's body. Individuals whose thermographic readings are asymmetrical (indicating imbalances and sensory interference) are prone to injury, says Dr. Schindler. Symmetrical patterns were achieved after 30 minutes in the aromaSpa.

According to Dammann, aroma steam therapy can also reduce lactic acid buildup in muscles following exercise, thereby preventing soreness. The approach may be effective in reducing cellulite (lumpy fat areas in the skin), especially when used with rosemary, sandalwood, juniper, geranium, or lemon essential oils. These can produce detoxifying and water-draining effects in only 10 minutes, compared to standard hot body wraps, which require 60 minutes, says Dammann.

Steam heat therapy may increase blood circulation and heighten immune response by stimulating white blood cell production, Dammann says. The aromaSpa is now being used experimentally by patients with chronic fatigue syndrome, she reports. According to Zand Gard, M.D., "the only detoxification program that has proven successful in removing fat-stored toxins from the body is hyperthermia." The use of the essential oils of clove, cinnamon, melissa, and lavender has been clinically shown to benefit bronchial conditions as effectively as antibiotics, especially when delivered by steam heat, Dammann says.

How to Use Aromatherapy

Aromatherapy uses essential oils to affect the body in several ways. The benefits of essential oils can be obtained through inhalation, external application, or ingestion.

■ Through a diffusor: Diffusors disperse microparticles of the essential oil into the air. They can be used to achieve beneficial results in respiratory conditions, or to simply change the air with the mood-lifting or calming qualities of the fragrance.

■ External application: Oils are readily absorbed through the skin. Convenient applications are baths, massages, hot and cold compresses, or a simple topical application of diluted oils.[12] Essential oils in a hot bath can stimulate the skin, induce relaxation, and energize the body. According to Debra Nuzzi St. Claire, M.H., an aromatherapist and herbalist from Boulder, Colorado, using certain essential oils, such as rosemary, in the bath can stimulate the elimination of toxins through the skin. In massage, the oils can be worked into the skin and, depending on the oil and the massage technique, can either calm or stimulate an individual. When used in compresses, essential oils soothe minor aches and pains, reduce swelling, and treat sprains.

■ Floral waters: These can be sprayed into the air or sprayed on skin that is too sensitive to the touch.

■ Internal application: For certain conditions (such as organ dysfunction/disorder), it can be advantageous to take oils internally. It is essential to receive proper medical guidance for internal use of oils. However, such professional guidance is difficult to obtain in the United States.

Purchasing Oils

Aromatherapy is ideally suited for home use. While it is true that irresponsible or ignorant use of essential oils may pose certain risks, these risks are small compared to the potential gain. Typical problems are caused by excessive use of potentially irritating or allergenic oils such as clove, cinnamon, oregano, or savory, but with proper knowledge these pitfalls are easily avoided.

Most health food stores now carry essential oils, and many even carry "starter kits" with selections of the most widely used essential oils. However, selecting essential oils from the many different offerings in the marketplace can be confusing. Vast differences in price exist for what seems to be the same oil. Inquiries are often met with the universal assurance that the oil is absolutely pure and natural. This is not always the case. Many suppliers do not verify the purity of the oils they distribute. When purchasing essential oils, it is important to take note of their purity, quality, and price.

"Pure essential oils are expensive," according to Dr. Schnaubelt. "Often 1,000 pounds of plant are needed to produce one pound of essence. This process involves manpower to cultivate and harvest the plant, and the energy cost for distillation. Because of the variations in these factors, the prices of essential oils can differ. If every oil in a line carries the same price tag, this is a sure sign of large-scale homogenization and adulteration for the production of sheer fragrance oils as opposed to essential oils.

"Essential oils should be called 'essential oils'. If names are used that sound evasive, such as 'pure botanical perfume' or 'pure fragrance essence,' this is an indication that the supplier is aware that the oils are

The greatest successes in controlling hypertension are with patients who combine biofeedback training with other forms of relaxation, visualization, exercise, and a low-salt diet.

not true essential oils," adds Dr. Schnaubelt. Oil essences are most commonly produced to create fragrances and to process food. The quality requirements of these oils are substantially lower than of those used for aromatherapy. Companies that concern themselves solely with aromatherapy will go to great lengths to ensure purity.

While pure, natural essential oils may seem expensive, the smallest amounts will go far, and this makes them cost-effective. In contrast, the effectiveness of lower-grade oils, or oils that are diluted, drastically diminishes over time due to a loss of their essential properties.

The best way to purchase essential oils for aromatherapy applications is from a supplier who specializes in essential aromatherapy oils.

Ayurvedic Medicine

Ayurvedic medicine treats hypertension according to metabolic type. According to Virender Sodhi, M.D. (Ayurveda), N.D., director of the American School of Ayurvedic Sciences in Bellevue, Washington, hypertension is found most often in *pitta* and *kapha* types and is usually due to a combination of genetics and lifestyle. Patients of Dr. Sodhi are put on a diet low in sodium, cholesterol, and triglycerides (the latter cause the blood to become viscous and therefore raise blood pressure).

Yogic breathing exercises help to relax the body and stimulate the cardiovascular system, effectively reducing hypertension, says Dr. Sodhi. "Breathing first with one nostril, then the other for ten to 15 minutes, two to three times a day is highly effective in lowering blood pressure. I have patients try this in the office, and after ten minutes, their blood pressure drops considerably," he adds.

Herbs also play an important role in treating hypertension. Herbs are usually used in combinations, depending on the patient's individual needs, and are often combined with rose water and minerals such as calcium, magnesium, silicon, and zinc.

According to Dr. Sodhi, the following herbs are indicated for hypertension: *Convolvulus pluricaulis* has a calming effect, reduces anxiety and anger, and lowers serum cholesterol while increasing high-density lipoproteins (this

For information about **Ayurvedic health products,** contact: Maharish Ayurvedic Products International, P.O. Box 49667, Colorado Springs, CO 80949-9667; tel: 719-260-5500 or 800-255-8332; fax: 719-260-7400.

helps to improve circulation and lower blood pressure). *Ashwaganda* also has a calming effect and helps to reduce stress and thus blood pressure. Coral in rose water is an excellent tonic for the heart, as it contains calcium and magnesium, which are usually deficient in hypertensives.

Biofeedback

The idea that a person can learn to modify his or her own vital functions is relatively new. Before the 1960s, most scientists believed that autonomic functions, such as heart rate and pulse, digestion, blood pressure, brain waves, and muscle behavior, could not be voluntarily controlled. Recently, biofeedback, along with other methods of self-regulation such as guided imagery, progressive relaxation, and meditation, has found widespread acceptance among physiologists and psychologists alike.

Biofeedback training is a method of learning how to consciously regulate normally unconscious bodily functions (such as heart rate, blood pressure, and breathing) in order to improve overall health. It refers to any process that measures and reports back immediate information about the biological system of the person being monitored so he or she can learn to consciously influence that system.

How Biofeedback Works

Instrumented biofeedback was pioneered by O. Hobart Mowrer in 1938, when he used an alarm system triggered by urine to stop bed-wetting in children. But it was not until the late 1960s, when Barbara Brown, Ph.D., of the Veterans Administration Hospital in Sepulveda, California, and Elmer Green, Ph.D., and Alyce Green of the Menninger Foundation in Topeka, Kansas, used EEG biofeedback to observe and record the altered states/self-regulation of yogis, that biofeedback began to attract widespread attention.

A person seeking to regulate his or her heart rate trains with a biofeedback device set up to transmit one blinking light or one audible beep per heartbeat. By learning to alter the rate of the flashes and beeps, the subject is subtly programmed to control the heart rate. "The self-regulation skills acquired through

QUICK DEFINITION

Ayurveda is the traditional medicine of India, based on many centuries of empirical use. Its name means "end of the Vedas" (which were India's sacred scripts), implying that a holistic medicine may be founded on spiritual principles. Ayurveda describes three metabolic, constitutional, and body types (*doshas*), in association with the basic elements of Nature— *vata, pitta,* and *kapha*—and uses them as the basis for prescribing individualized formulas of herbs, diet, massage, and detoxification techniques.

CAUTION

Rauwolfia and its extract, reserpine, are particularly useful in helping to regulate blood pressure. Care must be taken when prescribing rauwolfia and reserpine, however, because they can depress the central nervous system, and should not be given to patients suffering from depression.

By teaching self-regulation skills, biofeedback can allow patients to take more control of their health and help prevent disorders that can result in costly medical procedures.

biofeedback training are retained by the individual even after the feedback device is dispensed with," explains Patricia Norris, Ph.D., biofeedback specialist in private practice and former clinical director of the Biofeedback and Psychophysiology Clinic at the Center for Applied Psychophysiology at the Menninger Clinic in Topeka, Kansas. "In fact, with practice, biofeedback skills continue to improve. It is like taking tennis lessons. If you stop taking the lessons but continue playing, your game will improve. With biofeedback, it works the same way. The more you practice, the better you get."

The effects of biofeedback can be measured in a variety of ways: monitoring skin temperature (ST) influenced by blood flow beneath the skin; monitoring galvanic skin response (GSR), the electrical conductivity of the skin; observing muscle tension with an electromyogram (EMG); tracking heart rate with an electrocardiogram (EKG); and using an electroencephalogram (EEG) to monitor brain wave activity.

For biofeedback, electrodes are placed on the patient's skin (a simple, painless process). The patient is then instructed to use various techniques such as meditation, relaxation, and visualization to effect the desired response (muscle relaxation, lowered heart rate, or lowered temperature). The biofeedback device reports the patient's progress by a change in the speed of the beeps or flashes.

Normal, healthy, "relaxed" readings include fairly warm skin, low sweat gland activity (this keeps the skin's conductivity low), and a slow, even heart rate. Biofeedback technologies utilize computers to provide a rapid and detailed analysis of activities within the complex human system. Biofeedback practitioners interpret changes in these readings to help the patient learn to stabilize erratic and unhealthy biological functions.

Conditions Benefited by Biofeedback Training

Biofeedback training has a vast range of applications for health and prevention, particularly in cases where psychological factors play a role. Heart dysfunctions, loss of control due to brain or nerve damage, sleep disorders, hyperactivity in children, postural problems, back pain, and cerebral palsy have all shown improvement when patients undergo biofeedback training. Severe structural problems like broken bones and slipped discs are among the only conditions that don't respond to biofeedback.

One of the most common uses for biofeedback training is the treatment of stress and stress-related disorders, including hypertension, insomnia, migraines, asthma, gastrointestinal disorders, and muscular dysfunction. Teaching people self-regulation and relaxation through biofeedback helps lower blood pressure.[13] The greatest successes in controlling hypertension are with patients who combine biofeedback training with other forms of relaxation, visualization, exercise, and a low-salt diet. Through biofeedback, people become aware of their innate ability to regulate themselves and influence their health.

Your Heart Rate Can Tell You How Well a Medicine Works

Biofeedback and the monitoring of your heart rate can be used to obtain important information besides the health of your heart.

Physicians at The Royal Center of Advanced Medicine in Henderson, Nevada, report that a test called Heart Rate Variability (HRV), which has been in testing and development for several decades, is now available as a dependable means of showing how the nervous system responds to high-dilution medicines, typically homeopathic remedies. According to Daniel F. Royal, D.O., of The Royal Center of Advanced Medicine and Medi-Tec Systems, Inc., which distributes HRV technology, HRV testing can be used to monitor the way a patient's autonomic nervous system responds to any medical therapy. As such, it has the capacity to objectively demonstrate and thus *prove* the effectiveness of a given remedy, says Dr. Royal.

"As a diagnostic device, HRV could also supply the alternative medical community with a common testing procedure by which different approaches could be uniformly evaluated and compared," states Dr. Royal. HRV also has a treatment function: frequency information, originally obtained by HRV from the patient's nervous system, is returned (a biofeedback function) to the patient through light and sound waves generated in accordance with the specific rhythm of the heart. Over a 24-minute period, the time between human heartbeats varies somewhat; when measured, this variability in heart rate provides useful information about the state of the autonomic nervous system, which regulates about 87% of the body's functions.

Specifically, HRV is a computerized graph showing the shape of the pulse wave of the left versus the right carotid artery. The approach is called "noncognitive" biofeedback because it works without the conscious participation or awareness (cognition) of the patient; the HRV device talks

For more information about **HRV** equipment and training, contact: F. Fuller Royal, M.D., Medi-Tec Systems, Inc., 3663 Pecos McLeod, Las Vegas, NV 89121; tel: 702-732-1400; fax: 702-732-9661; website: www.nevadaclinic.com. For Daniel Royal, D.O., contact: The Royal Center of Advanced Medicine, 38 Diplomat Ct., Henderson, NV 89014; tel: 702-433-8800; fax: 702-269-6395.

directly with the subject's nervous system. When the heart rate shifts, these changes are routed, by computer, into audiovisual signals (light flashes and intermittent sounds); the patient becomes aware of these through headphones and a TV screen, and this triggers the autonomic nervous system to rebalance itself.

HRV testing can indicate an imbalance even when the patient reports feeling well, because an imbalance in the autonomic nervous system will eventually produce physical symptoms. On the other hand, if a patient reports still feeling sick, but the HRV shows improvement, this indicates that the treatment is still working at the level of the nervous system.

A statistical analysis of 12 years of Israeli clinical experience with HRV, used in 30,000 sessions, indicates that about 66% of the positive improvements from HRV sessions take place suddenly and dramatically, as if through major nervous system shifts, explains Dr. Royal. The Israeli study also suggested that over 50 common health problems (such as autism, hyperactivity, insomnia, chronic digestive complaints, psoriasis, stress, and poor circulation) were traceable to an inefficient nervous and regulatory system.

The advantage of HRV is speed and specificity. It normally takes about 72 hours for the autonomic nervous system to respond to a biofeedback stimulus, explains Dr. Royal; homeopathic remedies produce a much faster response. When this response occurs, it effects changes in several aspects of the nervous system and the heart rate. HRV can measure these subtle but important changes immediately after ingestion of the homeopathic remedy. HRV also improves communication between left and right brain hemispheres.

The minimum course of treatment is one weekly HRV session for 12 weeks. Each session is recorded on videocassettes that the patient watches privately at home twice weekly with a 48-hour gap in between each viewing. In effect, rewatching the video of the lights, sounds, and graph images helps the patient's autonomic nervous system reset itself in accordance with the more healthy pattern, says Dr. Royal.

For example, a woman, 56, had suffered with goiter for 30 years. After one dose of homeopathic *Iodum* 200C, the HRV registered an immediate positive effect; then, 24 hours later, Dr. Royal gave her a follow-up single dose of

QUICK DEFINITION

Standard anatomy describes two components to the nervous system. The **central nervous system** (CNS) comprises the spinal cord, containing millions of nerve fibers, and the brain, while the **peripheral nervous system** (PNS) is the network of nerves, estimated to extend 93,000 miles inside the body. The PNS is the sensory motor branch that pertains to the five senses and is how sensory information from the outside world gets translated into muscle movements.

The **autonomic nervous system** (ANS) involves elements of both the CNS and PNS, is controlled by the brain's hypothalamus gland, and pertains to the automatic regulation of all body processes, such as breathing, digestion, and heart rate. It can be likened to the body's automatic pilot, keeping you alive without your being aware of it or participating in its activities. Neural therapy focuses its injections of anesthetics into body structures whose nerve supply is linked with the autonomic nervous system.

homeopathic *Nux Vomica* 30C. Three months later, she reported she was feeling better; after 6 months, her improvement continues, states Dr. Royal. "HRV testing provides objective information which, in turn, enables the physician to choose the most effective therapeutic regimen for each patient as well as monitor the response to treatment," states Dr. Royal. This can include the patient's response to nutritional supplements, dental amalgam removals, chiropractic adjustments, and acupuncture treatments, for example.

Detoxification

Detoxification is the body's natural process of eliminating internal toxins, and is accomplished by the various systems and organs of the body, including the liver, kidneys, intestines, and skin, with toxins eliminated through urine, feces, and perspiration. Everyone has a specific level of tolerance to toxicity that cannot be exceeded if good health is to be maintained; if the system becomes overwhelmed, various symptoms can occur, including hypertension.

William Lee Cowden, M.D., puts hypertensive patients through a detoxification regimen consisting of daily saunas, homeopathic remedies, and a vegetarian diet supplemented with cayenne (*Capsicum annuum*) and garlic. "Cayenne mixed with vegetable juices or lemon juice is excellent for lowering blood pressure," says Dr. Cowden. He adds that after a few days of treatment, alternating cayenne/vegetable juice with cayenne/lemon juice, patients are often able to come off medication, because this regime helps to cleanse the body of toxins that may be causing the high blood pressure.

Dr. Cowden notes that individuals with hypertension often suffer from a liver insufficiency, in which the liver does not properly clear steroid hormones (sex hormones and hormones of the adrenal glands as well as other toxic substances) from the blood. Saunas and a vegetarian diet can help to restore liver function and lower blood pressure. (Patients with more severe hypertension should be medically supervised in their use of saunas.)

A toxic lymphatic system can also contribute to hypertension. Dr. Cowden suggests deep breathing exercises and dry brushing of the skin for three weeks, ten minutes daily. For this, brush the entire body using a dry brush with soft, natural vegetable fiber bristles. Move the brush toward the middle of the collarbone on each side of the body, as important lymph drainage sites are located here. Brush gently at first (some body parts are more sensitive than others) and build up

Research has shown that potassium supplementation can help reduce a patient's reliance on blood pressure medication or diuretic drugs.

to vigorous brushing. Dry brushing helps the skin detoxify, stimlates lymph drainage, and, by applying friction to acupuncture points on the skin, invigorates the entire nervous system.

Another way to stimulate the flow of lymph and to clear the lymph system of toxins is to use a small trampoline or rebounder for 20 minutes a day, says Dr. Cowden. One of rebounding's special benefits is its ability to improve flow in the lymphatic system. This is the body's primary system for collecting and eliminating wastes and toxins. "The lymphatic system is the metabolic garbage can of the body," says Morton Walker, D.P.M., in *Jumping for Health* (1989). "It rids the body of toxins, fatigue substances, dead cells, cancer cells, nitrogenous wastes, trapped protein, fatty globules, pathogenic bacteria, infectious viruses, foreign substances, heavy metals, and other assorted junk the cells cast off."

Stagnant or inadequate lymph flow is associated with the onset of many symptoms and illnesses, including bursitis in the shoulders, bunions, joint stiffness or soft tissue spasms, dry flaking skin, bad breath, body odors, lethargy, depression, and cancer. The lymph system lacks a pump such as the heart to move the fluid around. Instead, the lymphatic system must rely on physical movement and gravity to keep waste products from building up in the lymph glands and tissues. Aerobic exercise, and rebounding in particular, helps to keep the lymph flowing.

So, it is vital that the lymph fluids continue to flow in order to eliminate waste from the body. Lymph flow is dependent on muscle con-

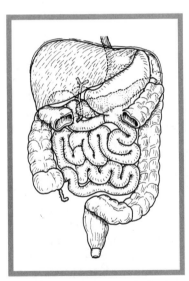

The intestines, when stretched out, are over 25 feet long. In fact, if the inner surface of the small intestines was smooth and flat rather than convoluted, they would stretch for 2¼ miles or completely cover an area the size of a tennis court. Once the bowel is toxic, it creates toxicity for the entire body and an inability to absorb the nutrients necessary for healing.

tractions and body movements, massage and other compression of the tissues, and gravity. Rebounding specifically stimulates the flow of lymph fluid. The change in gravitational forces experienced during rebounding allows for greater blood flow, which in turn increases the amount and movement of interstitial fluids, flushing the cells of waste products.

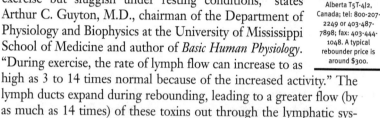

For information on **rebounders** and books and videos about rebounding exercise, check at your local fitness and sporting goods store, or contact: Best of Health (Needak® brand), Unit #1758 W.E. Mall 8770-170st, Edmonton, Alberta T5T-4J2, Canada; tel: 800-207-2249 or 403-487-7898; fax: 403-444-1048. A typical rebounder price is around $300.

"The lymphatic [flow] becomes very active during exercise but sluggish under resting conditions," states Arthur C. Guyton, M.D., chairman of the Department of Physiology and Biophysics at the University of Mississippi School of Medicine and author of *Basic Human Physiology*. "During exercise, the rate of lymph flow can increase to as high as 3 to 14 times normal because of the increased activity." The lymph ducts expand during rebounding, leading to a greater flow (by as much as 14 times) of these toxins out through the lymphatic system. Or, as Dr. Walker says, rebounding stimulates "an optimum drainage of the lymphatic circulation."

Dr. Cowden reports a case of a woman who was severely hypertensive, with blood pressure of 240/140. She had tried every prescription hypertensive drug and had adverse reactions to all of the medications. When she came to his office, Dr. Cowden found that, due to years of poor dietary habits and an unhealthy lifestyle, her system was highly toxic. He put her on a detoxification program that included a vegetarian diet, fasts of vegetable juice and lemon juice with garlic and cayenne, supplements of oral magnesium, saunas, simple stress-reduc-

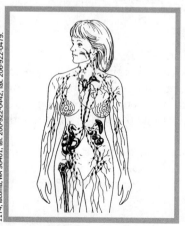

Reprinted with permission from Life Sciences Press. Appears in *The Health and Medical Use of Aloe Vera*. Cost: $29.95 + 2.50 S&H. To order: P.O. Box. 1174, Tacoma, WA 98401; tel: 206-922-0442; fax: 206-922-0479.

The lymphatic system consists of numerous lymph nodes. These are clusters of immune tissue that work as filters or "inspection stations" for detecting foreign and potentially harmful substances from the lymph. Acting like spongy filter bags, they are part of the lymphatic system, which is the body's master "drain." Cells inside the nodes examine the lymph fluid, as collected from body tissues, for foreign matter. While the body has many dozens of lymph nodes, they are mostly clustered in the neck, armpits, chest, groin, and abdomen. Lymph fluid (1-2 quarts) accounts for about 1% of body weight.

A study of 21 patients with hypertension found that daily supplementation with a combination of antioxidants and zinc lowered blood pressure from 165/89 to 160/85.5 in eight weeks.

tion techniques, and cranial electrotherapy stimulation. Within two weeks her blood pressure went down to a safe 140/80. She went off her hypertension medications, and her blood pressure continued to remain in that safe range during her follow-up visits over the next six months.

Nutritional Supplements

In addition to the supplements listed for general heart health (see Chapter 5), nonchloride potassium salts, calcium, and magnesium can help reduce hypertension. Other beneficial supplements include the antioxidant vitamins A, C, and E, niacin (vitamin B3), bioflavonoids (particularly rutin), and the amino acid taurine.[14]

Antioxidants and Zinc

Research has found that antioxidants are linked to an increase in nitric oxide activity.[15] Nitric oxide helps to open blood vessels, which in turn helps to lower blood pressure. Zinc activates SOD (superoxide dismutase, an antioxidant enzyme). A study of 21 patients with hypertension found that daily supplementation with a combination of antioxidants and zinc (500 mg of vitamin C, 50,000 IU of beta carotene, 600 IU of vitamin E, and 80 mg of zinc) lowered blood pressure from 165/89 to 160/85.5 in eight weeks.[16]

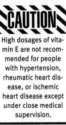

High dosages of vitamin E are not recommended for people with hypertension, rheumatic heart disease, or ischemic heart disease except under close medical supervision.

Calcium

A daily dosage of 1,000 mg of calcium has been shown to lower blood pressure in hypertensives.[17] Calcium can lower high blood pressure for both the contracting (systolic) and expanding (diastolic) phases of the heartbeat. When eight patients with high blood pressure took 1.4 g of calcium every day for 18 weeks, their blood pressure was significantly decreased.[18]

Many hypertensives have a lower daily calcium intake than people with normal blood pressure, so calcium-rich foods, including nuts and leafy green vegetables such as watercress and kale, are advisable as part of the diet.[19]

Magnesium

In one study, magnesium supplementation lowered blood pressure in 19 of 20 hypertensives, compared to none out of four in the control group.[20] Dietary magnesium is found in nuts (almonds, cashews, pecans), rice, bananas, potatoes, wheat germ, kidney and lima beans, soy products, and molasses.

Sodium and Potassium

As mentioned in Chapter 5, research has shown that potassium supplementation can help reduce a patient's reliance on blood pressure medication or diuretic drugs.[21] In order to reduce blood pressure, sodium intake must be restricted at the same time potassium intake is increased.[22] Individuals with high blood pressure should be aware of "hidden" salt in processed foods. Although their salt intake is comparable, vegetarians generally have less hypertension and cardiovascular disease than non-vegetarians do because their diets contain more potassium, complex carbohydrates, polyunsaturated fat, fiber, calcium, magnesium, and vitamins A and C.[23]

According to Dr. Cowden, regular consumption of potassium-rich fruits (such as avocados, bananas, cantaloupe, honeydew melon, grapefruit, nectarines, and oranges) and vegetables (such as asparagus, broccoli, cabbage, cauliflower, green peas, potatoes, and squash) can lower high blood pressure. Steaming rather than boiling vegetables helps prevent vital nutrient loss.

Additional Alternative Therapies

Self-Care

The following therapies for the treatment and prevention of hypertension can be undertaken at home under appropriate professional supervision:

- Fasting
- Yoga
- Hydrotherapy: Constitutional hydrotherapy—apply two to five times weekly.
- Juice Therapy: Celery, beet, and carrot or cucumber, spinach, and parsley. Add a little raw garlic to vegetable juices. Or, run a clove of garlic through a juicer, followed by enough carrots to make eight ounces of juice. Drink once per day.

Professional Care

The following therapies can only be provided by a qualified health professional:

- Acupuncture
- Chelation Therapy
- Environmental Medicine
- Hypnotherapy
- Orthomolecular Medicine
- Osteopathy
- Bodywork: acupressure, reflexology, *shiatsu*, massage, Rolfing, Feldenkrais, Alexander technique, therapeutic touch
- Magnetic Field Therapy: Recent studies from Russia show that magnetic treatments reduce blood pressure in certain patients with hypertension.[24]
- Cranial Electrical Stimulation: William Lee Cowden, M.D., uses cranial electrical stimulation to treat hypertensive patients, reporting that it can lower blood pressure and alleviate panic attacks within 30 to 40 minutes of treatment.

William Lee Cowden, M.D., puts hypertensive patients through a detoxification regimen consisting of daily saunas, homeopathic remedies, and a vegetarian diet supplemented with cayenne (*Capsicum annuum*) and garlic.

He says that after a few days of treatment, alternating cayenne/vegetable juice with cayenne/lemon juice, patients are often able to come off medication, because this regime helps to cleanse the body of toxins that may be causing the high blood pressure.

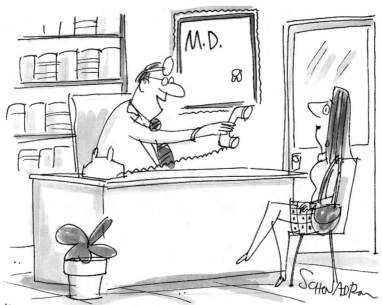

"I NOW OFFER NUTRITIONAL COUNSELING. HERE'S A RECORDING OF MY MOM'S RECIPE FOR CHICKEN SOUP."

PART THREE

Stroke

What Causes Stroke?

STROKE (or cerebrovascular accident) is the sudden disturbance of blood flow to the brain as a result of a clogged or burst artery. It is the third leading cause of death in the U.S. and the leading cause of adult disability, with an estimated annual medical cost of $30 billion. Approximately 500,000 Americans suffer a stroke each year. That's 200 out of every 100,000 people and the percentage is higher among men and the elderly. However, women who suffer a stroke die from it more often than men do.[1]

About 30% of strokes are fatal. In 1994, 154,350 people in the U.S. died from this "brain attack."[2] Among women 45-64 years old, stroke is the number two killer, causing more deaths in that age group than breast cancer.[3]

In the U.S., there are about 1.7 million stroke survivors at any given moment, and 75% of them are 55-84 years old.

In the U.S., there are about 1.7 million stroke survivors at any given moment, and 75% of them are 55-84 years old. Only about 10% of stroke survivors are fit enough to return to work without a disability; 40% have a mild disability, 40% are severely disabled, and 10% must be hospitalized.

By interrupting the flow of blood to a region of the brain, a stroke starves the brain cells of oxygen, thereby producing tissue death. Stroke symptoms may develop within a few minutes to over several days and can include loss of speech, physical movement, or eyesight, depending on the area of the brain affected. Headaches, dizziness, confusion, and difficulty swallowing are also associated symptoms.

Many people who become paralyzed by a stroke learn to walk again. However, lost intellectual functioning tends not to be recovered as fully. When the symptoms from a stroke last for 24 hours or less, followed by full recovery of lost functions, the episode is called a transient ischemic attack (TIA). TIAs are warning signals and the person who suffers such an attack would be well advised to begin taking some of the steps toward heart health detailed in this book.

What Causes a Stroke?

Arteriosclerosis (thickening and hardening of the lining of the arteries) is a major risk factor associated with stroke. Atherosclerosis (the most common form of arteriosclerosis; due to deposits of plaque composed of fatty substances on arterial walls) of the cerebral arteries can decrease blood flow to the brain and increase the likelihood of stroke.

Stroke caused by diminished blood supply to the brain is called an ischemic stroke and represents about 70% of all cases. In addition to

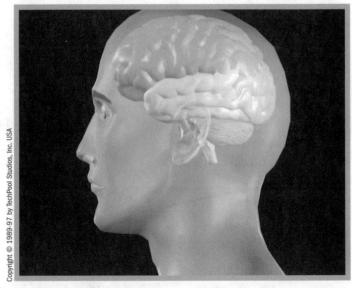

Copyright © 1989-97 by TechPool Studios, Inc. USA

The brain. A stroke, which involves the sudden disturbance of blood flow to brain tissues, can be described as a "heart attack" in the brain. Most commonly, an artery, blocked by a blood clot, interrupts the flow of blood and oxygen to a region of the brain, producing tissue death by starving the brain cells of oxygen.

The Five Warning Signs of Stroke

Many people can recite the seven warning signs of cancer, but do you know how to recognize when you've had or are having a stroke? Being aware of these five warning signs could save your life and reduce the damage inflicted by a stroke. Seek medical assistance immediately upon noticing one or more of these signs:

1. Numbness, weakness, or paralysis of the face, arm, or leg on one side of the body
2. Sudden blurring or loss of vision in one or both eyes
3. Difficulty speaking or comprehending simple statements
4. Unexplainable dizziness, loss of balance, or loss of coordination, especially when experienced with one of the other four signs
5. Sudden severe headache with no apparent cause—described by those who have suffered it as "the worst headache of your life"[4]

artery blockage produced by arteriosclerosis, blood flow to the brain can be impeded by a blood clot which, if the blockage is extensive enough, will result in a stroke. A blood clot that forms in an artery and is attached to the arterial wall is called a thrombus. A thrombus in itself is not life-threatening. In fact, it is lifesaving when it forms as the result of hemorrhage. But when it occurs in a narrow artery and blocks blood flow, a thrombus becomes dangerous. This condition is called thrombosis.

When a blood clot travels in the bloodstream from another part of the body, it is called an embolus. An embolus can also be a foreign object or an air or gas bubble traveling in the bloodstream. An embolus in the head, usually having arrived from the heart or from arteries of the neck, can produce a stroke.

Another cause of stroke is a blood vessel that ruptures (hemorrhage). Blood spills into the brain, not only damaging the brain cells directly, but producing further damage to brain tissue due to lack of oxygen when the blood supply is interrupted. This is known as a hemorrhagic stroke and can result from injury to the head or a burst aneurysm (bulging of a blood vessel due to disease in the arterial wall).

Who is Likely to Have a Stroke?

Once you have suffered one stroke or TIA, you are in the higher risk category. Inherited disorders, birth defects, and certain rare blood diseases are also linked to the occurrence of strokes.[5] Blood platelet stickiness, associated with a raised level of red blood cells (polycythemia) or with low levels of nutrients, such as vitamin B6, that prevent stickiness,

A study of 116,759 women, 30-55 years old, found that overweight women had a higher risk of ischemic stroke; extremely obese women more than doubled their stroke risk as compared to lean women; and those who had gained more than 24 pounds between the ages of 18 and 42 had almost twice the risk.

is another risk factor. In addition, the following increase your risk of having a stroke:
- smoking
- being over the age of 55
- high cholesterol
- a recent heart attack
- lack of exercise
- excessive consumption of alcohol
- diabetes
- history of a damaged heart valve
- obesity
- irregular heartbeat (atrial fibrillation)
- hypertension
- carotid artery disease
- overuse of decongestants[6]

A study of 116,759 women, 30-55 years old, found that overweight women had a higher risk of ischemic stroke; extremely obese women more than doubled their stroke risk as compared to lean women; and those who had gained more than 24 pounds between the ages of 18 and 42 had almost twice the risk.[7]

Various components in the blood have also been linked with an increased risk of stroke. These include lipoproteins, homocysteine, and fibrinogens.

Lipoproteins—Multiple studies have demonstrated the connection between lipoproteins (fat-carrying proteins) and stroke. Lipoproteins occur in two principal forms. Low-density lipoproteins (LDLs) are combination molecules of proteins and fats, particularly cholesterol. LDLs circulate in the blood and act as the primary carriers of cholesterol to the cells of the body. An elevated level of LDLs, the so-called bad cholesterol, is a contributing factor in causing atherosclerosis (plaque deposits on the inner walls of the arteries). A diet high in saturated fats can lead to an increase in the level of LDLs in the blood.

An excess of homocysteine, which increases the risk of stroke, is linked with deficiencies of folic acid and vitamins B12 and B6. Researchers state that elevated homocysteine levels can be reduced fairly easily with supplementation of these nutrients.

Low Iron is Better When It Comes to Stroke

One factor in how well or poorly a person fares after a stroke is the iron level in the blood. A study of 67 patients found that those with a poor outcome had elevated iron levels within the 24 hours following an ischemic stroke, while those with a good outcome did not.[11]

For more about **homocysteine**, see Chapter 1: What Causes Heart Disease?, pp. 33-37.

High-density lipoproteins (HDLs) are also fat-protein molecules in the blood, but contain a larger amount of protein and less fat than LDLs. HDLs are able to absorb cholesterol and related compounds in the blood and transport them to the liver for elimination. HDL, the so-called good cholesterol, may also be able to take cholesterol from plaque deposits on the artery walls, thus helping to reverse the process of atherosclerosis. A higher ratio of HDL to LDL cholesterol in the blood is associated with a reduced risk of cardiovascular disease.

The Copenhagen Heart Study of 693 stroke victims found that levels of triglyceride (a lipid or fat) were positively associated with risk of a nonhemorrhagic stroke; this means the higher your levels, the greater your risk. The study also showed a negative relationship between HDL cholesterol and nonhemorrhagic stroke risk; the more HDLs you have in your blood, the lower your risk.[8]

Another study found lipoprotein (a) levels to be a "critical risk factor" in ischemic stroke[9] and a third group of researchers demonstrated that a high lipoprotein (a) blood level was associated with a more than 20 times greater risk of cerebrovascular disease.[10] Lipoprotein (a) is a form of cholesterol.

Homocysteine—Homocysteine, an amino acid, is a normal by-product of protein metabolism; specifically, of the amino acid methionine, which is found in red meat, milk, and milk products and which does not create a problem when present in small amounts. Methionine is converted in the body to homocysteine, which is normally then converted to the harmless amino acid, cystathionine. But in individuals deficient in the enzyme necessary to convert homocysteine to cystathionine, homocysteine will be abnormally high. "Protein intoxication" starts damaging the cells and tissues of arteries, setting in motion the many processes that lead to loss of elasticity, hardening and calcification, narrowing of the lumen, and formation of blood clots within arteries. Homocysteine can, when allowed to accumulate to toxic levels, degenerate arteries and produce heart disease. The homocysteine theory suggests that heart disease is attributed to abnormal processing of protein in the body because of deficiencies of B vitamins in the diet.

An elevated blood level of homocysteine puts a person at risk for stroke, as it does for cardiovascular disease in general. In 107 cases of stroke in men, 40-59 years old, homocysteine levels were significantly higher than in the control group.[12]

In another study, patients with elevated homocysteine levels had two to three times the risk of recurrent thrombosis (blood clot blockage) in the veins.[13] An excess of homocysteine is also linked to deficiencies of folic acid and vitamins B12 and B6. On the positive side, researchers state that elevated homocysteine levels can be reduced fairly easily with supplementation of these nutrients.[14]

Bypass Surgery Can Cause a Stroke

A study reported in the *New England Journal of Medicine* reveals that the risk of suffering a stroke or other brain damage as a result of coronary artery bypass surgery is as much as ten times higher than previously thought. Of those who had bypass surgery, more than 6% had to have brain surgery afterward to address brain injury caused by the operation. This adds up to 25,000 patients in the U.S. and 50,000 worldwide. These numbers do not include all those patients who did not require further surgery but suffered strokes or other mental impairment, including difficulty remembering or thinking clearly.[15]

Fibrinogens—A high level of fibrinogens (protein in the blood that is converted into fibrin, which is vital for blood clotting) is considered by some researchers to be a far stronger stroke risk factor than cholesterol.[16] They suggest that this is because the higher levels may make the blood more sluggish and trigger plaque formation as well. One study of 140 stroke patients found that those with the higher degrees of artery blockage had higher levels of fibrinogens. The area of stroke damage in the brain was also significantly related to the fibrinogen level; in other words, higher levels of fibrinogens were associated with a larger area of damage.[17] Research has also found that elevated fibrinogen increases the risk in stroke survivors of a second stroke, heart attack, or other cardiovascular event.[18]

Hormones—Hormones are the chemical messengers of the endocrine system that impose order through an intricate communication system among the body's estimated 50 trillion cells. Examples include the "male" sex hormone (testosterone), the "female" sex hormones (estrogen and progesterone), melatonin (pineal), growth hormone (pituitary), and DHEA (adrenal).

The incidence and severity of stroke appear to be linked with hormones. For example, women under 50 who take oral contraceptives increase their risk of stroke. One study found, however, that low-estrogen oral contraceptives do not result in greater risk.[19] On the other hand, testosterone seems to have a protective effect. Men with decreased testosterone levels who had a stroke suffered greater damage and were more likely to die from the stroke than men with higher testosterone levels.[20]

Homocysteine can, when allowed
to accumulate to toxic levels,
degenerate arteries
and produce heart disease. The
homocysteine theory suggests
that heart disease is
attributed to abnormal
processing of protein in the body
because of deficiencies
of B vitamins in the diet.

Self-Care Essentials for Stroke

A S   W I T H   H E A R T   disease and high blood pressure, attention to diet, exercise, and lifestyle is essential in preventing the conditions that lead to stroke and in helping the body to recover if a stroke has occurred. Many of the recommendations in these areas for heart disease (see Chapter 2) and high blood pressure (see Chapter 9) apply to stroke as well, but the following are a few additional considerations.

Diet

A whole foods diet composed of whole grains, raw nuts and seeds, and plenty of fresh fruits and vegetables (all organically raised and pesticide-free) is recommended. Yellow and green fruits and vegetables, including broccoli, sprouts, and kelp, are particularly helpful. An emphasis on garlic, onions, and vitamin B6 is advisable, because all three tend to prevent platelets from sticking together. Fats (unprocessed only) should be limited to 10% to 15% of your total diet. Deep-fried foods, animal fats, and semi-solid fats should be avoided. Foods that are natural plant sources of estrogens, such as soybeans and peanuts, are also best to avoid, along with alcoholic beverages and especially alcoholic binges (four drinks or more in a short period of time).

Numerous studies have shown that eating fish, especially freshwater fish, can enhance blood circulation and reduce the risk of stroke. According to the *Harvard Heart Letter* (October 1994), moderate fish consumption leads to mild, beneficial blood "thinning," which helps prevent strokes. A study of 552 men, from 50 to 69

Increasing fruit and vegetable intake by three servings per day decreased the risk of having a stroke by 25%, and by 50% for hemorrhagic stroke in particular.

years old, found that eating at least one serving of fish a week is associated with less risk of stroke. Consuming too much fish, on the other hand, can be detrimental to health. Men who ate more than 35 g of fish daily had the highest stroke rates and more deaths from stroke than men who ate less fish.[1]

A second study of 4,410 whites and 782 blacks, 45 to 75 years old and with no stroke history, found that eating fish more than once a week cuts stroke risk in half for white and black women and black men. This study found no stroke protection for white men as a result of eating fish, but the kind of fish consumed was not studied and that may have had an effect on the results.[2]

The reason why fish intake reduces stroke risk may be because certain kinds of fish are high in alpha-linolenic acid (ALA), an omega-3 fatty acid. Remember, essential fatty acids contribute to heart health. One study increased the ALA intake of 96 stroke victims compared to 96 controls. Each 0.13% increase in the ALA level in the blood was associated with a 37% reduction in stroke risk. The study concluded that getting more omega-3 fatty acids in your diet from any source (fish, soybeans, walnuts, or leafy green vegetables) can help prevent stroke.

Eating more fruits and vegetables can also contribute to reducing your stroke risk. In one study of 832 middle-aged men, increasing fruit and vegetable intake by three servings per day decreased the risk of having a stroke by 25%, and by 50% for hemorrhagic stroke in particular.[3] This effect may be due to the concentration of flavonoids in fruits and vegetables. Flavonoids are plant pigments that are known to inhibit platelet clustering, a contributing factor in stroke.

According to one study, carrots and spinach may be especially useful in stroke prevention. The 87,000 female nurses who ate five or more servings of carrots per week had a 68% reduced risk of stroke compared to women eating one serving or less per month. The risk among those

QUICK DEFINITION

Omega-3 and **omega-6 oils** are the two principal types of essential fatty acids, which are unsaturated fats required in the diet. The digits "3" and "6" refer to differences in the oil's chemical structure with respect to its chain of carbon atoms and where they are bonded. A balance of these oils in the diet is required for good health. The primary omega-3 oil is called alpha-linolenic acid (ALA) and is found in flaxseed (58%), canola, pumpkin and walnut, and soybeans. Fish oils, such as salmon, cod, and mackerel, contain the other important omega-3 oils, DHA (docosahexaenoic acid) and EPA (eicosapentaenoic acid). Omega-3 oils help reduce the risk of heart disease. Linoleic acid or cis-linoleic acid is the main omega-6 oil and is found in most plant and vegetable oils, including safflower (73%), corn, peanut, and sesame. The most therapeutic form of omega-6 oil is gamma-linolenic acid (GLA), found in evening primrose, black currant, and borage oils. Once in the body, omega-6 is converted to prostaglandins, hormone-like substances that regulate many metabolic functions, particularly inflammatory processes.

Eating at least one serving of fish a week is associated with less risk of stroke.

who ate a daily serving of spinach was 43% lower.[4]

As mentioned in Chapter 2, eating onions and apples and drinking black tea can reduce the risk of cardiovascular disease. This holds true for stroke as well. The common denominator which onions, apples, and black tea share is quercetin, a dietary flavonoid. Quercetin helps prevent oxidation of LDL cholesterol, which in turn helps prevent atherosclerosis. One study of 552 men, 50 to 69 years old, found that higher intake of dietary flavonoids, mainly quercetin, was linked to lower incidence of stroke. For example, those men who drank more than 4.7 cups of black tea daily had 69% less risk of stroke than those who drank under 2.6 cups.[5]

Exercise

Exercise makes a significant contribution to both the prevention and treatment of stroke. Scientists found that in 906 men and women, 57-82 years old, who regularly had moderate to heavy exercise in the form of fast walking or calisthenics, there was a 63% reduction in the risk of stroke. Light exercise resulted in a 57% reduced chance of stroke, compared to inactivity. Nearly any form of physical activity can significantly reduce the risk,[6] but high levels of activity do not provide any more protection than medium levels.[7]

Another study produced similar results. Among 7,700 men, between 40 and 59 years old, with a history of heart disease, moderate exercise reduced the risk of stroke and heart attack by more than 50%. The exercises included bicycling, walking, running, playing golf or tennis, and gardening or doing other household jobs.[8]

Surprisingly, exercise in youth carries over to middle age in reducing stroke risk. A comparison between 125 men and women, 35-74 years old, who had suffered a first stroke, and 198 controls revealed that those who had exercised vigorously from the age of 15 to 25 reduced their risk of stroke by two-thirds over those who had not.[9] The exercises included swimming, bicycling, running, playing tennis or squash, and digging. In addition, the protection against stroke increased with the number of years the person exercised. For example, exercising between 15 and 40 brought the risk down to slightly over one-fifth the risk of those who were less active.

The study also demonstrated, however, that starting exercise later in life can still help in prevention. Those who had recently been exercising vigorously had two-fifths the risk of stroke than their less-active counterparts, and those who had taken at least a mile walk sometime in the previous month had two-thirds less chance of suffering a stroke than those who had not exerted themselves even that much.

The benefits of exercise as treatment for stroke are also evident. Aerobic exercise after suffering a stroke has been found to improve physical function (especially oxygen consumption), reduce cardiovascular risk, control blood pressure, prevent muscle atrophy, and boost self-confidence.[10]

Lifestyle

Probably the single greatest stroke risk factor among lifestyle habits is cigarette smoking. Research has clearly demonstrated the link. One study of 7,264 men, followed over 12 years, found that current smokers had a four times greater risk of stroke than those who had never smoked. Previous smokers had an increased risk as well, but it was lower than for those who were still smoking.

Probably the single greatest stroke risk factor among lifestyle habits is cigarette smoking.

In addition, contrary to what many might think, switching from cigarettes to a pipe or cigar made little difference in the risk level. Those who had been heavy cigarette smokers and quit were still twice as likely to have a stroke as those who had never smoked. However, ceasing to smoke had clear benefits, especially for those who smoked less than 20 cigarettes a day. For these men, their risk of stroke five years after quitting was comparable to that of those who had never smoked.[11]

Similarly, a study of 117,006 female nurses, between 30 and 55 years old, showed that the risk of stroke was over two-and-a-half times greater among current smokers, compared to those who had never smoked. The risk among former smokers was only slightly elevated and this difference for the most part disappeared after two to four years without smoking. This study found that the benefits of quitting were not dependent on the number of cigarettes the person previously smoked daily.

Finally, it appears you are at risk of a stroke if you are younger than 45, have migraines, and smoke cigarettes, according to research reported in the *British Medical Journal* (July 31, 1993). French doctors found in a study of 212 women that those under the age of 45 with a previous history of migraines had a significantly higher risk factor for stroke. If they smoked cigarettes, the risk was even higher. However, men of all ages and women older than 45 were not more likely to have a stroke if they had migraines.

Eleven Steps to Prevent Stroke

David A. Steenblock, M.S., D.O., of Mission Viejo, California, a specialist in alternative treatments (especially hyperbaric oxygen) for stroke, offers the following recommendations for stroke prevention:

1. Avoid tobacco smoke and alcohol.

2. Don't use amphetamines, cocaine, or other illicit drugs, as these can be harmful to the heart.

3. After age 50, have your carotid arteries checked every five years for atherosclerosis.

4. Monitor your blood pressure (normal=120/70).

5. Exercise daily.

6. Eat fresh, nonprocessed vegetables.

7. Eat a high-fiber diet.

8. Avoid fats, cholesterol, and sugar and keep your weight down to help prevent diabetes, which affects the heart.

9. Take magnesium, calcium, vitamins E and C, and bioflavonoids.

10. If you are a woman over 35, avoid birth control pills.

11. Quickly correct any medical problems that develop.

Two Ways to Check Your Heart Status—Here are two physician-delivered noninvasive ways of checking your heart status: Doppler Ultrasound and Diagnostic Thermography.

Doppler Ultrasound—This test uses a flowmeter to measure blood flow and transmits the information by sound frequency. Some of the sound waves emitted by the flowmeter are reflected back by the red blood cells; the difference in pitch between sound waves sent and received is indicative (and proportional to) the speed of blood flow. The flowmeter can be incorporated into a standard stethoscope, so that information about blood flow in selected veins and arteries may be obtained. The device can detect very rapid changes in flow as well as steady flow rates.

Diagnostic Thermography—This approach provides

For more information about **Diagnostic Thermography**, contact: Therma-Scan™ Inc., 26711 Woodward Avenue, Suite 203, Huntington Professional Building-South, Huntington Woods, MI 48070; tel: 810-544-7500.

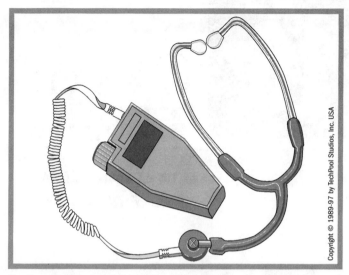

The Doppler Ultrasound test uses a *flowmeter* to measure blood flow and transmits the information by sound frequency.

a noninvasive cerebrovascular analysis. The Therma-Scan™ device measures infrared energy emissions from targeted areas of the body, including the heart. These emissions are the result of emanations of physiologic processes such as the flow of blood and nutrients. If this flow is deficient in a particular body area, such as the heart, the temperature value for that area will be abnormal and the diagnostic thermography read-out will indicate this in terms of different colors. Patterns of abnormal cooling (in blood vessels, as measured by the device) correlate directly with a diminished blood flow in that blood vessel.

Copyright © 1989-97 by TechPool Studios, Inc. USA

Oxygen Therapy

HOW IT CAN HELP STROKE RECOVERY

T HE MAJORITY of stroke victims in the U.S. spend many months working with physical therapists, sometimes recovering only minimal bodily function. Unfortunately, most are unaware that there is a far more effective alternative. It is called hyperbaric oxygen therapy (HBOT), and the results of treatment for stroke using this technique are dramatic.

Hyperbaric oxygen therapy has long been used on divers, but its application to stroke treatment is relatively recent. Researchers, particularly in Germany, recognized that the loss of functioning of an arm or leg after a stroke is similar to the symptoms of the "bends," a sometimes fatal affliction deep-sea divers get from ascending too quickly to the surface. Restoring the balance of nitrogen and oxygen in the blood via a hyperbaric oxygen chamber cured divers of the bends, and physicians suspected that victims of stroke or heart attack might be helped in the same way.

Hyperbaric oxygen therapy may be the single most effective technique, conventional or alternative, for reversing the damage caused by a stroke.

Their conjecture has proven correct and, today, hyperbaric oxygen therapy may be the single most effective technique, conventional or alternative, for reversing the damage caused by a stroke. Every emergency room in the United States should have a hyperbaric oxygen chamber, and every physician should be trained in its use, says David A. Steenblock, M.S., D.O., of Mission Viejo, California, who is well qualified to make this kind of sweeping statement. He is one of the country's leading practitioners in the therapeutic use of oxygen under pressure to dramatically reduce the effects of stroke and brain injury.

While drug companies continue to search for a "cure" for acute stroke, an effective way to restore a damaged brain to healthy function already exists: oxygen. "If you can get more oxygen to the brain within the first 24 hours of having a stroke, you can often stop most of the damage and salvage a great deal of brain tissue, eliminating 70% to 80% of the damage," Dr. Steenblock says. "Treating the patient by getting more oxygen to the brain during the first three weeks after the stroke makes it still possible to minimize the damage." In fact, Dr. Steenblock has produced unexpected positive outcomes when treating people as long as 15 years after their stroke.

Since 1971, over 1,000 cases demonstrating a 40%-100% rate of improvement for stroke victims receiving oxygen under pressure have been reported in scientific journals. Given the facts about positive outcomes, Dr. Steenblock encourages U.S. physicians to consider the merits of this approach as revealed in the following cases.

Moving Again After Right-Side Paralysis—Barbara, 62, had a stroke that completely paralyzed her right arm and left her severely bent over, limping, with pain in her right leg, and unable to control her urination. She had physical therapy and took conventional prescription medications, but nothing helped her. Barbara remained in this condition for 42 months before seeing Dr. Steenblock.

Over the course of 12 weeks, he started Barbara on a series of 60 treatments in a hyperbaric oxygen chamber (hyperbaric means pure oxygen under pressure). Oxygen is delivered to the body at an atmospheric pressure 1.5 to 1.75 times stronger than what we normally experience. During the treatment, Barbara wore an oxygen mask and laid down inside a sealed chamber that resembles a miniature submarine.

Barbara breathed pure oxygen for an hour. The higher

Hyperbaric oxygen therapy refers to pure oxygen delivered for 30 to 60 minutes to patients inside sealed chambers with high pressure (hence "hyperbaric" as in high barometric pressure), usually at 2.5 times higher than the atmospheric pressure at sea level. A monoplace chamber accommodates a single patient who absorbs the concentrated oxygen through the skin as well as through inhalation. A multiplace chamber services several people at once; patients wear oxygen masks.

According to Dr. Steenblock, if you can get more oxygen to the brain within the first 24 hours of having a stroke, you can often eliminate 70% to 80% of the damage.

For more on **chelation therapy**, see Chapter 3: Scrubbing the Arteries Naturally, pp. 70-92.

Due to its wide application for a number of conditions, oxygen therapy can save money in long-term health costs.

Barbara's Stroke Recovery Prescription

- N-acetyl carnitine: ¼ tsp, 2X daily, increasing to ½ tsp in water, 3X daily
- Cytidine disphosphate choline: 2 capsules, daily (A.M.)
- N-acetyl cysteine: 2 capsules, 3X daily
- Glycine: ¼ tsp, 2X daily, increasing to ½ tsp in water, 3X daily
- Super KMH (72 trace minerals, 18 herbs): 1 tsp, 2X daily
- Vitamin E: 400 IU, 3X daily
- Lipoic acid (an essential fatty acid): 1 capsule, 3X daily
- L-carnitine: 50 mg, daily
- Calcium magnesium potassium: 1 tablet, 3X daily
- Brewer's yeast: 2 tablets, 3X daily
- Aqua Flora (a homeopathic remedy for *Candida*): 2 tbsp, daily
- Calcium: 1,200 mg, daily
- Magnesium: 1,200 mg, daily
- Co-enzyme B complex: 1 capsule, daily
- Free Radical Quenchers: 2 capsules, 2X daily
- Zinc picolinate: 1 tablet, daily
- Low-fat, low-cholesterol diet
- Lescol (Fluvastatin, a conventional drug for lowering cholesterol)

atmospheric pressure inside the chamber literally forced more oxygen into her blood. In fact, hyperbaric oxygen can deliver eight to nine times more oxygen to the capillaries compared to breathing normal air, says Dr. Steenblock. "With 100% oxygen under pressure, oxygen is dissolved into the red blood cells and into body and brain fluids."

The goal is to get as much oxygen into the brain as possible. This helps to revive oxygen-starved brain tissue that was damaged but not entirely destroyed by the stroke, Dr. Steenblock explains. The principle holds true for traumatic brain injury as well, such as people sustain from accidents. Some of the brain tissue is irreversibly destroyed, as brain cells deprived of oxygen usually die within ten minutes, but a larger portion is potentially revivable.

A stroke produces most of its damage through swelling of and injury to surrounding brain tissue, yet this tissue lies dormant, not dead but not active either, surviving on as little as 15% to 20% of its normal oxygen supply. If you can restore blood flow and flood this area with oxygen, there is a strong likelihood of restoring these "hibernating" brain cells to function, five or even ten years after a stroke, says Dr. Steenblock.

For more information about **OPC-95** (for licensed practitioners only), contact: Jarrow Formulas, 1824 South Robertson Boulevard, Los Angeles, CA 90035; tel: 800-726-0886 or 310-204-6936; fax: 310-204-2520. To contact **Dr. Steenblock:** Health Restoration Medical Center, David Steenblock, D.O., Medical Director, 26381 Crown Valley Parkway, Suite 130, Mission Viejo, CA 92691; tel: 714-367-8870; fax: 714-367-9779. For a useful reference work: K.K. Jain, M.D., *Textbook of Hyperbaric Medicine*, 2nd Edition (1996), Hogrefe & Huber Publications, P.O. Box 2487, Kirkland, WA 98023; tel: 206-820-1500; fax: 206-823-8324.

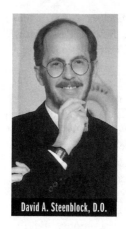

David A. Steenblock, D.O.

A stroke produces most of its damage through swelling of and damage to surrounding brain tissue, yet this tissue lies dormant. If you can restore blood flow and flood this area with oxygen, there is a strong likelihood of restoring these "hibernating" brain cells to function, five or even ten years after a stroke, says Dr. Steenblock.

Dr. Steenblock also gave Barbara a two-month course of chelation therapy, consisting of 23 infusions, to improve her general circulation. Her carotid artery, which is the main artery that passes through the neck, supplying blood to the brain, was about 50% blocked; in addition, Barbara had high blood pressure and atherosclerosis (arteries lined and clogged with deposits)—conditions that contributed strongly to her stroke, says Dr. Steenblock. Barbara also received about two hours of physical therapy five days a week and went on a nutritional supplementation program.

After one month of treatment, Barbara showed clear signs of improvement. Her walking improved noticeably and, instead of shuffling, she could raise her right heel off the ground and move with a smoother gait. Her posture was more erect. Barbara was able to open and close her right hand, and use it to grip and squeeze objects. She could also raise her arm to her chest level.

Hyperbaric oxygen, by restoring proper circulation to damaged brain tissues, can also stimulate the growth of new blood vessels and the repair

David's Stroke Recovery Prescription

- N-acetyl-carnitine: ½ tsp, 2X daily
- Cytidine choline: 1 capsule, 2X daily
- N-acetylcysteine: ½ tsp, 2X daily
- Melatonin: as needed for sleep
- Chlorella: 5 tablets, 2X daily
- OPC-95 (grape seed): 2X daily
- Juice Plus+™: Orchard Blend, 2X daily; Garden Blend, 2X daily
- Ginger root: 2 tablets, daily
- Pycnogenol: 10 tablets, daily
- Psyllium root powder: 2X, daily
- Goldenseal root: 2X, daily
- DHEA (hormone): 100 mg, daily

of damaged ones, but this takes time, Dr. Steenblock explains. "It may take upwards of two years of this therapy for all these cells to regrow, reconnect, and start to function again. But you're going to keep on seeing improvement."

A Quadriplegic Regains His Ability to Move—One day while getting up from a sofa in the lounge at chiropractic school, David, 25, fell over, unconscious. He had sustained a hemorrhagic stroke (caused by a burst aneurysm) that left him a quadriplegic. He could move only his eyelids and occasionally one eye. He ate by way of a stomach tube. He had to have everything done for him and was transported on an electric cart. David also suffered from a chronic cough and recurrent pneumonia. By the time David came to Dr. Steenblock, he had endured eight years of physical therapy and numerous other therapies, all of which failed to improve his condition.

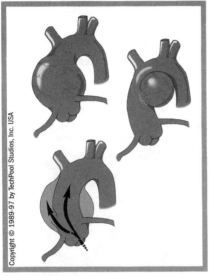

Copyright © 1989-97 by TechPool Studios, Inc. USA

An *aneurysm* is a problem in the cardiovascular system in which a sac is formed by the expansion of a wall in an artery, vein, or the heart; it is usually filled with fluid or clotted blood. The most common site for an aneurysm is the aorta. Aneurysms are usually associated with atherosclerosis (hardening of the arteries from plaque deposits); however, trauma and injury may also cause them. Over time, an aneurysm tends to increase in size and pose the danger of rupture. A ruptured aneurysm is usually accompanied by severe pain and blood loss, followed by shock; symptoms may resemble those associated with a stroke.

Dr. Steenblock started David on a two-month series of daily hyperbaric oxygen treatments. At the end of two months, David began regaining neck strength and right-side motion. He could stand, with support straps or parallel bars, for up to an hour and for three minutes without any assistance. Feeling started to return on his right side. He could sit up in his wheelchair and hold his head erect. His constant drooling started to diminish and his swallowing became easier. His eyes were able to track objects normally and his facial muscles filled out. For the first time in eight years, David was able to feed himself.

Since 1971, over 1,000 cases demonstrating a 40%-100% rate of improvement for stroke victims receiving oxygen under pressure have been reported in scientific journals.

David also received regular physical therapy, biofeedback, and a nutritional prescription (see sidebar). After four months on this program, David regained full hearing in his right ear; since childhood, he had had only 70% of hearing capacity in that ear. "He's gradually getting better, and his voice is starting to come back, but it's a slow process when somebody has that level of damage," says Dr. Steenblock.

David works out regularly with weights and is able to lift about 100 pounds with his legs and 60 pounds with his arms. "And his brain is fine," adds Dr. Steenblock.

Out of the Wheelchair in Just Fifteen Treatments—Ten years prior to seeking treatment with Dr. Steenblock, Sonya had suffered a stroke that left her confined to a wheelchair and unable to take care of herself. After consulting 22 doctors for her paralysis and severe pain, she was no better and despairing. Dr. Steenblock gave Sonya ten treatments with hyperbaric oxygen. At nine times the level provided to her body's capillaries by breathing normal air, the oxygen began to revive brain tissue that hadn't functioned since the stroke. Her pain subsided. After another five treatments, Sonya was able to walk again and begin taking care of herself.

All About HBOT

Hyperbaric oxygen therapy dates back to the beginning of this century, although its modern use in the United States dates only to the formation of the Undersea Medical Society in 1967. HBOT may be administered in individual oxygen chambers that consist of acrylic tubes about seven feet long and 25 inches in diameter. The patient lies on a stretcher that slides into the tube. The entry is sealed and the tube is pressurized with pure oxygen for 30 to 120 minutes.

The increased pressure makes it possible to breathe oxygen at a concentration higher than that allowed by any

QUICK DEFINITION

Oxygen therapies involve the use of oxygen and can be used in various forms to promote healing and to destroy pathogens in the body. Oxygen-based therapies treat a variety of conditions, including cancer, infections, circulatory problems, chronic fatigue syndrome, arthritis, allergies, and multiple sclerosis. There are 2 principal types of oxygen therapy, classified according to the chemical process involved. *Oxygenation* is the process of enriching the oxygen content of the blood or tissues. One oxygenation therapy is called hyperbaric oxygen therapy, which introduces oxygen to the body in a pressurized chamber.

Oxygenation employed under strictly controlled conditions can have positive therapeutic effects. The second type of oxygen therapy is called *oxidation*, which is a chemical reaction occurring when electrons (electrically-charged particles; frequently, but not always, oxygen) are transferred from one molecule to another. Although uncontrolled oxidation can be destructive—as is the case when free radicals are produced in excess—it can also be therapeutic when carefully used on weak and devitalized cells as the targets.

other means. After treatment, the chamber is depressurized slowly with the patient resting inside. Most of the hyperbaric facilities in the United States are either part of, or affiliated with, American hospitals or the military.

Multiplace chambers can accommodate many patients at once and the oxygen is delivered by mask. These chambers allow nurses and technical personnel to attend to patients during the treatment. An added advantage of multiplace chambers is that a patient can be removed immediately if problems arise, whereas in individual chambers, the patient cannot be removed until the entire chamber is depressurized.

Conditions Benefited
by Hyperbaric Oxygen Therapy

The use of oxygen under pressure to treat serious health conditions including stroke is medically well-established, though not yet widely used in this country. There are only 300 hyperbaric oxygen chambers in the U.S., while in Russia, for example, there are 2,000. HBOT is primarily used in the U.S. for traumas such as crash injuries, burns, wounds, gangrene, carbon monoxide poisoning, bed sores, stasis (the stagnation of the normal flow of fluids), radiation

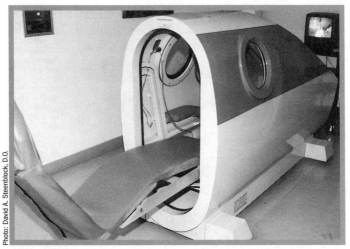

HBOT may be administered in individual oxygen chambers that consist of acrylic tubes about seven feet long and 25 inches in diameter. The patient lies on a stretcher which slides into the tube. The entry is sealed and the tube that is pressurized with pure oxygen for 30 to 120 minutes.

In West Germany, HBOT has been used extensively to treat stroke victims, and government sponsorship of HBOT has reduced aftercare costs for stroke victims by 71%.

necrosis (death of an area of tissue or bone surrounded by healthy parts), and skin grafting that doesn't take. Some microsurgical procedures for the repair and restoration of severed limbs are made possible only by the use of HBOT during the surgery.

CAUTION
Hyperbaric oxygen therapy may cause problems for those with a history of middle-ear infection, emphysema, or spontaneous pneumonia, due to the pressure it requires.

"In West Germany, HBOT has been used extensively to treat stroke victims, and government sponsorship of HBOT has reduced aftercare costs for stroke victims by 71%," reports David Hughes, Ph.D., of the Hyperbaric Oxygen Institute in San Bernardino, California. A landmark 1971 study showed that hyperbaric oxygen treatment of 40 stroke patients produced moderate to significant improvement in 80% of patients.

"In France," says Dr. Hughes, "HBOT is employed for peripheral vascular and arterial problems, and in Russia, it is used in drug and alcohol detoxification. In Japan, the medical establishment boasts that no citizen is ever more than half an hour away from a hyperbaric chamber." In Great Britain, more than 25,000 multiple sclerosis patients have benefited from HBOT.[1] HBOT is gaining acceptance and is utilized by both alternative and conventional physicians. Its broad spectrum of applications gives it enormous potential for more widespread therapeutic use and accessibility.

Oxygen Therapy

Hyperbaric oxygen therapy is one in a wide range of therapies utilizing oxygen in various forms to promote healing and destroy pathogens (disease-producing microorganisms and toxins) in the body. These therapies are grouped according to the type of chemical process involved: the addition of oxygen to the blood or tissues is called "oxygenation," and "oxidation" is the reaction of splitting off electrons (electrically-charged particles) from any chemical molecule. Oxidation may or may not involve oxygen (oxidation refers to the chemical reaction and not to oxygen itself).

Hyperbaric oxygen therapy utilizes the oxygenation process. Hydrogen peroxide therapy, on the other hand, uses the process of oxidation. Ozone therapy utilizes both of these chemical processes.

The Suppression of Hyperbaric Oxygen Therapy: State Raids Dr. Steenblock's Clinic

During the Communist era, political dissidents were routinely arrested, subjected to mock trials, imprisoned, and often murdered in the remote Gulag Archipelago of the Soviet Union. Thanks to the Food and Drug Administration (FDA), conventional medicine trade groups, state medical boards, and the big drug companies, America has its own "Gulag" for doctors who deviate from the enforced norms and who practice alternative medicine. What the Soviet Union accomplished through state-imposed tyranny, American medicine accomplishes through licensing, regulations, and the FDA—the suppression of your freedom of choice in medical care.

Our American Gulag ruins alternative doctors through suppression, harassment, indictments, licensure revocation, and bankruptcy. David A. Steenblock, D.O., M.S., is one physician who has endured this political intimidation. Here is his story:

Dr. Steenblock was forced into bankruptcy in September 1995 when state medical authorities confiscated six FDA-approved hyperbaric oxygen machines, worth $600,000, which he used to treat patients who had had strokes and heart attacks. No patient complaints were registered, but 30 very ill patients were forced to wait two months for treatment, and one died the day after being grilled by state medical authorities. The embargo was lifted in November 1995 and the clinic struggles on.

Research is needed on the effects of hyperbaric oxygen therapy for the treatment of early complications of stroke. This type of therapy could prove revolutionary by preventing permanent damage to stroke patients and could be a great money saver.

Although various oxygen therapies have been employed in Europe for many years for a wide range of conditions, in the United States most remain controversial and are currently unapproved by the FDA (Food and Drug Administration). Legality of oxygen therapies varies from state to state.

How Oxygenation Therapy Works

All human cells, tissues, and organs need oxygen to function. Oxygenation saturates the body with oxygen in the form of gas, sometimes at high pressure (hyperbaric), increasing the total amount of available oxygen in the body. Insufficient oxygenation may promote the growth of pathogens, whereas excessive oxygenation may damage normal tissues. Oxygenation employed under strictly controlled conditions can have very positive therapeutic effects.

Otto Warburg, former Director of the Max Planck Institute for

Cell Physiology in Germany and a two-time Nobel laureate, proposed that a lack of oxygen at the cellular level may be the prime cause of cancer, and that oxygen therapy could be an effective treatment for it.[2] He showed that normal cells in tissue culture, when deprived of oxygen, become cancer cells, and that oxygen can kill cancer cells in tissue cultures.

Oxygen therapy may be professionally administered in many ways: orally, rectally, vaginally, intravenously (into a vein), intra-arterially (into an artery), through inhalation, or by absorption through the skin. High concentrations of oxygen gas can also be given orally through masks or tubes, via oxygen tents, or within pressurized hyperbaric chambers. Oxygen may also be injected subcutaneously (beneath the skin). Ionized oxygen, both positively and negatively charged, is administered by inhalation or dissolved in drinking or bath water.

How Oxidation Therapy Works

The word oxidation refers to a chemical reaction whereby electrons are transferred from one molecule to another. Oxygen molecules are frequently, but not always, involved in these reactions. The molecules that "donate" electrons are said to be oxidized, whereas the molecules that accept electrons are called oxidants.

CAUTION

Oxidation therapy needs to be administered under clinical supervision, since uncontrolled oxidation may be destructive to the body.

A healthy state of oxidative balance is necessary for optimal function of the body, but when the body is exposed to repeated environmental stresses, its oxidative function is weakened. When oxidation is partially blocked by toxicity in the body or by pathological (disease-causing) organisms, oxidation therapy may help by "jump-starting" the body's oxidative processes and returning them to normal,[3] according to Charles Farr, M.D., Ph.D., of Oklahoma City, Oklahoma.

When properly administered, oxidation therapy selectively destroys pathogenic (disease-producing) bacteria, viruses, and other invading microbial organisms, and deactivates toxic substances without injury to healthy tissues or cells.[4] For example, if diluted hydrogen peroxide is placed on a wound, the normal cells thrive while the pathogens die.

Oxidation therapy must be administered under clinical supervision, since uncontrolled oxidation may be destructive to the body. Oxidation therapy may be given intravenously, orally, rectal-

According to Dr. Farr, arteriosclerosis and strokes may also benefit from hydrogen peroxide therapy. Infusing highly diluted *medical-grade* 35% hydrogen peroxide into the bloodstream brings oxygen to the tissues (as does hyperbaric oxygen therapy), which is what produces beneficial results in the case of stroke.

There are few side effects with hydrogen peroxide therapy. In rare cases, a problem involving inflammation of veins at the site of injection will occur. Hydrogen peroxide should not be taken orally, as it causes nausea and vomiting, and rectal administration can lead to inflammation of the lower intestinal tract. Other side effects observed include temporary faintness, fatigue, headaches, and chest pain. Most problems stem from an inappropriate administration route, administration above patient tolerance, the mixing of oxidative chemicals with other substances, or using oxidative chemicals in too great a concentration, reports Dr. Farr.

ly by enema, vaginally, or transcutaneously (absorbed through the skin).

Hydrogen Peroxide Therapy

Hydrogen peroxide is a liquid with the molecular structure of two atoms of hydrogen and two atoms of oxygen (H_2O_2). Because it is less stable than water (H_2O), hydrogen peroxide readily enters into oxidative reactions, ultimately becoming oxygen in water. It was Dr. Farr who, in 1984, first characterized the oxidative effects of hydrogen peroxide in humans.[5] Today, the use of hydrogen peroxide for its oxidative effects has spread to over 38 countries, and remains one of the least expensive, yet effective, oxidation therapies.

Oxidation administered through hydrogen peroxide therapy regulates tissue repair, cellular respiration, growth, immune functions, the energy system, most hormone systems, and the production of cytokines (chemical messengers that are involved in the regulation of almost every system in the body). Oxidation therapy can also work as a defense system, directly destroying invading bacteria, viruses, yeast, and parasites, according to Dr. Farr.

Conditions Benefited by Hydrogen Peroxide Therapy

Dr. Farr uses hydrogen peroxide for a variety of health problems, including AIDS, arthritis, cancer, candidiasis, chronic fatigue syndrome, depression, lupus erythematosus (a chronic inflammatory disease with symptoms including arthritis, fatigue, and skin lesions), emphysema, multiple sclerosis, varicose veins, and fractures.

According to Dr. Farr, arteriosclerosis and strokes may also benefit from hydrogen peroxide therapy.[6] Infusing highly diluted *medical-grade* 35% hydrogen peroxide into the bloodstream brings oxygen to the tissues (as does hyperbaric oxygen therapy), which is what produces beneficial results in the case of stroke. Concerning arteriosclerosis, hydrogen peroxide has been shown to dissolve fats (lipids) from the arterial walls.[7]

Research is needed into the many conditions oxygen therapy can benefit. Because oxygen therapy can help the body repair itself, it is an ideal treatment to integrate into a comprehensive health care system.

Ozone Therapy

Ozone therapy relies on the process of oxidation as well as oxygenation. Approximately one-fifth of the air humans breathe is comprised of two atoms of oxygen (O_2). Ozone (O_3) contains three oxygen atoms and is a less stable form of molecular oxygen. Due to this added molecule, ozone is more reactive than oxygen and readily enters into reactions to oxidize other chemicals. During oxidation in the body, the extra oxygen molecule in ozone breaks away, leaving a normal O_2 molecule. This increases the oxygen content of the blood or tissues. For this reason, ozone therapy is a combination of both oxygenation therapy and oxidation therapy.

Ozone is a common substance in nature, but can also be a source of air pollution when produced by man-made combustion. Medical-grade ozone is made from pure oxygen. Used therapeutically, ozone increases local oxygen supply to lesions, improves and accelerates wound healing, deactivates viruses and bacteria, and increases local tissue temperature, thus enhancing local metabolic processes, according to Gerard Sunnen, M.D., of New York City.

Ozone therapy can be used to treat arterial circulatory disturbances and to dissolve atherosclerotic plaque. Typically, intra-arterial injection (injection into an artery) is the method employed for this type of treatment.

Since the FDA has not approved the practice of ozone therapy in the United States, it is difficult to get data on its use. For fear of FDA reprisals, many physicians use ozone therapy without calling attention to themselves. However, numerous patient anecdotes are available.

Like many oxygen therapies, ozone therapy is widely employed and practiced in Europe, but still not readily available in the United States. According to Dr. Sunnen, prospective patients and doctors in America must await two further animal studies before the FDA sanctions a phase-one clinical trial with humans, and ultimately approves the therapeutic use of ozone.

The Future of Oxygen Therapy

The main stumbling blocks for all oxygen therapies, according to Dr. Hughes, are the FDA, health insurance companies, and the entrenched medical establishment. "The problem is that most areas of conventional medicine in this country are driven by the pharmaceutical companies," he says. "The incentive is always to sell pills, and you can't sell oxygen pills. This tends to hold it back, especially since a very large percentage of the research that's done at universities is funded by pharmaceutical companies."

Despite this fact, as Dr. Farr points out, the medical profession is becoming more receptive to oxygen therapy's potential benefits. For example, 10 to 12 years ago there were only eight locations in America for the use of hyperbaric oxygen. Now, according to Dr. Hughes, there are 28, and that number is increasing all the time. "More and more people are becoming familiar with HBOT, and we're getting more and more requests from the medical profession about what other conditions it can help."

"Treating the patient by getting more oxygen to the brain during the first three weeks after the stroke makes it still possible to minimize the damage," says David A. Steenblock, M.S., D.O. In fact, Dr. Steenblock has produced unexpected positive outcomes when treating people as long as 15 years after their stroke.

More Options for Treating Stroke

MANY OF THE THERAPIES discussed in Part One (Heart Disease) and Part Two (High Blood Pressure) are applicable to stroke as well. The following additional alternative medicine techniques have proven particularly useful in preventing or treating stroke.

Lasers

Margaret A. Naeser, Ph.D., associate research professor of neurology at Boston University School of Medicine and a licensed acupuncturist in Massachusetts, has conducted research on the use of low-energy lasers (20 milliwatt red-to-infrared laser light) in the treatment of paralysis from stroke. Five of her six subjects showed improvement, and patients with mild to moderate paralysis responded better than those with severe paralysis, according to Dr. Naeser. The improvements were observed even when treatments were begun three or four years after the stroke.

Neuropathways EEG Imaging

California therapist Margaret Ayers has been researching brain biofeedback for 20 years, a study that led her to invent a new form of therapeutic neurofeedback she calls Neuropathways EEG Imaging™. Ayers' brain research has shown that Neuropathways EEG Imaging

Research has shown that Neuropathways EEG Imaging may be an effective adjunct in the treatment of numerous serious brain disorders and injuries, including stroke.

may be an effective adjunct in the treatment of numerous serious brain disorders and injuries, including stroke, oxygen deprivation (anoxia), epileptic seizures, depression, and closed head injury, among others.

The device used in this technique displays the shape and electrical strength of a patient's brain waves on a computer screen and enables a person to interact, in real time, with the brain-wave pattern. Ayers has brought five patients out of Level Two coma using this device. (Level Two means the patient is unable to respond to sound, verbal commands, light, touch, or pressure.) Although a coma is not exactly like a stroke, some of the damage to the brain that can produce a coma is similar to the damage suffered in some strokes. The following examples will give you an idea of how the treatment works and how it could be used to regain movement and skills impaired by stroke.

Collin, 21, had spent two years in a coma following a motorcycle accident. He came out of his coma after two 1-hour treatments, states Ayers. Peter, 30, had been in a coma for three months following eight brain surgeries to remove a baseball-sized tumor. After a 60-minute session, in which Peter's brain was trained to make small responses to electrical stimulation, he snapped out of his coma, opened his eyes, and kissed his wife. After four more one-hour sessions, spaced one month apart, Peter was able to speak, eat, and move one side of his body.

A study Ayers conducted in 1987 with 250 individuals with closed head injuries (concussions), showed that long-term brain wave abnormalities resulting from the injury could be improved within six treatments, and entirely corrected within 24 sessions.

The brain constantly emits electrical impulses, registered as waves, that indicate the state of health and activity of the brain. In Neuropathways EEG Imaging, gold-plated cup electrodes are placed on certain areas of the head, corresponding to the brain regions whose waves the patient wishes to bring into balance. In effect, the brain is trained—this is the neuro (brain cells) feedback function—to replace abnormal waves with normal rhythmic patterns, explains

For more about **biofeedback**, see Chapter 13: Alternative Medicine Options for Lowering High Blood Pressure, pp. 217-221.

QUICK DEFINITION

Biofeedback training is a method of learning how to consciously regulate normally unconscious bodily functions (such as heart rate, blood pressure, and breathing). It uses a monitoring device to measure and report back immediate information about the heart rate, for example, transmitting one blinking light or beep per heartbeat. The person being monitored learns techniques such as meditation, relaxation, and visualization to slow their heart rate and then uses the flashes or beeps to check their progress and make adjustments accordingly.

Ayers. The brain is encouraged to recognize the normal, healthy brain waves as the computer produces audio and visual reinforcements when these desired waves are achieved.

According to Ayers, once the brain learns how to change its beat, the new wave patterns are permanent. Mastering neurofeedback is a lot like learning to ride a bicycle; once learned, it's a skill never forgotten. Demonstrated benefits include improvements in short-term memory, concentration, speech, motor skills, energy level, sleep regularity, and emotional balance.[1]

Nutritional Supplements

The nutritional supplements discussed here are specific to stroke and may be considered along with the supplements recommended for maintaining general heart and circulatory health. As mentioned previously, excess homocysteine in the blood has been linked to stroke and is also associated with deficiencies of folic acid and vitamins B12 and B6. Therefore, supplementation with these nutrients may be advisable. Since low blood levels of the antioxidant vitamins C and E and beta carotene have also been linked to stroke,[2] supplementation can be preventive. As always, it is best to consult a health practitioner for assistance in designing the optimum supplement program for your individual biochemistry and health status.

As part of a stroke prevention regimen, coenzyme Q10, lipoic acid (especially if you are diabetic and eat lots of sweets or drink fruit juices), selenium, chromium GTF, and magnesium are also useful, reports David A. Steenblock, M.S., D.O. Vitamin B complex, *Ginkgo biloba*, and superoxide dismutase (SOD, an antioxidant enzyme) can be beneficial as well. In addition, vitamin E and essential fatty acids are important nutritional components for stroke prevention and recovery.

Vitamin E

According to Dr. Steenblock, vitamin E has been shown to reduce the damage from a stroke or transient ischemic attack. If you are at risk of a stroke, supplementing with this vitamin may therefore be a wise precaution.

When consumed in doses higher than 1,200 IU daily, vitamin E can have anticoagulant effects. This means it will increase your tendency to have a hemorrhagic stroke; especially if you have high blood pressure, do not have atherosclerosis (cholesterol deposits on the arterial walls) or arteriosclerosis (hardened arteries, reduced blood flow), and are female, frail, or have dry and brittle ("friable") blood vessels.

On the other hand, if you are of a stout build and have significant atherosclerosis or diabetes, or both, you probably would do well with higher doses of vitamin E, in the range of 1,200 to 2,000 IU daily, says Dr. Steenblock. At this dosage, the vitamin can act as a blood thinner (preventing blood clots) and may also decrease or stop atherosclerosis by stopping the spread of certain cells. Additionally, it can slow down or even prevent the production of harmful free radicals in the arterial walls. This is very important for diabetics since it stops a process in which sugars become attached to proteins when the blood sugar level is too high. These "sugar-proteins" are thought to be one of the main mechanisms of aging and atherosclerosis.

A daily dose of 400 to 800 IU of mixed tocopherols should be good for almost everyone, states Dr. Steenblock. These are various fat-soluble compounds with vitamin E antioxidant activity. Reliance on only one antioxidant (to neutralize free radicals) for stroke prevention is incorrect, he says. As always, he cautions, consult with your own qualified health professional before commencing any treatment.

Essential Fatty Acids

Research has shown that supplementation with EPA (eicosapentaenoic acid, an omega-3 essential fatty acid) from fish oil significantly reduces fibrinogen,[3] high levels of which can contribute to stroke.

William Lee Cowden, M.D., has noticed that if patients can be treated within the first 12 hours after a stroke with a combination of essential fatty acids, a high antioxidant intake, and either hyperbaric oxygen therapy or ozone therapy (see Chapter 16), a dramatic regression of symptoms of stroke can occur. Patients regain sensation, strength, and mental clarity, as well as motor and sensory skills and orientation. In his treatment, Dr. Cowden uses the antioxidants vitamin E, beta carotene, ascorbyl palmitate (a fat-soluble form of vitamin C), and pycnogenol (a fat-soluble antioxidant found in grape seeds and pine bark), along with the essential fatty acids EPA and DHA (docosahexaenoic acid, from fish oil) to help prevent damage to the fatty-acid membranes in brain cells.

QUICK DEFINITION

A **free radical** is an unstable molecule with an unpaired electron that steals an electron from another molecule and produces harmful effects. Free radicals are formed when molecules within cells react with oxygen (oxidize) as part of normal metabolic processes. Free radicals then begin to break down cells, especially if there are not enough free-radical quenching nutrients, such as vitamins C and E, in the cell. While free radicals are normal products of metabolism, uncontrolled free-radical production plays a major role in the development of degenerative disease, including cancer and heart disease. Free radicals harmfully alter important molecules, such as proteins, enzymes, fats, even DNA. Other sources of free radicals include pesticides, industrial pollutants, smoking, alcohol, viruses, most infections, allergies, stress, even certain foods and excessive exercise.

Additional Alternative Therapies

Self-Care

QUICK DEFINITION

DHA (docosa-hexaenoic acid), is the primary structural fatty acid in the retina of the eye and the most abundant fat in the gray matter of the brain. (DHA, which is an omega-3 long-chain fatty acid, is unrelated to DHEA, which is a hormone.) Adequate levels of DHA are required for proper brain and eye development and function. DHA is important for signal transmission in the brain, eye, and nervous system. Research has shown that DHA has benefits for patients with depression, Alzheimer's, or attention deficit disorder, and for pregnant and lactating women. Initially, DHA is obtained fetally through the placenta; after birth, DHA comes from breast milk, then later from dietary sources such as fish (tuna, salmon, and sardines, or fish oils), red meats, animal organs, and eggs. DHA is also available in capsule form from a single nutrient source: microalgae, the fish's original source.

The following therapies can be undertaken at home under appropriate professional supervision:

- Flower Remedies
- Guided Imagery
- Massage
- Meditation
- Qigong
- Yoga
- Aromatherapy: For muscular paralysis, use lavender—Rub the spinal column and paralyzed area with a mixture of one quart of rubbing alcohol and one ounce each of essence of lavender, essence of rosemary, and essence of basil.
- Herbs: To improve circulation to extremities—elder flowers, hyssop, rosemary, yarrow. To nourish the nervous system—damiana, lavender, rosemary, Siberian ginseng. Consult a trained herbalist.
- Hydrotherapy: Constitutional hydrotherapy—apply two to five times weekly.
- Swimming to restore strength
- Reflexology: tip of big toe (opposite side from paralysis), other toes, reflexes to affected areas

Professional Care

The following therapies should only be provided by a qualified health professional:

- Chelation Therapy
- Hypnotherapy
- Light Therapy
- Magnetic Field Therapy
- Naturopathic Medicine
- Osteopathy
- Sound Therapy
- Traditional Chinese Medicine
- Reconstructive Therapy
- Bodywork: Feldenkrais
- Vision Therapy: Vision therapy may be an important ingredient in rehabilitation. Victims suffer impairment in aim, focus, and eye movement, as well as visual-field and perceptual defects. Without

William Lee Cowden, M.D., has noticed that if patients can be treated within the first 12 hours after a stroke with a combination of essential fatty acids, a high antioxidant intake, and either hyperbaric oxygen therapy or ozone therapy, a dramatic regression of symptoms of stroke can occur.

evaluation by a behavioral optometrist, these can be overlooked and recovery hindered. Therapy includes awareness training, visual/motor exercises, and lenses and prisms. Gross and fine movement control, hand-eye coordination, attention, memory, and learning skills improve dramatically.

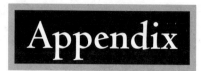

Where to Find Help

For additional information and referrals concerning treatment for heart disease, hypertension, and stroke, contact the following organizations:

American Academy of Environmental Medicine
P.O. Box 1001-8001
New Hope, Pennsylvania 18938
(215) 862-4544
(215) 862-4583 (Fax)
The academy offers extensive training for physicians interested in learning more about environmental medicine. For information on physicians practicing environmental medicine send a self-addressed, stamped envelope along with your request.

American Holistic Medical Association
4101 Lake Boone Trail, Suite 201
Raleigh, North Carolina 27607
(919) 787-5181
A professional organization for holistic practitioners, the AHMA offers information and services for its members and lobbies for holistic issues. It also provides referrals for the public; requests must be in writing.

Aromatherapy

The Pacific Institute of Aromatherapy
P.O. Box 6723
San Rafael, California 94903
(415) 479-9121
(415) 479-0119 (Fax)
The Pacific Institute of Aromatherapy offers courses to individuals and companies interested in learning about, or becoming certified in, the practice of aromatherapy. Call for a brochure and course listing.

Aromatherapy Seminars
117 N. Robertson Blvd.
Los Angeles, California 90048
(800) 677-2368

(310) 276-1191
(310) 276-1156 (Fax)
Provides programs to become a certified aromatherapist, locally or through a correspondence course. They offer specialty classes for those already certified and have available videotapes, audiotapes and blending materials.

Lotus Light
P.O. Box 1008
Silver Lake, Wisconsin 53170
(414) 889-8501
(414) 889-8591 (Fax)
Provides mail order distribution of aromatherapy videotapes, books, and materials.

Ayurvedic Medicine

American School of Ayurvedic Sciences
2115 112th Avenue NE
Bellevue, Washington 98004
(206) 453-8022
This college provides medical training for physicians and health care practitioners, as well as individual courses for lay people. Dr. Virender Sodhi's Ayurvedic, Naturopathic Medical Clinic is also located at this address.

Ayurvedic Institute
11311 Menaul NE
Albuquerque, New Mexico 87112
(505) 291-9698
(505) 294-7572 (Fax)
The institute, directed by Dr. Vasant Lad, trains people from all walks of life in most of the aspects of Ayurveda.

The College of Maharishi Ayur-Veda Medical Center
P.O. Box 282
Fairfield, Iowa 52556
(515) 472-8477
The center provides referrals to health centers which offer methods of prevention and treatment of a broad range of illnesses. They also

train practitioners and provide information to the lay public.

Biofeedback

Association for Applied Psychophysiology and Biofeedback
10200 West 44th Avenue, Suite 304
Wheat Ridge, Colorado 80033
(303) 422-8436
(303) 422-8894 (Fax)
Provides names and phone numbers of chapters in your state (formerly Biofeedback Society of America).

Biofeedback Certification Institute of America
10200 West 44th Avenue, Suite 304
Wheat Ridge, Colorado 80033
(303) 420-2902
Runs the major certification program for biofeedback practitioners and provides information about certified local practitioners.

Tools for Exploration
47 Paul Drive
San Rafael, California 94903
(415) 499-9050
(415) 499-9047 (Fax)
Carries home biofeedback devices. Call for catalog.

Biological Dentistry

American Academy of Biological Dentistry
P.O. Box 856
Carmel Valley, California 93924
(408) 659-5385
(408) 659-2417 (Fax)
The purpose of the AABD is to promote biological dental medicine, which uses nontoxic diagnostic and therapeutic approaches in the field of clinical dentistry. They publish a quarterly journal, *Focus*, and hold regular seminars on biological diagnosis and therapy.

The Safe Water Coalition
5615 West Lyons Court
Spokane, Washington 99208
(509) 328-6704
The purpose of this organization is to educate legislators and the public on the hazards of fluoridation.

Chelation Therapy

American College of Advancement in Medicine
P.O. Box 3427
Laguna Hills, California 92654
(714) 583-7666
ACAM seeks to establish certification and standards of practice for chelation therapy. It provides training and education, and sponsors semiannual conferences for physicians and scientists. It provides referrals and informational material, including a directory listing of all physicians worldwide who have been trained in preventive medicine as well as in the ACAM protocol. The directory is updated monthly. The organization also provides a copy of the ACAM protocol for chelation to the public. For more information, send a stamped, self-addressed envelope along with your request.

The Rheumatoid Disease Foundation
5106 Old Harding Road
Franklin, Tennessee 37064
(615) 646-1030
This nonprofit, charitable organization has a listing of physicians who perform chelation therapy. Send a legal-size, stamped, self-addressed envelope, along with a donation, when requesting information.

Herbal Medicine

American Botanical Council
P.O. Box 201660
Austin, Texas 78720
(800) 373-7105
Nonprofit research and education organization. Publishes *HerbalGram* magazine, booklets on herbs, and reprints of scientific articles.

The American Herbalists Guild
P.O. Box 746555
Arvada, Colorado 80006
(303) 423-8800
(303) 402-1564 (Fax)
The Guild, with members ranging from clinical practitioners to ethnobotanists, has become an important influence in the reemergence of medical herbalism in the United States. A directory of schools and teachers is available.

Herb Research Foundation
1007 Pearl Street, Suite 200
Boulder, Colorado 80302
(303) 449-2265
(303) 449-2265 (Fax)
Co-publishes *HerbalGram* with ABC. Provides research materials for consumers, pharmacists, physicians, scientists, and industry.

Magnetic Field Therapy

Bio-Electro-Magnetics Institute
2490 West Moana Lane
Reno, Nevada 89509-3936
(702) 827-9099
A private, nonprofit organization established to provide research, education, support, and technical assistance in matters relating to bioelectromagnetics. A national clearinghouse for information relating to both health risks from power line magnetic fields and the health benefits from magnetic therapy.

Enviro-Tech Products
17171 Southeast 29th Street
Choctaw, Oklahoma 73020
(405) 390-3499
(405) 390-8934 (Fax)
This service includes self-help information, information for physicians, and information and guidance for research projects under the Institutional Review Board of the Bio-Electro-Magnetics Institute of Reno, Nevada.

Dr. Wolfgang Ludwig
Silcherstrasse 21
Horb A.N.1, Germany
011-49-7451-8648 (Fax)
For information regarding German instruments utilizing magnetic energy and pulsing frequencies, such as Endomet and Magnetron.

Prometheus Italia SrL
Centro Commerciale, VR-EST
Viale del Lavoro 45
I-36037, S. Martino B.A. (VR), Italy
This company produces magnetic blankets according to Dr. Ludwig's design.

Nutritional Supplements

American College of Advancement in Medicine
P.O. Box 3427

Laguna Hills, California 92654
(714) 583-7666
ACAM provides a directory listing of physicians worldwide who have been trained in nutritional and preventative medicine. The directory also provides an extensive list of books and articles on nutritional supplementation.

Oxygen Therapy

The American College of Hyperbaric Medicine
Ocean Medical Center
4001 Ocean Drive, Suite 105
Lauderdale-by-the-Sea, Florida 33308
(954) 771-4000
(954) 776-0670 (Fax)
A group of physicians dedicated to the clinical aspects of hyperbaric medicine. Their purpose is to foster ethical growth and development of the science and practice of hyperbaric oxygen therapy. Promotes research and education.

International Bio-oxidative Medicine Foundation
P.O. Box 891954
Oklahoma City, Oklahoma 73189
(405) 478-IBOM Ext. 4266
(405) 623-7320 (Fax)
The foundation publishes and distributes a newsletter as well as scientific research data. Supports educational programs that highlight current research and the therapeutic use of oxidative therapies. Encourages basic and clinical research. Membership available.

International Ozone Association
31 Strawberry Hill Avenue
Stamford, Connecticut 06902
(203) 348-3542
A professional scientific organization disseminating information on use and production of ozone through meetings, synopses, and world congresses. Publishes books and journals on ozone.

Medical Society for Ozone Therapy
Klagen Furtestrasse 4
D. 7000 Stuttgart 30, Germany
An excellent informational resource for the public and professionals. Addresses the differences between free ozone and medical ozone. The Society can explain how medical ozone is used to treat diseases, provide treat-

ment applications, and explain where and why medical ozone is used.

Medizone International, Inc.

123 East 54th Street
New York, New York 10022
(212) 421-0303
Developers of ozone-based blood purification systems and treatments for diseases caused by lipid-enveloped viruses, including AIDS, hepatitis B, and herpes.

Carolina Center for Alternative and Nutritional Medicine

4505 Fair Meadow Lane, Suite 111
Raleigh, North Carolina 27607
(800) 473-9812 (U.S. and Canada)
(407) 967-6466 (outside North America)
Outpatient facility which focuses on metabolic and intestinal detoxification. Comprehensive and synergistic treatment regimens for each patient are developed utilizing therapies such as colon hydrotherapy, intravenous therapies (including ozone), and external ozone hydrotherapy. Supportive elements such as acupuncture and lymphatic massage, as well as techniques to address the psychological/emotional components of health and illness are also part of the program.

Traditional Chinese Medicine

American Association of Oriental Medicine

433 Front Street
Catasauqua, Pennsylvania 18032
(610) 266-1433
(610) 264-2768 (Fax)
The association (formerly AAAOM) is a national professional trade organization of acupuncturists who meet acceptable standards of competency and can provide you with the names and locations of local members. Referrals by written request only.

Endnotes

Chapter I
What Causes Heart Disease?

1 Privitera, James R., M.D. *Clots: Life's Biggest Killer* Unpublished manuscript. Covina, CA (1992).

2 American Heart Association Internet web site http://www.amhrt.org/hs96/has.html.

3 CASS Principal Investigators and Associates. "Myocardial Infarction and Mortality in the Coronary Artery Surgery Study (CASS) Randomized Trial." *New England Journal of Medicine* 310:12 (March 1984), 750-758.

4 McTaggart, Lynn. *What Doctors Don't Tell You* (San Francisco: Thorsons/HarperCollins, 1996). For her newsletter, *What Doctors Don't Tell You:* 4 Wallace Road, London, N12PG, England.

5 "Study Suggests Common Heart Test May Harm Patients." Internet: CNN Interactive Heath Page (September 16, 1996).

6 Robbins, S. L., R. S. Cotran, and V. Kumar, eds. *Pathological Basis of Disease* (New York: W.B. Saunders, 1984).

7 This report is based solely on product labeling as published by PDR®. Copyright © 1993 by Medical Economics Data, a division of Medical Economics Company, Inc. All rights reserved. There is no affiliation between Medical Economics Company, Inc., and Future Medicine Publishing, Inc.

8 Jaffe, D., et al. "Coronary Arteries in Newborn Children: Intimal Variations in Longitudinal Sections and Their Relationships to Clinical and Experimental Data." *Acta Paediatrica Scandinavica Suppl.* 219 (1971), 3-28.

9 Rath, Matthias, M.D. *Eradicating Heart Disease* (San Francisco: Health Now, 1993). Available from: Health Now, 387 Ivy Street, San Francisco, CA 94102; tel 800-624-2442.

10 Ibid.

11 Kostner, G. M., et al. "The Interaction of Human Plasma Low Density Lipoproteins with Glycosamino-Glycans: Influence of the Chemical Composition." *Lipids* 20:1 (January 1985), 24-28.

12 Passwater, Richard. *Supernutrition for Healthy Hearts* (New York: Dial Press, 1977); Gordon, T., et al. *American Journal of Medicine* 62 (1977), 707-714; Williams, P. et al. *The Lancet*

1 (1979), 72-75.

13 Gruberg, E. R., and S.A. Raymond. *Beyond Cholesterol: Vitamin B6, Arteriosclerosis, and Your Heart* (New York: St. Martin's Press, 1981), 34-35.

14 *British Heart Journal* 29:337 (1967).

15 Kostner, G. M., et al. "HMG CoA Reductase Inhibitors Lower LDL Cholesterol Without Reducing Lp(a) Levels." *Circulation* 80:5 (1989), 1313-1319.

16 Strandberg, T. E., et al. "Long-term Mortality after 5-year Multi-Factorial Primary Prevention of Cardiovascular Diseases in Middle-Aged Men." *Journal of the American Medical Association* 266:9 (September 1991),1225-1229.

17 Folkers, K., et al. "Lovastatin Decreases Coenzyme-Q Levels in Humans." *Proceedings of the National Academy of Sciences of the USA* 87:22 (November 1990), 8931-8934.

18 Public Citizen Health Research Group. *Health Letter* (April 1994).

19 Morris, R. D., et al. "Chlorination, Chlorination Byproducts, and Cancer: A Meta-Analysis." *American Journal of Public Health* 82:7 (July 1992), 955-963.

20 Morin, R. J., and S.K. Peng. "The Role of Cholesterol Oxidation Products in the Pathogenesis of Atherosclerosis." *Annals of Clinical and Laboratory Science* 19:4 (July/August 1989), 225-237.

21 Hattersley, J. G. "Acquired Atherosclerosis: Theories of Causation, Novel Therapies." *Journal of Orthomolecular Medicine* 6:2 (1991), 83-98.

22 Morin, R. J., and S.K. Peng. "The Role of Cholesterol Oxidation Products in the Pathogenesis of Atherosclerosis." *Annals of Clinical and Laboratory Science* 19:4 (July/August 1989), 225-237.

23 McCully, K. S. "Homocysteine Theory of Arteriosclerosis: Development and Current Status." *Atherosclerosis Reviews* 11 (1983), 157-246.

24 Morris, R. D., et al. "Chlorination, Chlorination Byproducts, and Cancer: A Meta-Analysis." *American Journal of Public Health* 82:7 (July 1992), 955-963; Yiamouiannis, J. *Fluoride: The Aging Factor: How to Recognize and Avoid the*

Devastating Effects of Fluoride (Delaware, OH: Health Action Press, 1986).

25 McCully, K. S. "Homocysteine Theory of Arteriosclerosis: Development and Current Status." *Atherosclerosis Reviews* 11 (1983), 157-246.

26 Morin, R. J., and S.K. Peng. "The Role of Cholesterol Oxidation Products in the Pathogenesis of Atherosclerosis." *Annals of Clinical and Laboratory Science* 19:4 (July/August 1989), 225-237.

27 Malinow, M. R. "Risk for Arterial Occlusive Disease: Is Hyperhomocysteinemia an Innocent Bystander?" *Canadian Journal of Cardiology* 17 (1989), x-xi; Stampfer, M. J., et al. "A Prospective Study of Plasma Homocysteine and Risk of Myocardial Infarction in U.S. Physicians." *Journal of the American Medical Association* 268:7 (August 1992), 877-881.

28 Barnes, Broda O., M.D., and Lawrence Galton. *Hypothyroidism: The Unsuspected Illness* (New York: Harper & Row, 1976).

29 Peng, S. K. and C.B. Taylor. "Cholesterol Autooxidation, Health and Arteriosclerosis." *World Reviews of Nutrition and Diet* 44 (1984), 117-154.

30 McCully, Kilmer S., M.D. *The Homocysteine Revolution: Medicine for the New Millennium* (New Canaan, CT: Keats Publishing, 1997).

31 Nehler, Mark, M.D., et al., "Homocysteinemia as a Risk Factor for Atherosclerosis: A Review." *Cardiovascular Pathology* 6 (1997), 1-9.

32 Queen, H.L. *Chronic Mercury Toxicity: New Hope Against an Endemic Disease* (Colorado Springs, CO: Queen and Company, 1988).

Chapter 2

Caring for Yourself: Use Diet, Exercise, and Lifestyle Changes to Improve Your Heart Fitness

1 *Circulation* 89:94 (January 1994).

2 *Science* 264:532 (April 22, 1994).

3 *American Journal of Clinical Nutrition* 59:861 (April 1994); *Medical Journal of Australia* 156:Suppl. (May 4, 1992), S9-S16.

4 Schwartz, Elizabeth. "Misunderstood Soy May Lower Cholesterol." Internet: CNN Interactive Fitness & Heath Page (August 2, 1996).

5 "Veggies Fight Heart Disease, Cancer, Study Finds," Internet: Reuters via Individual, Inc. (June 20, 1997).

6 Ornish, Dean, M.D. *Dr. Dean Ornish's Program for Reversing Heart Disease* (New York: Ballantine, 1990).

7 Ibid.

8 "Chocolate May Help Reduce Heart Disease, Study Suggests." Internet: CNN Interactive Heath Page (September 20, 1996).

9 *The Lancet* 344:8933 (November 1994), 1356.

10 Hertog, M.G., et al. "Antioxidant Flavonols and Coronary Heart Disease Risk." *The Lancet* 349:699 (1997).

11 Nash, David T. "Grapeseed Oil Increases High Density Lipoprotein Cholesterol Levels in Dyslipidemic Subjects with Initially Low Levels." *Arteriosclerosis* 10:6 (Nov/Dec 1990). Nash, David T. et al. "Grapeseed Oil, A Natural Agent Which Raises Serum HDL Levels." *Journal of the American College of Cardiology* (March 1993). Huttunen, Jussi K., et al. "The Helsinki Heart Study: Central Findings and Clinical Implications." *Annals of Medicine* 23 (1991), 155-159. Feldman, Henry A. et al. "Impotence and Its Medical and Psychosocial Correlates: Results of the Massachusetts Male Aging Study." *Journal of Urology* 151 (January 1994), 54-61. Humer, Valentin. "Grapeseed Oil: The Champagne of Cooking Oils." *Healthy & Natural Journal* 2:3 (1995), 74-76. Kamen, Betty, Ph.D., "Natural Nutrition: Grapeseed Oil." *Let's Live* 62:12 (December 1994).

12 *American College of Cardiology*, March 14-18, 1993.

13 "Special Report: Olive Oil." *UC Berkeley Wellness Letter* (June 1995), 6. Sinatra, Stephen T., M.D. *Optimum Health: A Natural Lifesaving Prescription for Your Body and Mind* (New York: Bantam Books, 1997). Visioli, Francesco, et al. "Low Density Lipoprotein Oxidation is Inhibited In Vitro by Olive Oil Constituents." *Atherosclerosis* 117 (1995), 25-32. Staninger, Hildegarde L.A., Ph.D. *Olive Oil: Its Medicinal Uses for a Healthier You*. Monograph, (1996). Sharhil, Ltd., International Institute of Medical Toxicology, 2699 Lee Road, Suite 303, Winter Park, FL 32789; tel: 407-628-3399; fax: 407-628-1061.

14 Key, Timothy J.A., et al. "Dietary Habits and Mortality in 11,000 Vegetarians and Health Conscious People: Results of a 17-Year Follow Up." *British Medical Journal* 313 (1996), 775-779.

15 Gruberg, E. R., and S.A. Raymond. *Beyond Cholesterol: Vitamin B6, Arteriosclerosis, and Your Heart* (New York: St.Martin's Press, 1981).

16 Ornish, Dean, M.D., et al. "Can Lifestyle Changes Reverse Coronary Heart Disease? The Lifestyle Heart Trial." *The Lancet* 336:8708 (July 1990), 129-133.

17 Halsey, Eugenia. "Researchers Pinpoint Link Between Smoking and Heart Disease." Internet: CNN Interactive Main Food & Heath Page (May 3, 1996).

18 Ciampa, Linda. "Study: Passive Smoke and Even Greater Risk." Internet: CNN Interactive Heath Page (May 19, 1997).

19 Halsey, Eugenia. "Researchers Pinpoint Link Between Smoking and Heart Disease." Internet: CNN Interactive Main Food & Heath Page (May 3, 1996).

20 Hinman, Al. "Studies Show Wine, Beer and Grape Juice Help Prevent Heart Disease." Internet: CNN Interactive Fitness and Health Page (March 18, 1997).

21 Ibid.

22 Stuttaford, Thomas, M.D. "Exercise is at the Heart of the Matter." *The Times* (April 17, 1997).

23 Kahn, Jason. "Study Says Reduced Exercise, Not Age, Hurts Heart." *Medical Tribune News Service* (April 18, 1996).

24 Verrill, David E., and Paul M. Ribisl. "Resistive Exercise Training and Cardiac Rehabilitation." *Sports Medicine* 21:5 (May 1996), 347-383.

25 Woolf-May, Kathryn, et al. "Effects of an 18-Week Walking Programme on Cardiac Function in Previously Sedentary or Relatively Inactive Adults." *British Journal of Sports Medicine* 31 (1997), 48-53.

26 *Journal of the American Medical Association* 275:18 (May 8, 1996).

27 Lomama, E., et al. "Rehabilitation of Aged Patients with Bicycle Ergometer after Coronary Surgery." *Archives des Maladies du Coeur et des Vaisseaux* 89:11 (1996), 1351-1355.

28 Meyer, Katharina, Ph.D. "Effects of Short-Term Exercise Training and Activity Restriction on Functional Capacity in Patients with Severe Chronic Congestive Heart Failure." *American Journal of Cardiology* 78 (November 1, 1996), 1017-1022.

29 Rafoth, Richard, M.D. *Bicycling Fuel* (Osceola, WI: Bicycle Books, 1988); Robertson, Gary. "Exercise Goes High-Tech." *Richmond Times-Dispatch* (February 6, 1997).

Chapter 3

Scrubbing the Arteries Naturally: How Chelation Therapy Can Help Prevent and Treat Heart Disease

1 Farr, C. H., M.D., R. White, and M. Schachter, M.D. "Chronological History of EDTA Chelation Therapy." Presented to the American College of Advancement in Medicine, Houston, TX (May 1993).

2 Olszewer, E., and J. Carter. "EDTA Chelation Therapy: A Retrospective Study of 2,870 Patients." *Journal of Advancement in Medicine* Special Issue 2:1-2 (1989), 209.

3 McDonagh, E., C. Rudolph, and E. Cheraskin. "An Oculocerebrovasculometric Analysis of the Improvement in Arterial Stenosis Following EDTA Chelation Therapy." *Journal of Advancement in Medicine* Special Issue 2:1-2 (1989), 155.

4 Chappell, L. Terry, M.D., and John P. Stahl, Ph.D. *Questions from the Heart* (Charlottesville, VA: Hampton Roads Publishing, 1996).

5 Olszewer, E., and J. Carter. "EDTA Chelation Therapy: A Retrospective Study of 2,870 Patients." *Journal of Advancement in Medicine* Special Issue 2:1-2 (1989), 183.

6 Walker, M., and G. Gordon. *The Chelation Answer: How to Prevent Hardening of the Arteries and Rejuvenate Your Cardiovascular System* (New York: M. Evans and Company, 1982).

7 Olszewer, E., and J.P. Carter. "EDTA Chelation Therapy in Chronic Degenerative Disease." *Medical Hypotheses* 27:1 (September 1988), 41-49.

8 Cranton, E. M., M.D. "Protocol of the American College of Advancement in Medicine for the Safe and Effective Administration of Intravenous EDTA Chelation Therapy." *Journal of Advancement in Medicine* Special Issue 2:1-2 (1989), 269-305.

9 Walker, M. *Chelation Therapy* (Stamford, CT: New Way of Life, 1984).

10 Olszewer, E., and J. Carter. "EDTA Chelation Therapy: A Retrospective Study of 2,870 Patients." *Journal of Advancement in Medicine* Special Issue 2:1-2 (1989), 197-211.

11 Ibid.

12 McDonagh, E. W., C. J. Rudolph, and E. Cheraskin, M.D. "An Oculocerebrovasculometric Analysis of the Improvement in Arterial Stenosis Following EDTA Chelation Therapy." *Journal of Advancement in Medicine* Special Issue 2:1-2 (1989), 155-166.

13 Alsleben, H. R., M.D., and W. E. Shute, M.D. *How to Survive the New Health Catastrophes* (Anaheim, CA: Survival Publications, 1973).

14 McDonagh, E. W., C. J. Rudolph, and E. Cheraskin, M.D. "An Oculocerebrovasculometric Analysis of the Improvement in Arterial Stenosis Following EDTA Chelation Therapy." *Journal of Advancement in Medicine* Special Issue 2:1-2 (1989), 155-166.

15 Casdorph, H. R., M.D. "EDTA Chelation Therapy: Efficacy in Brain Disorders." *Journal of Advancement in Medicine* Special Issue 2:1-2 (1989), 131-153.

16 Alsleben, H. R., M.D., and W. E. Shute, M.D. *How to Survive the New Health Catastrophes* (Anaheim, CA: Survival Publications, 1973).

17 Blumer, W., M.D., and E. M. Cranton, M.D. "Ninety Percent Reduction in Cancer Mortality After Chelation Therapy with EDTA." *Journal of Advancement in Medicine* Special Issue 2:1-2 (1989), 183.

18 Alsleben, H. R., M.D., and W. E. Shute, M.D. *How to Survive the New Health Catastrophes* (Anaheim, CA: Survival Publications, 1973).

19 Ibid.

20 Chappel, T. L., M.D. "Preliminary Findings From the Media Analysis Study of EDTA Chelation Therapy." Presented to the American College of Advancement in Medicine, Houston, TX (May 5-9, 1993).

21 Walker, M., and G. Gordon. *The Chelation Answer* (New York: M. Evans and Company, 1982), 175.

22 Tu, Jack V., et al. "Use of Cardiac Procedures and Outcomes in Elderly Patients with Myocardial Infarction in the United States and Canada." *New England Journal of Medicine* 336:21 (May 22, 1997).

23 Maugh, T.H. "Invasive Heart Attack Treatment Questioned." *Los Angeles Times (*March 20, 1997).

24 Whitaker, Julian, M.D., "Heart Surgery Does More Harm Than Good." *Dr. Julian Whitaker's Health & Healing* 7:5 (May 1997), 1-3.

25 Strauts, Z., M.D. "Correspondence Re: Berkeley Wellness Letter and Chelation Therapy." *Townsend Letter for Doctors* 106 (May 1992), 382-383.

Chapter 4

The Dental Connection: Problems With Your Teeth Can Affect Your Heart— and How to Reverse Them

1 Neuner, O. "The Diagnosis and Therapy of Focal and Field Disorders." *Raum & Zeit* 2:4 (1991), 38-42.

2 Price, W. A. *Dental Infections Volume 1: Oral and Systemic* (Cleveland, OH: Benton Publishing, 1973).

3 Strauss, F. G., and D. W. Eggleston. "IgA Nephropathy Associated with Dental Nickel Alloy Sensitization." *American Journal of Nephrology* 5 (1985), 395-397.

4 "Dental Mercury Hygiene: Summary of Recommendations in 1990." *Journal of the American Dental Association* 122 (August 1991), 112.

5 "Dental Amalgam: A Scientific Review and Recommended Public Health Service Strategy for Research, Education and Regulation." *Final Report of the Subcommittee on Risk Management of the Committee to Coordinate Environmental Health and Related Programs* (Washington: U.S. Public Health Service, 1993).

6 "Dental Mercury Hygiene: Summary of Recommendations in 1990." *Journal of the American Dental Association* 122 (August 1991), 112.

7 Melillo, W. "How Safe is Mercury in Dentistry?" *The Washington Post Weekly Journal of Medicine, Science and Society* (September 1991), 4.

8 World Health Organization. *Environmental Health Criteria for Inorganic Mercury* 118 (Geneva: World Health Organization, 1991).

9 Hahn, L. J., et al. "Dental 'Silver' Tooth Fillings: A Source of Mercury Exposure Revealed by Whole-Body Image Scan and Tissue Analysis." *FASEB Journal* 3 (1989), 2641-2646; Hahn, L. J., et al. "Whole-Body Imaging of the Distribution of Mercury Released from Dental Fillings into Monkey Tissues." *FASEB Journal* 4 (1990), 3256-3260.

10 Vimy, M. J., et al. "Maternal-Fetal Distribution of Mercury Released from Dental Amalgam Fillings." *American Physiological Society* 258 (1990), R939-R945.

11 For the key research on mercury dental amalgam toxicity, consult: Lorscheider, Fritz, et al. "Mercury Exposure from 'Silver' Tooth Fillings: Emerging Evidence Questions a Traditional Dental Paradigm," *FASEB Journal* 9 (1995), 504-508. Huggins, Hal, D.D.S. *Coors Study: A Landmark in Dental Research*, a video, P.O. Box 49145, Colorado Springs, CO 80949; tel: 719-522-0566; fax: 719-548-8220; website: http://www.hugnet.com. Lichtenberg, H. "Mercury Vapor in the Oral Cavity in Relation to the Number of Amalgam Surfaces and the Classic Symptoms of Chronic Mercury Poisoning." *Journal of Orthomolecular Medicine* 11:2 (Second Quarter 1996), 87-94. See all issues of *Heavy Metal Bulletin: International Forum Focusing on Immuno-Toxic Effects of*

Dental Fillings and Related Disorders (Lilla Aspuddvs. 10, S-12649 Hägersten, Stockholm, Sweden; tel & fax: 46-8-184086; $65 U.S./3 issues). Richardson, G. Mark, Ph.D. *Assessment of Mercury Exposure and Risks from Dental Amalgam* (Medical Devices Bureau, Environmental Health Directorate, Health Canada, August 18, 1995).

12 Ziff, S. "Consolidated Symptom Analysis of 1,569 Patients." *Bio-Probe Newsletter* 9:2 (March 1993), 7-8.

13 Grandjean, P., M.D. "Reference Intervals for Trace Elements in Blood: Significance of Risk Factors." *Scandinavian Journal of Clinical and Laboratory Investigation* 2 (June 1992), 321-337; Schiele, R., et al. *Studies on the Mercury Content in Brain and Kidney Related to Number and Condition of Amalgam Fillings* (Nurnberg, West Germany: Institution of Occupational and Social Medicine, University Erlangen, 1984); Boyd, N. D., et al. "Mercury from Dental 'Silver' Tooth Fillings Impairs Sheep Kidney Function." *American Physiological Society* 261 (1991), R1010-R1014.

Chapter 5

Nutritional Supplements: How They Can Benefit Your Heart

1 Street, D. A., et al. "A Population-Based Case Control Study of the Association of Serum Antioxidants and Myocardial Infarction." *American Journal of Epidemiology* 131 (1991), 719-720.

2 Harvard Physicians Study. Ongoing.

3 Berge, K. G., and P. L. Canner. "Coronary Drug Project: Experience with Niacin. Coronary Drug Project Research Group." *European Journal of Clinical Pharmacology* 40:Suppl.1 (1991), S49-S51; Luria, M. H. "Effect of Low-Dose Niacin on High-Density Lipoprotein Cholesterol and Total Cholesterol/High-Density Lipoprotein Ratio." *Archives of Internal Medicine* 148:11 (November 1988), 2493-2495.

4 Canner, P. L., et al. "Fifteen Year Mortality in Coronary Drug Project Patients; Long-Term Benefit with Niacin." *Journal of the American College of Cardiology* 8:6 (December 1986), 1245-1255.

5 Hattersley, J. G. "Heart Attacks and Strokes." *Townsend Letter for Doctors* 104 (February/March 1992).

6 Berge, K. G., and P. L. Canner. "Coronary Drug Project: Experience with Niacin. Coronary Drug Project Research Group." *European Journal of*

Clinical Pharmacology 40:Suppl.1 (1991), S49-S51.

7 Olszewski, A. J., et al. "Reduction of Plasma Lipid and Homocysteine Levels by Pyridoxine, Folate, Cobalamin, Choline, Riboflavin, and Troxerutin in Atherosclerosis." *Atherosclerosis* 75:1 (January 1989), 1-6.

8 Mudd, S. H., et al. "The Natural History of Homocystinuria Due to Cystathionine Beta-Synthose Deficiency." *American Journal of Human Genetics* 37:1 (January 1985), 1-31.

9 Editorial. "Is Vitamin B6 an Antithrombotic Agent?" *The Lancet* 1:8233 (June 1981),1299-1300.

10 Suzman, M. M. "Effect of Pyridoxine and Low Animal Protein Diet in Coronary Artery Disease." *Circulation* Suppl. IV-254 (October 1973), Abstracts of the 46th Scientific Sessions.

11 Ibid.

12 McCully, K. S. "Homocysteine Theory of Arteriosclerosis: Development and Current Status." *Atherosclerosis Reviews* 11 (1983), 157-246.

13 Ibid.

14 Brattstrom, L., et al. "Higher Total Plasma Homocysteine Due to Cystathionine Beta-Synthase Deficiency." *Metabolism: Clinical and Experimental* 37:2 (February 1988), 175-178.

15 Ibid.

16 Olszewski, A. J., et al. "Reduction of Plasma Lipid and Homocysteine Levels by Pyridoxine, Folate, Cobalamin, Choline, Riboflavin, and Troxerutin in Atherosclerosis." *Atherosclerosis* 75:1 (January 1989),1-6.

17 Brattstrom, L., et al. "Impaired Homocysteine Metabolism in Early-Onset Cerebral and Peripheral Occlusive Artery Disease. Effects of Pyridoxine and Folic Acid Treatment." *Atherosclerosis* 81:1 (1990), 51-60; Olszewski, A. J., et al. "Reduction of Plasma Lipid and Homocysteine Levels by Pyridoxine, Folate, Cobalamin, Choline, Riboflavin, and Troxerutin in Atherosclerosis." *Atherosclerosis* 75:1 (January 1989), 1-6.

18 Rimm, E., et al. "Vitamin E Consumption and the Risk of Coronary Heart Disease in Men." *New England Journal of Medicine* 328:20 (May 1993), 1450-1456; Stampfer, M. J., et al. "Vitamin E Consumption and the Risk of Coronary Heart Disease in Women." *New England Journal of Medicine* 328:20 (May 1993), 1444-1449.

19 McCully, K. S. "Homocysteine Metabolism in Scurvy, Growth, and Arteriosclerosis." *Nature*

231:5302 (June 1971), 391-392.

20 Rath, M., and L. Pauling. "Hypothesis: Lipoprotein(a) is a Surrogate for Ascorbate." *Proceedings of the National Academy of Sciences of the U.S.A.* 87:16 (August 1990), 6204-6207.

21 Ginter, E. R., et al. "Vitamin C in the Control of Hypercholesterolemia in Man." *International Journal for Vitamin and Nutrition Research* 23:Suppl. (1982), 137-152.

22 Rath, M., and L. Pauling. "Solution to the Puzzle of Human Cardiovascular Disease: Its Primary Cause is Ascorbate Deficiency Leading to the Deposition of Lipoprotein(a) and Fibrinogen/Fibrin in the Vascular Wall." *Journal of Orthomolecular Medicine* 6 (1991), 125-134.

23 Rath, M., and L. Pauling. "Hypothesis: Lipoprotein(a) is a Surrogate for Ascorbate." *Proceedings of the National Academy of Sciences of the U.S.A.* 87:16 (August 1990), 6204-6207.

24 Rath, M., and L. Pauling. "Solution to the Puzzle of Human Cardiovascular Disease: Its Primary Cause is Ascorbate Deficiency Leading to the Deposition of Lipoprotein(a) and Fibrinogen/Fibrin in the Vascular Wall." *Journal of Orthomolecular Medicine* 6 (1991), 125-134.

25 Enstrom, J. E., et al. "Vitamin C Intake and Mortality Among a Sample of the United States Population." *Epidemiology* 3 (1992), 194-202.

26 Sahyoun, Nadine R., et al. "Carotenoids, Vitamins C and E and Mortality in an Elderly Population." *American Journal of Epidemiology* 144:5 (September 1, 1996), 501-511.

27 Jialal, I., and S. M. Grundy. "Effect of Dietary Supplementation with Alpha-Tocopherol on the Oxidative Modification of Low Density Lipoprotein." *Journal of Lipid Research* 33:6 (June 1992), 899-906; Steiner, M. "Influence of Vitamin E on Platelet Function in Humans." *Journal of the American College of Nutrition* 10:5 (October 1991), 466-473.

28 Boscoboinik, D., et al. "Alpha-Tocopherol (Vitamin E) Regulates Vascular Smooth Muscle Cell Proliferation and Protein Kinase C Activity." *Archives of Biochemistry and Biophysics* 286:1 (April 1991), 264-269; Hennig, B., et al. "Protective Effects of Vitamin E in Age-Related Endothelial Cell Injury." *International Journal of Vitamin and Nutrition Research* 59 (1989), 273-279.

29 Rimm, E., et al. "Vitamin E Consumption and the Risk of Coronary Heart Disease in Men." *New England Journal of Medicine* 328:20 (May 1993), 1450-1456; Stampfer, M. J., et al. "Vitamin E Consumption and the Risk of Coronary Heart Disease in Women." *New England Journal of Medicine* 328:20 (May 1993), 1444-1449.

30 Stampfer, M., et al. "Vitamin E and Heart Disease Incidence in the Nurses Health Study." American Heart Association Annual Meeting. New Orleans, LA (November 18, 1992).

31 Rimm, E., et al. "Vitamin E and Heart Disease Incidence in the Health Professionals Study." American Heart Association Annual Meeting, New Orleans, LA (November 18, 1992).

32 Kushi, L.H., et al. "Dietary Antioxidant Vitamins and Death from Coronary Heart Disease in Postmenopausal Women" *New England Journal of Medicine* 334:18 (May 2, 1996), 1156-1162.

33 Gey, K. F., et al. "Inverse Correlation Between Plasma Vitamin E and Mortality from Ischemic Heart Disease in Cross-Cultural Epidemiology." *American Journal of Clinical Nutrition* 53:Suppl. 1 (January 1991), 326S-334S.

34 Stephens, Nigel G., et al. "Randomized Controlled Trial of Vitamin E in Patients with Coronary Artery Disease: Cambridge Heart Antioxidant Study (CHAOS)." *The Lancet* (March 23, 1996), 781-786.

35 Jialal, I., et al. "The Effect of Alpha-Tocopherol Supplementation on LDL Oxidation: A Dose-Response Study." *Arteriosclerosis, Thrombosis, and Vascular Biology* 15 (1995), 190-198.

36 *The Diet-Heart Newsletter* 7:1 (Winter 1994), 2.

37 Karanja, N., et al. "Plasma Lipids and Hypertension: Response to Calcium Supplementation." *American Journal of Clinical Nutrition* 45:1 (January 1987), 60-65.

38 Leifsson, Bjorn G., M.D., and Bo Ahren. "Serum Calcium and Survival in a Large Health Screening Program." *Journal of Clinical Endocrinology and Metabolism* 81:6 (1996), 2149-2153.

39 Simonoff, M, et al. "Low Plasma Chromium in Patients with Coronary Artery and Heart Diseases." *Biological Trace Elements Research* 6:5 (October 1984), 431-439; Newman, H. A., et al. "Serum Chromium and Angiographically Determined Coronary Artery Disease." *Clinical Chemistry* 24:4 (April 1978), 541-544.

40 Press, R. I., et al. "The Effect of Chromium Picolinate on Serum Cholesterol and Apolipoprotein Fractions in Human Subjects."

Western Journal of Medicine 152:1 (January 1990), 41-45.

41 Urberg, M., et al. "Hypercholesterolemic Effects of Nicotinic Acid and Chromium Supplementation." Journal of Family Practice 27:6 (December 1988), 603-606.

42 Wood, D. A., et al. "Adipose Tissue and Platelet Fatty Acids and Coronary Heart Disease in Scottish Men." The Lancet 2:8395 (July 1984), 117-121.

43 Ferneandes, J.S., et al. "Therapeutic Effect of a Magnesium Salt in Patients Suffering from Mitral Valvular Prolapse and Latent Tentany." Magnesium 4 (1985), 283-290.

44 Lichodziejewsa, B., et al. "Clinical Symptoms of Mitral Valve Prolapse Are Related to Hypomagnesemia and Attenuated by Magnesium Supplementation." American Journal of Cardiology 79 (1997), 768-772.

45 Seelig, M. S., and H. A. Heggtveit. "Magnesium Interrelationships in Ischemic Heart Disease: A Review." American Journal of Clinical Nutrition 27:1 (January 1974), 59-79; Davis, W. H., et al. "Monotherapy with Magnesium Increases Abnormally Low Density Lipoprotein Cholesterol: A Clinical Assay." Current Therapeutic Research 36:2 (August 1984), 341.

46 Northeast Center for Environmental Medicine Health Letter (Fall 1992).

47 Salonen, J. T., et al. "Interactions of Serum Copper, Selenium and Low Density Lipoprotein Cholesterol in Atherogenesis." British Medical Journal 302:6779 (March 1991), 756-760.

48 Stead, N. W., et al. "Effect of Selenium Supplementation on Selenium Balance in the Dependent Elderly." American Journal of the Medical Sciences 290:6 (December 1985), 228-233.

49 Koifman, Bella, M.D. "Improvement of Cardiac Performance by Intravenous Infusion of L-Arginine in Patients with Moderate Congestive Heart Failure." Journal of the American College of Cardiology 26:5 (November 1, 1995), 1251-1256.

50 Singh, R. B. "A Randomized, Double-Blind, Placebo-Controlled Trial of L-Carnitine in Suspected Acute Myocardial Infarction." Postgraduate Medical Journal (1995).

51 Iliceto, Sabino, M.D. "Effects of L-Carnitine Administration on Left Ventricular Remodeling after Acute Anterior Myocardial Infarction." American Journal of Cardiology 26:2 (1995), 380-387.

52 Kneki, Paul. "Flavonoid Intake and Coronary Mortality in Finland: A Cohort Study." British Medical Journal 312 (1996), 478-481.

53 Hanaki, Y., S. Sugiyama, and T. Ozawa. "Ratio of Low-Density Lipoprotein Cholesterol to Ubiquinone as a Coronary Risk Factor." New England Journal of Medicine 325:11 (September 1991), 814-815; Frei, B., et al. "Ubiquinol-10 Is an Effective Lipid-Soluble Antioxidant at Physiological Concentrations." Proceedings of the National Academy of Sciences of the U.S.A. 87:12 (1990), 4879-4883.

54 The Energy Times (January/February 1995), 12, 56; Cancer Communication Newsletter 1:1 (February 1995), 11; Information provided by Michael B. Schacter, M.D. Dr. Jonathan Wright's Nutrition & Healing Newsletter 1:1 (August 1994), 3-4.

55 New England Journal of Medicine 312 (1985), 1250-1259.

56 Atherosclerosis 63 (1987), 137-143; Hypertension 4:Suppl. (1982), iii-34.

57 Olszewski, A. J., and K. S. McCully. "Fish Oil Decreases Serum Homocysteine in Hyperlipemic Men." Coronary Artery Disease 4 (1993), 53-60.

58 Kromhout, D., et al. "The Inverse Relation Between Fish Consumption and 20-Year Mortality From Coronary Heart Disease." New England Journal of Medicine 312:19 (May 1985), 1205-1209.

59 Renaud, S., and A. Nordy. "'Small is Beautiful': Alpha-Linoleic Acid and Eicosapentaenoic Acid in Man." The Lancet 1:8334 (May 1983), 1169.

60 Rosenbaum, M. E., M.D., and D. Bosco. Super Fitness Beyond Vitamins: The Bible of Super Supplements (New York: New American Library, 1987).

61 Crayhon, Robert. Health Benefits of FOS (New Canaan, CT: Keats Publishing, 1995).

62 Pao, E. M., and S. Mickle. "Problem Nutrients in the United States." Food Technology (September 1981), 58-79.

63 "Dietary Intake Source Data: U.S. 1976-1980." Data from the National Health Survey Series 11 #231. (DHHS Publication (PHS) 8361, March 1983).

64 Yankelovich, Clancy, and Schulman. "Survey for Nutritional Health Alliance 1992." Whole Foods Magazine 16:3 (March 1993), 55.

Chapter 6

How Herbs Can Aid Your Heart

1 Herb Trade Association. Definition of "Herb." (Austin, TX: Herb Trade Association, 1977).

2 Henry, C. J., and B. Emery. "Effect of Spiced Food on Metabolic Rate. Human Nutrition." *Clinical Nutrition* 40:2 (March 1986), 165-168.

3 Glatzel, H. "Blood Circulation Effectiveness of Natural Spices." *Medizinische Klinik* 62:51 (December 1967), 1987-1989. (Published in German).

4 Barrie, S. A., J. V. Wright, M.D., and J. E. Pizzorno. "Effect of Garlic Oil on Platelet Aggregation, Serum Lipids and Blood Pressure in Humans." *Journal of Orthomolecular Medicine* 2:1 (1987), 15-21.

5 Shoji, N., et al. "Cardiotonic Principles of Ginger (Zingiber officinale Roscoe)." *Journal of Pharmaceutical Sciences* 71:10 (October 1982), 1174-1175.

6 Srivastava, K. C. "Effects of Aqueous Extracts of Onion, Garlic and Ginger on Platelet Aggregation and Metabolism of Arachidonic Acid in the Blood Vascular System." *Prostaglandins Leukotrienes and Medicine* 13 (1984), 227-235.

7 Foster, S. *Ginkgo. Botanical Series 304* (Austin, TX: American Botanical Council, 1991).

8 Kleijnen, J., and P. Knipschild. "*Ginkgo biloba.*" *The Lancet* 340:8828 (November 1992), 1136-1139.

9 Braquet, P., ed. *Ginkgolides—Chemistry, Biology, Pharmacology and Clinical Perspectives*, Volume 1 (Barcelona, Spain: J. Prous Science Publishers, 1988) and Volume 2 (1989); Fungfeld, E. W., ed. *Rokan: Ginkgo biloba* (New York: Springer-Verlag, 1988).

10 *Arzneimittel-Forschung* 43:9 (September 1993), 978.

11 Weiss, R. F. *Herbal Medicine* (Gothenburg, Sweden: A. B. Arcanum, 1988).

12 Walker, Morton, D.P.M. "Antimicrobial Attributes of Olive Leaf Extract." *Townsend Letter for Doctors & Patients* (July 1996), 80-85; Renis, Harold E. "In Vitro Antiviral Activity of Calcium Elenolate." *Antimicrobial Agents and Chemotherapy-1969* (1970), 167-171; Juven, B., et al. "Studies on the Mechanism of the Antimicrobial Action of Oleuropein." *Journal of Applied Bacteriology* 35 (1972), 559-567; Konlee, Mark. "The Olive Leaf: A Sign from Above?" *Positive Health News* 11 (May 1996) [from: Keep Hope Alive, P.O. Box 27041, West Allis, WI 53227; tel: 414-548-4344].

13 Ficarra, Paola, and Rita Ficarra. "HPLC Analysis of Oleuropein and Some Flavonoids in Leaf and Bud of *Olea Europea L.*" *Il Farmaco* 46:6 (1991), 803-815.

14 Visioli, Francesco, and Claudio Gaili. "Oleuropein Protects Low Density Lipoprotein from Oxidation." *Life Sciences* 55:24 (1994), 1965-1971.

15 Farnsworth, N. R., et. al. "Medicinal Plants in Therapy." *Bulletin of the World Health Organization* 63:6 (1985), 965-981; reprinted in *Classic Botanical Reprint* 212 (Austin, Texas: American Botanical Council).

16 Ibid.

17 "New Health and Medical Findings from Around the World." *Life Extension Magazine* 14:12 (December 1994), 99-103.

Chapter 7

Other Alternatives for Heart Health

1 Becker, R. O., M.D. *Cross Currents: The Promise of Electromedicine, The Perils of Electropollution* (Los Angeles: Jeremy P. Tarcher, 1990).

2 Davis, A. R., and W. C. Rawls. *Magnetism and Its Effects on the Living System* (New York: Exposition Press, 1974).

3 Becker, R. O., M.D. *Cross Currents: The Promise of Electromedicine, The Perils of Electropollution* (Los Angeles: Jeremy P. Tarcher, 1990), 187.

4 Nakagawa, K., M.D. "Magnetic Field Deficiency Syndrome and Magnetic Treatment." *Japan Medical Journal* 2745 (December 1976).

5 Philpott, William H., M.D. *Diabetes Mellitus: A Reversible Disease* (an unpublished monograph).

6 Philpott, W., and S. Taplin. *Biomagnetic Handbook* (Choctaw, OK: Enviro-Tech Products, 1990).

7 Farr, C. H. *The Therapeutic Use of Intravenous Hydrogen Peroxide* Monograph. (Oklahoma City, OK: Genesis Medical Center, 1987).

8 Ibid.

9 Chung, H. Y. "Treatment of 103 Cases of Coronary Diseases with *Ilex pubescens.*" *Chinese Medical Journal* 1 (1973), 64.

Chapter 8

What Causes High Blood Pressure?

1 American Heart Association Internet web site: http://www.amhrt.org/hs96/hbps.html.

2 Havlik, R. J., et al. "Weight and Hypertension." *Annals of Internal Medicine* 98:5 pt. 2 (May 1983), 855-859.

3 Egan, K. J., et al. "The Impact of Psychological Distress on the Control of Hypertension." *Journal of Human Stress* 9:4 (December 1983), 4-10.

4 Gruchow, H. W., et al. "Alcohol, Nutrient Intake, and Hypertension in U.S. Adults." *Journal of the American Medical Association* 253:11 (March

1985), 1567-1570.

5 Pizzorno, J. E., and M. T. Murray, eds. "Hypertension." *A Textbook of Natural Medicine* (Seattle, WA: John Bastyr Publications, 1988).

6 Chow, H. Y., et al. "Cardiovascular Effects of Gardenia Florida L. (*Gardenie Fructus*) Extract." *American Journal of Chinese Medicine* 4:1 (1976), 47-51; Brewer, G. J. "Molecular Mechanisms of Zinc Action on Cells." *Agents and Actions* 8:Suppl. (1981), 37-49; Bennett, A. E., et al. "Sugar Consumption and Cigarette Smoking." *The Lancet* 1 (May 1970), 1011-1014; Kershbaum, A., et al. "Effects of Smoking and Nicotine on Adrenocortical Secretion." *Journal of the American Medical Association* 203:4 (January 1968), 275-278; Fortmann, S. P., et al. "The Association of Blood Pressure and Dietary Alcohol: Differences by Age, Sex and Estrogen Use." *American Journal of Epidemiology* 118:4 (October 1983), 497-507.

7 Pizzorno, J. E., and M. T. Murray, eds. "Hypertension." *A Textbook of Natural Medicine* (Seattle, WA: John Bastyr Publications, 1988).

8 He, J., et al. "Effect of Migration on Blood Pressure: The Yi People Study." *Epidemiology* 2:2 (March 1991), 88-97; Poulter, N. R., et al. "The Kenyan Luo Migration Study: Observations on the Initiation of a Rise in Blood Pressure." *British Medical Journal* 300:6730 (April 1990), 967-972; Salmond, C. E., et al. "Blood Pressure Patterns and Migration: A 14-Year Cohort Study of Adult Tokelauans." *American Journal of Epidemiology* 130:1 (July 1989), 37-52.

9 Meneely, G. R., and H. D. Battarbee. "High Sodium-Low Potassium Environment and Hypertension." *American Journal of Cardiology* 38:6 (November 1976), 768-785; Resnick, L. M., et al. "Intracellular Free Magnesium in Erythrocytes of Essential Hypertension: Relationship to Blood Pressure and Serum Divalent Cations." *Proceedings of the National Academy of Sciences of the U.S.A.* 81:20 (October 1984), 6511-6515.

10 Lang, T., et al. "Relation Between Coffee Drinking and Blood Pressure: Analysis of 6,321 Subjects in the Paris Region." *American Journal of Cardiology* 52:10 (December 1983), 1238-1242.

11 Fortmann, S. P., et al. "The Association of Blood Pressure and Dietary Alcohol: Differences by Age, Sex and Estrogen Use." *American Journal of Epidemiology* 118:4 (October 1983), 497-507; Gruchow, H. W., et al. "Alcohol, Nutrient Intake, and Hypertension in U.S. Adults." *Journal of the American Medical Association* 253:11 (March 1985), 1567-1570.

12 Bennett, A. E., et al. "Sugar Consumption and Cigarette Smoking." *The Lancet* 1 (May 1970), 1011-1014.

13 Schroeder, K. L., and M. S. Chen, Jr. "Smokeless Tobacco and Blood Pressure." *New England Journal of Medicine* 312:14 (April 1985), 919; Hampson, N. B. "Smokeless is Not Saltless." *New England Journal of Medicine* 312:14 (April 1985), 919-920.

14 Pirkle, J. L., et al. "The Relationship Between Blood Lead Levels and its Cardiovascular Risk Implications." *American Journal of Epidemiology* 121:2 (February 1985), 246-258.

15 Glauser, S. C., et al. "Blood-Cadmium Levels in Normotensive and Untreated Hypertensive Humans." *The Lancet* 1 (April 1976), 717-718.

16 *Science News* 148 (October 21, 1995), 268.

17 Barnes, Broda O., M.D., and Lawrence Galton. *Hypothyroidism: The Unsuspected Illness* (New York: Harper & Row, 1976).

Chapter 9

Self-Care Options: How to Use Diet, Exercise, and Lifestyle Changes to Lower Your Blood Pressure

1 Resnick, L. M., R. K. Gupta, and J. H. Laragh. "Intracellular Free Magnesium in Erythrocytes of Essential Hypertension: Relationship to Blood Pressure and Serum Divalent Cations." *Proceedings of the National Academy of Sciences of the U.S.A.* 81:20 (October 1984), 6511-6515.

2 Foushee, D. B., J. Ruffin, and U. Banerjee. "Garlic as a Natural Agent for the Treatment of Hypertension: A Preliminary Report." *Cytobios* 34:135-136 (1982), 145-152.

3 "Reducing Hypertension: Is Diet Better Than Drugs?" *Alternative & Complementary Therapies* 3:1 (February 1997), 3. (Available from: Mary Ann Liebert, Inc., 2 Madison Avenue, Larchmont, NY 10538; tel: 914-834-3100; fax: 914-834-3582; 6 issues/$79).

4 *Hypertension* 22:3 (September 1993), 371-379.

5 Gordon, Laura. "Exercise and Salt Restriction May Be Enough for Mildly High Blood Pressure." *Medical Tribune* 8 (December 21, 1995).

6 Merlo, Juan, et al. "Incidence of Myocardial Infarction in Elderly Men Being Treated with Antihypertensive Drugs: Population Based Cohort Study." *British Medical Journal* 313

(August 24, 1996), 457-461.

7 Altman, Lawrence K. "Use of Heart Drug Is Found To Increase the Risk of Death." *The New York Times* (November 1, 1995).

8 He, Jiang, et al. "Oats and Buckwheat Intakes and Cardiovascular Disease Risk Factors in an Ethnic Minority of China." *American Journal of Clinical Nutrition* 61 (1995), 366-372.

9 Pietinen, P., et al. "Intake of Dietary Fiber and Risk of Coronary Heart Disease in a Cohort of Finnish Men." *Circulation* 94:11 (December 1996), 2720-2727.

10 Davidson, M. H., et al. "The Hypocholesterolemic Effects of Beta-Glucan in Oatmeal and Oat Bran." *Journal of the American Medical Association* 265:14 (April 10, 1991), 1833-1839.

11 Van Horn, L.V., et al. "Serum Lipid Response to Oat Product Intake with a Fat-Modified Diet." *Journal of the American Dietetic Association* 86:6 (June 1986), 759-764.

12 Pick, Mary E., et al. "Oat Bran Concentrate Bread Products Improve Long-Term Control of Diabetes: A Pilot Study." *Journal of the American Dietetic Association* 96:12 (1996), 1254-1261.

13 Goldstein, I. B., et al. "Home Relaxation Techniques for Essential Hypertension." *Psychosomatic Medicine* 46:5 (September/October 1984), 398-414; Brassard, C., and R. T. Couture. "Biofeedback and Relaxation for Patients with Hypertension." *Canadian Nurse* 89:1 (January 1993), 49-52; Whyte, H. M. "NHMRC Workshop on Non-Pharmacological Methods of Lowering Blood Pressure." *Medical Journal of Australia* 2:1 Suppl. (July 1983), S13-S16; Blanchard, E.B., et al. "Preliminary Results from a Controlled Evaluation of Thermal Biofeedback as a Treatment for Essential Hypertension." *Biofeedback and Self Regulation* 9:4 (December 1984), 471-495.

14 The Joint National Committee on Detection, Evaluation, and Treatment of High Blood Pressure. "The 1988 Report of the Joint National Committee of the American Medical Association." *Archives of Internal Medicine* 148 (1988), 1023-1038.

15 McGrady, A., et al. "Sustained Effects of Biofeedback-Assisted Relaxation Therapy in Essential Hypertension." *Biofeedback and Self-Regulation* 16:4 (December 1991), 399-411.

16 Aivazyan, T. A., et al. "Efficacy of Relaxation Techniques in Hypertensive Patients." *Health Psychology* 7 Suppl. (1988), 193-200.

17 Yen, Lee-Lan. "Comparison of Relaxation Techniques, Routine Blood Pressure Measurements, and Self-Learning Packages in Hypertension Control." *Preventive Medicine* 25:3 (May/June 1996), 339-345.

18 Gordon, N. F., and C. B. Scott. "Exercise and Mild Essential Hypertension." *Primary Care Clinics in Office Practice* 18:3 (September 1991), 683-694.

19 Grimm, Richard H., Jr., M.D., Ph.D., et al., *Journal of the American Medical Association* 275:20 (May 22/29, 1996), 1549-1556.

20 Hirofumi Tanaka, David R., et al., "Swimming Training Lowers the Resting Blood Pressure in Individuals with Hypertension," *Journal of Hypertension* 15:6, 0651-0657.

21 Murray, Michael T., N.D. *Natural Alternatives to Over-the-Counter and Prescription Drugs* (New York: William Morrow, 1994).

Chapter 11

Chinese Medicine: How It Can Help Reverse High Blood Pressure

1 *A Proposed Standard International Acupuncture Nomenclature: Report of a World Health Organization Scientific Group* (Geneva, Switzerland: World Health Organization, 1991).

2 Kaptchuk, T. J. *The Web that Has No Weaver* (Chicago: Congdon & Weed, 1983).

3 It would be impossible to cite every study from every journal around the world that might be relevant. A sampling of a few articles include: Tani, T. "Treatment of Type I Allergic Disease with Chinese Herbal formulas: Minor Blue Dragon Combination and Minor Bupleurum Combination." *International Journal of Oriental Medicine* 14:3 (September 1989), 155-166; Chen, A., M.D. "Effective Acupuncture Therapy for Migraine: Review and Comparison of Prescriptions with Recommendations for Improved Results." *American Journal of Acupuncture* 17:4 (1989), 305-316; Chen, G. S. "The Effect of Acupuncture Treatment on Carpal Tunnel Syndrome." *American Journal of Acupuncture* 18:1 (1990), 5-10; Chen, K., and H. Liang. "Progress of Geriatrics Research in Chinese Medicine." *International Journal of Oriental Medicine* 14:1 (March 1989), 49-56.

4 Zhuang, H., et al. "Effects of *Radix Salviae Miltiorrhizae* Extract Injection on Survival of Allogenic Heart Transplantation." *Journal of Traditional Chinese Medicine* 10:4 (December 1990), 276-281; Lu, W. "Treatment of AIDS by TCM and Materia Medica."

Journal of Traditional Chinese Medicine 11:4 (December 1991), 249-252; Di Concetto, G., M.D., and L. Sotte. "Treatment of Headaches by Acupuncture and Chinese Herbal Therapy: Conclusive Data Concerning 1,000 Patients." *Journal of Traditional Chinese Medicine* 2:3 (September 1991), 174-176.

Chapter 12
Lower Your Blood Pressure With Herbs

1 ESCOP, European Scientific Cooperative for Phytotherapy. (Meppel, The Netherlands: European Scientific Cooperative for Phytotherapy, 1992).

2 German Ministry of Health. Commission E. *Monographs for Phytomedicines* (Bonn, Germany: German Ministry of Health, 1989).

3 Lau, Benjamin H.S., M.D., Ph.D. "Effects of an Odor-Modified Garlic Preparation on Blood Lipids." *Nutrition Research* 7 (1987), 131-149.

4 Mindell, Earl L., R.Ph., Ph.D. *Garlic: The Miracle Nutrient* (New Canaan, CT: Keats Publishing, 1996).

5 Foster, S. *Garlic*. Botanical Series 311 (Austin, TX: American Botanical Council, 1991); Kleijnen, J., et al. "Garlic, Onions and Cardiovascular Risk Factors: A Review of the Evidence from Human Experiments with Emphasis on Commercially Available Preparations." *British Journal of Clinical Pharmacology* 28:5 (November 1989), 535-544.

6 Shibata, S., et al. " Chemistry and Pharmacology of Panax." *Economic and Medicinal Plant Research* 1 (1985), 217-284.

7 Brekhman, I. I., and I. V. Dardymov. "Pharmacological Investigation of Glycosides From Ginseng and Eleutherococcus." *Lloydia* 32 (1969), 46-51.

8 Bombardelli, E., et al. "The Effect of Acute and Chronic (Panax) Ginseng Saponins Treatment on Adrenal Function, Biochemical and Pharmacological." *Proceedings of the 3rd International Ginseng Symposium* 1 (1980), 9-16; Fulder, S. J. "Ginseng and the Hypothalamic-Pituitary Control of Stress." *American Journal of Chinese Medicine* 9 (1981), 112-118.

9 Joo, C. N. "The Preventative Effect of Korean (P. Ginseng) Saponins on Aortic Atheroma Formation in Prolonged Cholesterol-Fed Rabbits." *Proceedings of the 3rd International Ginseng Symposium* (1980), 27-36.

10 Hobbs, C. "Hawthorn: A Literature Review." *HerbalGram* 21 (1990), 19-33.

11 German Ministry of Health. Commission E. *Monographs for Phytomedicines* (Bonn, Germany: German Ministry of Health, 1989).

12 Reuter, H.D. "Crataegus Hawthorn: A Botanical Cardiac Agent." *Quarterly Review of Natural Medicine* (Summer 1995), 107-117. (Available from Natural Product Research Consultants, Inc., 600 First Avenue, Suite 205, Seattle, WA 98104; tel: 206-623-2520; fax: 206-623-6340; $79/4 issues).

13 Berdyshev, V. V. "Effect of the Long-Term Intake of Eleutherococcus on the Adaptation of Sailors in the Tropics." *Voenno Meditsinskii Zhurnal* 5 (May 1981), 57-58. (Published in Russian).

14 German Ministry of Health. Commission E. *Valerian. Monographs for Phytomedicines* (Bonn, Germany: German Ministry of Health, 1985).

15 ESCOP, European Scientific Cooperative for Phytotherapy. *Valerian Root* (Meppel, The Netherlands: European Scientific Cooperative for Phytotherapy, 1990).

16 Hobbs, C. "Valerian: A Literature Review." *HerbalGram* 21 (1989), 19-34.

17 *Townsend Letter for Doctors* (May 1994), 432-434; *Explore! for the Professional* 4:5 (1993), 17-19.

18 Jin, H. et al. "Treatment of Hypertension by *Ling zhi* Combined with Hypotensor and Its Effects on Arterial, Arteriolar, and Capillary Pressure and Microcirculation." *Microcirculatory Approach to Asian Traditional Medicine,* edited by Nimmi, H., et al. (New York: Elsevier Science, 1996), 131-138.

Chapter 13
Alternative Medicine Options for Lowering High Blood Pressure

1 Wagner, H., and L. Sprinkmeier. "Uber die phar-makologischen Wirkungen von Melissengeist." *Deutsche Apotheker Zeitung* 113 (1973), 1159.

2 Franchomme, P., and D. Penoel. *Aromatherapie Exactement* (Limoges: Roger Jollois, 1990).

3 Tisserand, R. B. *The Art of Aromatherapy* (Rochester, VT: Healing Arts Press, 1977).

4 Czygan, F. C. "Essential Oils: Aspects of History of Civilization." *Atherische öle, Analytik, Physiologie, Zusammensetzung,* edited by K. H. Kubeczka, (Stuttgart, New York: Georg Thieme Verlag, 1982).

5 Dodd, G. H. "Receptor Events in Perfumery." *Perfumery: The Psychology and Biology of Fragrance* edited by van Toller, S., and G. H. Dodd (London: Chapman and Hall, 1988).

6 Steele, J. "Brain Research and Essential Oils."

Aromatherapy Quarterly 3 (Spring 1984), 5.

7 Lorig, T. S., et al. "The Effects of Low Concentration Odors on EEG Activity and Behavior." *Journal of Psychophysiology* 5 (1991), 69-77.

8 Belaiche, P. *Traite de Phytotherapie et d'aromatherapie Tome I: L'aromatogramme* (Paris: Maloine S.A., 1979).

9 Woolfson, A. "Intensive Aromacare." *International Journal of Aromatherapy* 4:2 (1992), 12-13.

10 Keller, W., and W. Kober. "Moglickeiten der Verwendung atherischer åle zur Raundesinfektion I." *Arzneimittelforschung* 5 (1955), 224; Keller, W., and W. Kober. "Moglickeiten der Verwendung atherischer åle zur Raundesinfektion II." *Arzneimittelforschung* 6 (1955), 768.

11 "Aromatherapy on the Wards: Lavendar Beats Benzodiazepines." *International Journal of Aromatherapy* 1:2 (1988), 1.

12 Tisserand, R. B. *The Art of Aromatherapy* (Rochester, VT: Healing Arts Press, 1977).

13 Fahrion, S. L. "Hypertension and Biofeedback." *Primary Care Clinics in Office Practice* 3 (September 1991), 663-682.

14 Namba, K., et al. "Effect of Taurine Concentration on Platelet Aggregation in Gestosis Patients with Edema, Proteinuria, and Hypertension." *Acta Medica Okayama* 46:4 (August 1992), 241-247; Ceriello, A., et al. "Anti-Oxidants Show an Anti-Hypertensive Effect in Diabetic and Hypertensive Subjects." *Clinical Science* 81:6 (December 1991), 739-742; Maxwell, S. R. "Can Anti-Oxidants Prevent Ischemic Heart Disease?" *Journal of Clinical Pharmacy and Therapeutics* 18:2 (April 1993), 85-95.

15 Galley, H.F., et al. "Regulation of Nitric Oxide Synthase Activity in Cultured Human Endothelial Cells: Effect of Antioxidants." *Free Radical Biology and Medicine* 21 (1996), 97-101.

16 Galley, H.F., et al. "Combination Oral Antioxidant Supplementation Reduces Blood Pressure." *Clinical Science* 92 (1997), 361-365.

17 Henry, H. J., et al. "Increasing Calcium Intake Lowers Blood Pressure: The Literature Reviewed." *Journal of the American Dietetic Association* 85:2 (February 1985), 182-185; Belizam, J. M., et al. "Reduction of Blood Pressure with Calcium Supplementation in Young Adults." *Journal of the American Medical Association* 249:9 (March 1983), 1161-1165.

18 Wimaladwansa, S., et al. "Mechanisms of Antihypertensive Effects of Dietary Calcium and

Role of Calcitonin-Gene-Related Peptide in Hypertension." *Canadian Journal of Physiology and Pharmacology* 73:7 (1995), 981-985.

19 McCarron, D. A., et al. "Dietary Calcium in Human Hypertension." *Science* 217:4556 (1982), 267-269.

20 Dyckner, T., and P. O. Wester. "Effect of Magnesium on Blood Pressure." *British Medical Journal* 286:6381 (January 1983), 1847-1849.

21 *Northeast Center for Environmental Medicine Health Letter* (Fall 1992).

22 Skrabal, F., et al. "Low Sodium/High Potassium Diet for Prevention of Hypertension: Probable Mechanisms of Action." *The Lancet* 2:8252 (October 1981), 895-900.

23 Armstrong, B., et al. "Urinary Sodium and Blood Pressure in Vegetarians." *American Journal of Clinical Nutrition* 32:12 (December 1979), 2472-2476; Rouse, I. L., et al. "Vegetarian Diet and Blood Pressure." *The Lancet* 2:8352 (1983), 742-743.

24 Ivanov, S. G., et al. "The Magnetotherapy of Hypertension Patients." *Terapevticheskii Arkhiv* 62:9 (1990), 71-74.

Chapter 14
What Causes Stroke?

1 "Stroke Statistics." National Stroke Association Internet web site: http://www.stroke.org/.

2 American Heart Association Internet web site: http://www.amhrt.org/hs96/strokes.html.

3 "Stroke Statistics." National Stroke Association Internet web site: http://www.stroke.org/.

4 Ibid.

5 U. S. Department of Health and Human Services. Public Health Service, National Institutes of Health. *Stroke: Hope Through Research* (Pub. No. 83-2222, August 1983).

6 Levine, Jeff. "Study: Some People Risk a Stroke by Overusing Decongestants." Internet: CNN Interactive Heath Page (April 16, 1997).

7 "Study: Overweight Women at Greater Risk of Stroke." Internet: CNN Interactive Heath Page (May 20, 1997).

8 Kindenstrom, Ewa, et al. "Influence of Total Cholesterol, High Density Lipoprotein Cholesterol, and Triglycerides on Risk of Cerebrovascular Disease: The Copenhagen City Heart Study." *British Medical Journal* 433:309 (1994), 11-15.

9 Nagayama, Masao, M.D., Ph.D., et al. "Lipoprotein (a) and Ischemic Cerebrovascular Disease in

Young Adults." *Stroke* 25 (1994), 74-78.

10 Peck, Peggy. "Elevated Lipoprotein (a) May Be the Strongest Predictor of Cerebrovascular Disease." *Family Practice News* (April 15, 1994), 2.

11 Davalos, Antonio, M.D., et al. "Iron-Related Damage in Acute Ischemic Stroke." *Stroke* 25:8 (1994), 1543-1546.

12 Perry, I.J., et al. "Prospective Study of Serum Total Homocysteine Concentration and Risk of Stroke in Middle-Aged British Men." *The Lancet* 346 (November 25, 1995), 1395-1398.

13 den Heijer, M., et al. "Is Hyperhomocysteinaemia a Risk Factor for Recurrent Venous Thrombosis?" *The Lancet* 345 (1995), 882-885.

14 Lalouschek, W., et al. "Hyperhomocysteinemia: An Independent Risk Factor for Stroke." *Fortschritte der Neurologie Psychiatic* 64 (1996), 271-277.

15 "Bypass Surgery Some Risk to the Brain." Internet: CNN Interactive Heath Page (December 18, 1996).

16 Phillips, Pat. "Fibrinogen Linked to Carotid Stenosis, Stroke." *Medical Tribune* (March 11, 1993), 3.

17 Ibid.

18 Resch, Karl L., M.D., et al. "Fibrinogen and Viscosity as Risk Factors for Subsequent Cardiovascular Events in Stroke Survivors." *Annals of Internal Medicine* 117:5 (September 1, 1992), 371-375.

19 Petitti, Diana B., M.D., et al. "Stroke in Users of Low-Dose Oral Contraceptives." *New England Journal of Medicine* 335:1 (July 1996), 8-15.

20 Jeppesen, Lise Leth, et al. "Decreased Serum Testosterone in Men with Acute Ischemic Stroke." *Arteriosclerosis, Thrombosis and Vascular Disease* 16:6 (June 1996), 749-754.

Chapter 15
Self-Care Essentials for Stroke

1 Orencia, Anthony J., M.D., Ph.D., et al. "Fish Consumption and Stroke in Men: 30-Year Findings of the Chicago Western Electric Study." *Stroke* 27:2 (February 1996), 204-209.

2 Gillum, R.F., et al. "The Relationship Between Fish Consumption and Stroke Incidence." *Archives of Internal Medicine* 156 (1996), 537-542.

3 Gillman, Matthew W., M.D., et al. "A Protective Effect of Fruits and Vegetables on Development of Stroke in Men." *Journal of the American Medical Association* 273:14 (April 12, 1995), 1113-1117.

4 "Carrots, Spinach and Diet Tied to Lower Stroke Risk." *Medical Tribune* (April 8, 1993), 7.

5 Keli, Sirving O., M.D., Ph.D., et al. "Dietary Flavonoids, Antioxidant Vitamins, and Incidence of Stroke: The Zupthen Study." *Archives of Internal Medicine* 157 (March 25, 1996), 637-642.

6 Mann, Denise. "Any Exercise at All Decreases Stroke Risk in Elderly." *Medical Tribune* (May 2, 1996).

7 Kiely, Dan K., et al. "Physical Activity and Stroke Risk: The Framingham Study." *American Journal of Epidemiology* 149:7 (1994), 608-620.

8 "Moderate Exercise Cuts Vessel Disease." *Medical Tribune* (March 26, 1992), 10.

9 Laino, Charlene. "Exercise from 25 On Guards Against Stroke." *Family Practice News* (August 26, 1993), 20.

10 Potempa, Kathleen, et al. "Benefits of Aerobic Exercise after Stroke." *Sports Medicine* 21:5 (May 1996), 337-346; Potempa, Kathleen, et al. "Physiological Outcomes of Aerobic Exercise Training in Hemiparetic Stroke Patients." *Stroke* 26:1 (January 1995), 101-105.

11 Wannamethee, S. Goya, Ph.D., et al. *Journal of the American Medical Association* 274:12 (July 12, 1995), 155-160.

Chapter 16
Oxygen Therapy: How It Can Help Stroke Recovery

1 Perrin, D. 1993 study in Great Britain (unpublished).

2 Warburg, O. "The Prime Cause and Prevention of Cancer." Revised lecture at the Meeting of the Nobel-laureates on June 30, 1966 (Bethesda, MD: National Cancer Institute, 1967).

3 Farr, C. H. Presented at the Fourth International Conference on Bio-Oxidative Medicine. Reston, VA (April 1-4, 1993).

4 Farr, C. H. "Workbook on Free Radical Chemistry and Hydrogen Peroxide Metabolism Including Protocol for the Intravenous Administration of Hydrogen Peroxide." Contains 32 citations with references in the workbook, and 123 in the protocol (1992). (Available from: International Bio-Oxidative Medicine Foundation. P.O. Box 13205, Oklahoma City, OK, 73113).

5 Farr, C. H. *The Therapeutic Use of Intravenous Hydrogen Peroxide* Monograph. (Oklahoma City, OK: Genesis Medical Center, 1987).

6 Farr, C. H. "Workbook on Free Radical Chemistry and Hydrogen Peroxide Metabolism Including Protocol for the Intravenous Administration of Hydrogen Peroxide." Contains 32 citations with references in

the workbook, and 123 in the protocol (1992).
(Available from: International Bio-Oxidative
Medicine Foundation. P.O. Box 13205, Oklahoma
City, OK, 73113).

7 Farr, C. H. *The Therapeutic Use of Intravenous
Hydrogen Peroxide* Monograph. (Oklahoma City,
OK: Genesis Medical Center, 1987); Baker, E. *The
Unmedical Miracle—Oxygen* (Indianola, WA:
Drelwood Communications, 1991).

Chapter 17
More Options for Treating Stroke

1 Ayers, Margaret E., M.A. "EEG Neurofeedback to Bring
Individuals Out of Level-Two Coma." *Biofeedback
and Self-Regulation* 20:3 (September 1995);
Ayers, Margaret E., M.A. "Electroencephalic
Neurofeedback and Closed Head Injury of 250
Individuals." *Head Injury Frontiers* (1987), 380.

2 Gey, K.F., et al. "Poor Plasma Status of Carotene and
Vitamin C is Associated with Higher Mortality from
Ischemic Heart Disease and Stroke: Basal
Prospective Study." *Clinical Investigator* 71 (1993),
3-6.

3 Clark, Wayne M., M.D., et al. "Need for Treatment of
Elevated Plasma Fibrinogen Levels in
Cerebrovascular Disease." *Heart Disease and
Stroke* (Available from Dr. Wayne M. Clark,
Department of Neurology L226, Oregon Health
Sciences University, 3181 SW Sam Jackson Park
Road, Portland, OR 97201).

Index

THIS BOOK COULD...

LEARN WAYS TO REVERSE AND PREVENT CANCER

Some of the Doctors in *An Alternative Medicine Definitive Guide to Cancer*:

Robert Atkins, M.D.
New York, NY
Learn about Dr. Atkins' multifaceted program to help the body overcome cancer.

Keith Block, M.D.
Chicago, IL
Dr. Block combines conventional therapy with immune-enhancing, detoxifying treatments to maximize cancer survival.

James W. Forsythe, M.D., H.M.D.
Reno, NV
An oncologist explains his use of immune-stimulating therapies.

Robert A. Nagourney, M.D.
Long Beach, CA
For those who are thinking of using chemotherapy, this oncologist can test for drug effectiveness first.

Jesse Stoff, M.D.
Tucson, AZ
All aspects of a patient's life—body, mind, and emotions—must receive therapeutic attention. Learn how.

Vincent Speckhart, M.D., M.D.H. Norfolk, VA
An oncologist for 22 years, Dr. Speckhart explains how he reverses cancer by removing toxins and repairing the immune system.

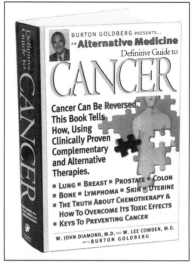

BURTON GOLDBERG PRESENTS...
AN **Alternative Medicine**
Definitive Guide to
CANCER

Cancer Can Be Reversed.
This Book Tells How, Using Clinically Proven Complementary and Alternative Therapies.

■ LUNG ■ BREAST ■ PROSTATE ■ COLON
■ BONE ■ LYMPHOMA ■ SKIN ■ UTERINE
■ THE TRUTH ABOUT CHEMOTHERAPY & HOW TO OVERCOME ITS TOXIC EFFECTS
■ KEYS TO PREVENTING CANCER

W. JOHN DIAMOND, M.D. AND W. LEE COWDEN, M.D.
WITH BURTON GOLDBERG

©1997 by Future Medicine Publishing, Inc.
Publishers of *Alternative Medicine: The Definitive Guide* and the bimonthly magazine *Alternative Medicine Digest*

THIS 1,116-PAGE BOOK ILLUSTRATES MANY SUCCESSFUL ALTERNATIVES TO CONVENTIONAL CARE THAT CAN REMOVE THE ROOT CAUSES OF CANCER AND RESTORE YOU TO HEALTH WITHOUT FURTHER POISONING OR DAMAGING YOUR BODY.

CALL FOR YOUR COPY TODAY.
BUY A COPY FOR YOUR ONCOLOGIST AND INSIST THAT IT BE READ.

CALL 800-333-HEAL

Valuable Information Featured in *An Alternative Medicine Definitive Guide to Cancer*:

• Cancer patients treated with nontoxic botanicals had twice the survival rate after 1 year, and 4 times the survival rate after 2 years, compared to chemotherapy patients. Readers are unlikely ever to see such results published in American medical journals, which receive their primary financial support from the pharmaceutical industry.

• The medical director of a prestigious clinic reports that in 90% of his breast cancer patients there is a dental factor.

SAVE YOUR LIFE

The single most important, lifesaving book on cancer ever published—37 top physicians explain their proven, safe, nontoxic, and successful treatments for reversing cancer.

From W. John Diamond, M.D., director of the Triad Medical Center in Reno, Nevada, and W. Lee Cowden, M.D., cardiologist and consultant to the Conservative Medicine Institute in Richardson, Texas, comes the book that finally tells you how to be cancer free for life.

The book guides you through the safest and most effective treatment alternatives known today. Learn how leading practitioners use herbs, nutrition and diet, supplements, oxygen, enzymes, glandular extracts, homeopathic remedies, plus specialized substances such as Ukrain, Essiac, Carnivora, Iscador, 714X, shark cartilage, and many others to prevent and reverse cancers. Learn why the mammoth U.S. cancer industry does not want you to know about these successful alternatives. See the proof of treatment success in 55 documented patient case histories demonstrating how alternative approaches to cancer can make the difference between life and death—as these people found out:

It was a marvelous feeling. I was blossoming like a flower. After a short time, I regained my appetite, went on shopping sprees with my daughter, even went to shows. I began to live again! Can I ever repay Dr. Atkins for giving me the gift of life? Perhaps not. But if I stay well and healthy, I think that will be his greatest reward.

CLAUDETTE, 52—Metastatic ovarian cancer reversed

I'm well aware of what eating a proper diet has done for me. It not only cured me of cancer, but controlled my weight and relieved my hypertension, for which I had been on medication for 42 years.

ETHAN, 66—14 years after metastatic prostate cancer diagnosis

TO ORDER, CALL 800-333-HEAL

CURE YOUR HEADACHES...

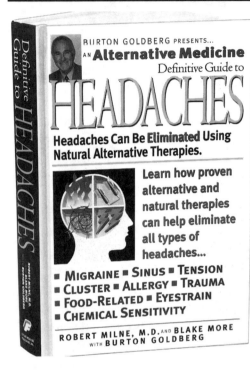

BURTON GOLDBERG PRESENTS...

AN **Alternative Medicine**
Definitive Guide to

HEADACHES

Headaches Can Be Eliminated Using Natural Alternative Therapies.

Learn how proven alternative and natural therapies can help eliminate all types of headaches...

- MIGRAINE ■ SINUS ■ TENSION
- CLUSTER ■ ALLERGY ■ TRAUMA
- FOOD-RELATED ■ EYESTRAIN
- CHEMICAL SENSITIVITY

ROBERT MILNE, M.D. AND BLAKE MORE
WITH BURTON GOLDBERG

If you suffer from headaches, this book could change your life. It is entirely possible that with this invaluable practical information, you may well put headaches behind you as something you once suffered from, but no more.

Robert Milne, M.D., and Blake More expertly guide you through the root causes and multiple treatment options for 11 major types of headaches, from sinus to migraine, cluster to tension.

We have made every effort possible to make this book practical and user-friendly for you. For a quick reference to headache types, symptoms, treatment options, use our Master Symptom Chart. If you suffer from tension headaches, turn directly to Chapter 6; if migraines are your millstone, see Chapter 7; and if you're not sure what type of headache you have, study the symptoms list in the Master Symptom Chart until you find the clinical term that best matches your condition.

No matter what kind of headache you used to have, after reading this book your head may never pain you again.

Hardcover ■ ISBN 1-887299-03-3
■ 6" x 9" ■ 525 pages

TO ORDER, CALL 800-333-HEAL

USING NATURAL THERAPIES

Say goodbye to headaches for the rest of your life. No matter what kind of headache you suffer from, thanks to the proven and effective health information in this book, your head may never pain you again.

Your headaches, whether migraine, tension, sinus, cluster, or any of the 11 different types covered in this book, can be eliminated for good. Drawing on the entire field of alternative medicine, Robert Milne, M.D., Blake More, and Burton Goldberg tell you how, using chiropractic, herbalism, acupuncture, homeopathy, nutrition, bodywork, biofeedback, aromatherapy, and more, plus extensive self-care suggestions—all from leading experts in the field. In dozens of real-life success stories, learn how headache sufferers used these techniques and are now headache free.

Unlike any other headache book, *An Alternative Medicine Definitive Guide to Headaches* gives you the cutting-edge, practical, and easy-to-understand medical advice you need to make your headaches a pain of the past. Here's how the invaluable advice in this book helped these people become headache free:

It was so easy. To think of all those years I spent in pain, bouncing from one prescription to another, when all I had to do was stop eating sugar and dairy products for my headaches to go away.

—SUSAN, A FORMER MIGRAINER

I had thousands of dollars' worth of tests—CAT scans, MRIs, all kinds of things—but they didn't cure anything. Then with a nutritional supplement called essential fatty acids, I was handed the key to ending my headaches. —ROBERT, A REAL ESTATE BROKER

Decongestants only offered temporary relief of my sinus headaches. A naturopath gently massaged my face, neck, and stomach, then gave me homeopathy, herbs, and nutritional supplements. Within a week, I began to feel myself again, and now, 8 months later, my sinus headaches are completely gone.

—KATHERINE, A MASSAGE THERAPIST

TO ORDER, CALL 800-333-HEAL

ALTERNATIVE
MEDICINE DIGEST

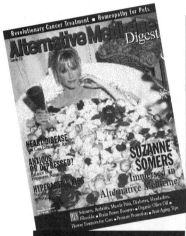

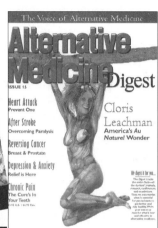

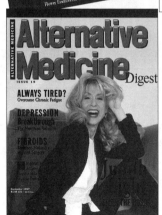

ORDER A
SUBSCRIPTION
TO THE
BIMONTHLY
ALTERNATIVE
MEDICINE
DIGEST
TODAY.

TO ORDER, CALL 800-333-HEAL

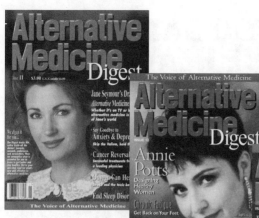

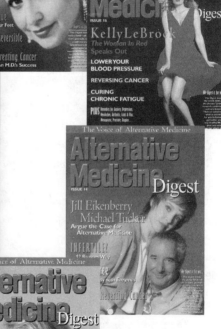

We digest it for you—The *Digest* tracks the entire field—all the doctor's journals, research, conferences, and newsletters. Then we summarize what is essential for you to know to get better and stay healthy. We're your one-stop read for what's new and effective in alternative medicine.

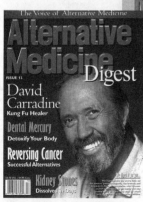

TO ORDER, CALL 800-333-HEAL

ARE YOU SATISFIED WITH THE HEALTH CARE YOU'RE GETTING?

INVEST IN YOUR HEALTH

No household should be without *Alternative Medicine: The Definitive Guide*. Over 380 leading edge physicians explain their treatments. In this remarkable 1,068-page resource book, you will have a single, authoritative source of information on 43 alternative therapies, including diet and nutrition. After each one, there are resource lists— "Where to Find Help" and "Recommended Reading"—related to the therapy described. You can look up specific problems and find natural remedies and therapies to help heal them. Health conditions and alternative therapies are described in detail, in clear, understandable language.

There is no substitute for this valuable resource book.

Chelation therapy v.s. bypass surgery and angioplasty page 128

Stretching for relief of back pain page 548

A quick fix for migraine headaches page 696

Using herbs to stop smoking page 491

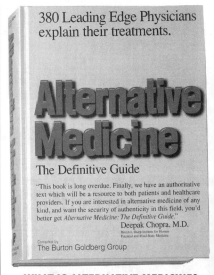

380 Leading Edge Physicians explain their treatments.

Alternative Medicine

The Definitive Guide

"This book is long overdue. Finally, we have an authoritative text which will be a resource to both patients and healthcare providers. If you are interested in alternative medicine of any kind, and want the security of authenticity in this field, you'd better get *Alternative Medicine: The Definitive Guide*."

Deepak Chopra, M.D.
Director, Sharp Institute for Human Potential and Mind-Body Medicine

Compiled by
The Burton Goldberg Group

WHAT IS ALTERNATIVE MEDICINE?

Alternative medicine is an umbrella term used to describe a wide range of health-care approaches, including acupuncture, homeopathy, herbal medicine, chiropractic, and others that differ from the more commonly known, conventional medical treatments. Whereas conventional medicine primarily approaches problems from the outside in...often in a way that is drug-based and symptom-driven...alternative medical therapies work from the inside out, in a sensitive, balanced approach to whole-body health.

EASY TO READ—FULL OF INFORMATION THAT COULD SAVE YOUR LIFE
NO OTHER BOOK LIKE IT IN PRINT
ORDER YOUR COPY TODAY
800-333-HEAL

ALSO AVAILABLE FROM FUTURE MEDICINE

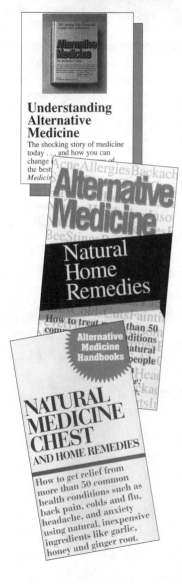

Understanding Alternative Medicine

The shocking story of medicine today . . . and how you can change i_____ of the best_____
Medicin_

Alternative Medicine

Natural Home Remedies

How to treat_____ than 50
comm_____ditions
_____atural
_____people_

Alternative Medicine Handbooks

NATURAL MEDICINE CHEST AND HOME REMEDIES

How to get relief from more than 50 common health conditions such as back pain, colds and flu, headache, and anxiety using natural, inexpensive ingredients like garlic, honey and ginger root.

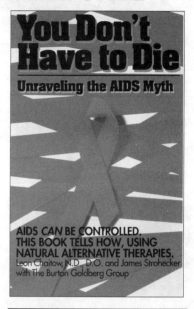

You Don't Have to Die

Unraveling the AIDS Myth

AIDS *CAN* BE CONTROLLED. THIS BOOK TELLS HOW, USING NATURAL ALTERNATIVE THERAPIES.
Leon Chaitow, N.D., D.O. and James Strohecker with The Burton Goldberg Group

- **You Don't Have to Die—Unraveling the AIDS Myth**
  319 pages, 5 1/4" x 8 1/4"
  ISBN 0-9636334-4-9

- **Understanding Alternative Medicine**
  Audio tape
  ISBN 0-9636334-6-5

- **Natural Home Remedies and Medicine Chest**
  72 pages, 4" x 7 1/2"
  ISBN 0-9636334-8-1

- **Natural Home Remedies**
  Video
  ISBN 0-9636334-7-3

TO ORDER, CALL 800-333-HEAL

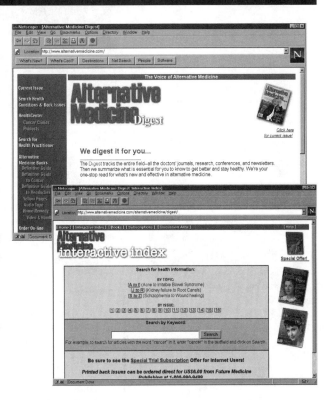

www.alternativemedicine.com

LOG ON to your one-stop information source for the best and boldest in alternative medicine. Find the answer to your health problem fast with our Interactive Index. Study the medical information you need to know by accessing our reference work, *Alternative Medicine: The Definitive Guide*. Browse all the back issues of *Alternative Medicine Digest* or hyperlink to our newest issue—before it hits the newsstands. Network worldwide with other enthusiasts in our chat room.

Alternative Medicine YELLOW PAGES

The comprehensive guide to the new world of health.

Become an active participant in your own well-being with the most complete directory of alternative therapies, health practitioners and products conveniently listed by type of therapy and location.

The perfect companion to the best-selling
Alternative Medicine: The Definitive Guide.

Put a one-stop telephone directory of 17,000 practitioners of alternative medicine around the U.S. at your fingertips. Find the alternative specialist by state and city, type of therapy, and health problem. Listings span back pain to weight management, arthritis to thyroid disorders. Learn even more about how alternative medicine can help end your health problem by browsing the hundreds of informative display ads throughout the book.

TO ORDER, CALL 800-333-HEAL

THE BOOK
THAT EVERYONE WITH
CANCER NEEDS

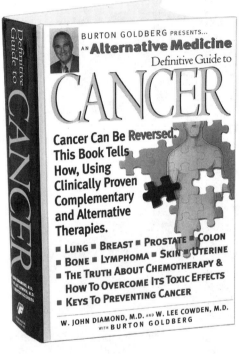

There has never been a book like this about cancer. The message is simple, direct, and lifesaving: cancer can be successfully reversed using alternative medicine. This book shows how.

The clinical proof is in the words and recommendations of 37 leading physicians who treat and restore life to thousands of cancer patients. Read 55 documented patient case histories and see how alternative approaches to cancer can make the difference between life and death. Learn about the 33 contributing causes to cancer.

These doctors bring to alternative cancer care decades of careful study and practice. They know that there is no magic bullet cure for cancer. They also know that many factors contribute to the development of cancer and many modalities and substances must be used to reverse it.

Hardcover ■ ISBN 1-887299-01-7 ■ 6" x 9" ■ 1,116 pages

TO ORDER, CALL 800-333-HEAL

PART FOUR

Alternative Practitioner Listings

Understanding
Alternative Medicine

In the face of an increasingly inadequate system of conventional medicine, a growing number of people are turning to alternative medicine to address their needs. The general public is starting to recognize the effectiveness of alternative medicine's approach to health, which blends body and mind, science and experience, and traditional and cross-cultural avenues of diagnosis and treatment. In fact, a recent study published in the *New England Journal of Medicine* found that over one-third of those surveyed chose alternative medicine over conventional methods, because of the medical establishment's emphasis on diagnostic testing and treatment with drugs without focusing on the patient as a whole. It is obvious that what was once considered a "fringe" interest is now on its way to becoming the primary medical approach of the next millennium.

The Crisis in Modern Medicine

It is no secret that the current United States medical system is in a state of terrible disarray. Though conventional medicine excels in the management of medical emergencies, certain bacterial infections, trauma care, and many, often heroically complex surgical techniques, it seems to have failed miserably in the areas of disease prevention and the management of the myriad new and chronic illnesses presently filling our hospitals and physicians' offices. In addition, as a nation we pay more for our medical care and accomplish less than most other nations of comparable living standards, while health care costs continue to spiral out of control.

Treatment of chronic disease currently accounts for 85% of the national health care bill. This state of affairs is due to the fact that we spend almost nothing to treat the causes of chronic disease before major illness develops, according to a report from the American Association of Naturopathic Physicians. "We wait for [illness] to develop and then spend huge sums on heroic measures, even then ignoring the underlying lifestyle-related causes. This is the equivalent of waiting for a leaky roof to destroy the infrastructure of a house and then repairing the damage without fixing the leak. This is naturally expensive and ineffective.

"Perhaps the greatest evidence of the depth of the crisis is that we have come to accept such levels of chronic disease as normal, despite evidence that much of it is preventable. Former Surgeon General C. Everett Koop, in his 1988 Report on Nutrition and Health, points out that 'dietary imbalances' are the leading preventable contributors to premature death in the U.S. and recommends the expansion of nutrition and lifestyle-modification education for all health care professionals." This is borne out by the Centers for Disease Control, which state that 54% of heart disease, 37 of cancer, 50% of cerebrovascular disease, and 49% of atherosclerosis (hardening of the arteries) is preventable through lifestyle modification.

The changes that are necessary, however, will not be implemented as long as physicians earn their living and win renown primarily by delivering rescue medicine (interventions that simply treat symptoms), since it is in this area and not prevention that they benefit most. If the United States is to be saved from catastrophic health care costs, it is time to take a good look at the wisdom and cost-effectiveness of alternative medicine.

Doctors are confronted daily with patients suffering from illnesses for which conventional medicine offers only superficial treatment of symptoms. The magic of antibiotics is vanishing as a host of resistant infections emerge; diseases such as AIDS and chronic fatigue syndrome have shown us clearly that our present treatments are simply not effective and hint at new health problems which may lie ahead.

The metaphor of a modern plague may be appropriate. Growing numbers of people lack vitality and suffer from a host of complaints difficult to define. Most adults, and many children, today suffer from complaints including allergies, headaches, lack of energy, excessive fatigue, and various digestive and respiratory disorders, along with a variety of emotional states ranging from mild depression to mood swings and anxiety.

They are manifesting what Jeffrey Bland, Ph.D., of Gig Harbor, Washington, calls a state of "vertical ill-health." "They are not sick enough to lie down (in which case they would become 'horizontally ill') and yet consider themselves 'normal' because most of the people they know are equally unhealthy," explains Leon Chaitow, N.D., D.O., of London, England. "They derive only limited benefit from the flood of tranquilizers, antidepressants, analgesics, and anti-inflammatory drugs they are commonly prescribed, while the side effects they develop from these drugs just add to their list of woes."

Thoughtful physicians are becoming increasingly aware that something is wrong with their patients' immune systems, since they continue to suffer from illnesses which normal immune function should be able to deal with. Yet this decline in immune efficiency is something contemporary medical treatments seem unable to do anything about. Doctors and patients alike are perplexed by this failure of drug-based therapies to bring relief. As a result, patients often become trapped in a cycle of dependency on physicians to monitor and constantly adjust their medications rather than becoming empowered to change lifestyle factors that might allow their body to regain its healthful potential.

"Most over-the-counter and almost all prescribed drug treatments merely mask symptoms or control health problems, or in some way alter the way organs or systems such as the circulatory system work," states John R. Lee, M.D., of Sebastopol, California. "Drugs almost never deal with the reasons why these problems exist, while they frequently create new health problems as side effects of their activities.

"People realize that their headaches are not due to aspirin deficiency or that their hypertension is not being properly addressed by prescriptions of drugs that merely induce diuresis [excessive urine excretion]. They are seeking answers that address the root causes of their health problems and aid in restoring normal, healthy body function. This is not to say that treatment of the symptoms of a condition is wrong. What would be wrong would be to think that by eliminating the symptom we have dealt with the problem itself."

Roots of the Crisis

The underlying concepts of alternative medicine are not new. They represent a return to the principles that have been part of human understanding of health and disease for thousands of years. Over the centuries, medical wisdom evolved within a framework which linked health to a state of harmony or balance, and disease to a state of disharmony or imbalance, and took into account the factors that contributed to both.

"The genius of the ancient Greek physician Hippocrates, the father of Western medicine, was not in the drugs he used or his diagnostic skills," Dr. Lee points out, "but in his insight that the elements which were needed to produce and maintain health were natural, and that they included hygiene, a calm balanced mental state, proper diet, a sound work and home environment, and physical conditioning. In addition, he recognized the life forces that pervade all of nature, and which have multiple expressions—some known, some theorized, and many unknown. He taught that health depended upon living in harmony with these forces." Recognition of these life forces is also vital to traditional Chinese medicine and Ayurvedic medicine from India.

A Dangerous Detour

In the mid-nineteenth century, following the discovery of disease-causing microbes, a departure from this philosophy of health occurred due to rival theories concerning the cause of disease. One theory was that infecting microbes called germs (viruses, bacteria, and fungi) were the cause of illness. The opposing theory maintained that these microbes only became infectious if conditions inside the body were right for them. According to this theory, by keeping the internal environment of the body healthy, these potential agents of infection will remain dormant.

When the germ theory of disease became dominant, the birth of contemporary medicine, with its emphasis on infectious causes of diseases rather than physiologic balance or harmony, occurred. This provided medical science with the opportunity to greatly expand its role in the treatment of illness. This was followed by the rapid development of microscopy, bacterial cultures, vaccines, X ray, and, in the 1930s, the discovery of antibacterial drugs such as penicillin and sulfa drugs. However, the more that medical science embraced the germ theory of disease, the more it also superseded the individual's role in his or her own health.

The Purpose of Medicine: War or Repair?

The thrust of twentieth century medicine can be described by the metaphor of war. Disease is considered an invasion by an enemy and treatment is aimed at developing "magic bullets" in the form of drugs and vaccines to eliminate that enemy. We have seen, for example, a failed "war on cancer," a proliferation of antibiotics, and a growing number of surgical procedures, cell-killing radiation treatments, and chemical medications (such as chemotherapy), all of which do harm to the body, in one form or another, in their attempts to restore health.

Lost in this approach is the concept of repairing the imbalances which allow the illnesses to occur in the first place. Medical science has become one-sided in its focus, increasingly losing sight of the whole person in its attempt to treat the body's individual parts.

"A more useful metaphor for medicine would be repair, not war," says Dr. Lee. "If we think of the body as a house, we see that problems lie in the gaps and breakdowns that occur in the foundation, allowing various pests to make their way inside. The contemporary physician addresses this problem by selling you poisons or traps to kill or catch the pests. But this still doesn't prevent other undesirables from coming in through the gaps in the future. How much better it would be for your physician to learn where the holes are and help you to repair them, while teaching you how to prevent them from occurring again."

Because the emphasis of conventional medicine remains upon war and not repair, it has led to the organization of medical schools with their various departments, such as cardiology, nephrology, neurology, dermatology, orthopedics, and psychiatry. This forces students to focus their study on one organ system at a time as if each bodily organ functioned independently of all the others; or to choose one for exclusive study in preparation for a career in medicine as a "specialist" in that organ system. "Our system of disease classification is based on specific organs as well," notes Dr. Lee. "We name our diseases by the organ that is being affected. Thus we have arthritis, ton-sillitis, appendicitis, heart or gallbladder disease, colitis, prostatitis, and many other examples. We even name the cancer we get by the organ it affects. This diverts attention away from the intrinsic interrelatedness of all parts of our body and the complex dynamism of life forces. It is no wonder that our 'modern' doctors understand so little of holistic concepts of health."

Why Are We Ill?

Health is far more than the absence of disease. When we are healthy all our bodily systems and functions are harmoniously balanced and integrated with each other and we are also in balance with our environment. In this state of equilibrium our defense mechanisms and our immune system can efficiently handle most of the hazards that life presents, whether these are pathogenic (disease-causing) organisms, toxic substances, or stress factors of various kinds.

Foundations of Health

According to Dr. Chaitow, positive health depends upon three factors, which are interconnected. The first of these is the body's structural system, including all of the muscles, bones, ligaments, nerves, blood vessels, and organs, and their functions. The second factor is the body's biochemical processes, which involve the absorption and utilization of nutrients, and the elimination of wastes, along with the complicated biochemical relationships which are the key to cellular function and health. The third factor comprises the mind and emotions, as well as the spiritual dimension of each person.

"When there is a balanced, energetic, interplay between these three components, we have health," Dr. Chaitow says. "But when imbalances exist within any of these factors, or in their relationships with each other, ill-health occurs."

Homeostasis

In a state of health, if we cut ourselves, we heal. If we are bruised, strained, or suffer a broken bone, healing starts immediately. If we are exposed to infection our immune system deals with it. These examples are illustrations of the body's natural tendency towards repairing itself. This tendency is known as homeostasis, the maintenance of the body's internal organs and defenses to compensate for external health hazards.

When homeostasis is called into play to handle a "crisis," its activity is usually experienced as "symptoms." For example, when you are exposed to an infection your body will mount an aggressive defensive response which might result in fever. Or, should you injure yourself, the healing process which starts immediately might involve inflammation and swelling of the traumatized area. In other words, under normal conditions, the body will attempt to heal itself without help, and the symptoms produced will indicate what sort of healing process is going on. Unfortunately many people, including all too many physicians, rather than respecting these homeostatic processes and simply waiting for them to finish their tasks, will actively try to suppress the symptoms of self-repair, whether this be a raised temperature or inflammation in an injured area. When this occurs, we are in effect saying that we know more than our body's innate intelligence about what is good for it.

In order to maintain good health, therefore, it is important to recognize that many symptoms are actually evidence that healing is underway, and that, unless they are actually unbearable or dangerous, the symptoms should be left alone so that the repair processes can be completed.

Stress Adaptation

The late Canadian physiologist Hans Selye developed a model of how the body copes with stress which he called the general adaptation syndrome (GAS). The three stages of GAS offer a clear explanation of how and why nearly all forms of illness develop.

In Dr. Selye's model, the initial acute reaction to any irritant or stress factor is called the Alarm Stage. An example of this stage occurs when a muscle in the body is overworked. Soreness will follow, and the muscle may even become inflamed. In a state of health, such symptoms will quickly pass, and the muscle will return to its normal state within a day or two as the self-regulating, balancing mechanisms of homeostasis do their work.

However, if the muscle is continuously overworked, or exposed to additional strains from other stress factors, it will eventually start to adapt and accommodate itself to the repetitive stress factor in order to cope with the demands of the stress in ways beyond those of the Alarm Stage. Eventually, the body as a whole will also begin adapting itself in this same manner, at which point, the second, or Resistance Stage comes into play.

This stage is usually without symptoms at first, and it can last for many years. In fact, Resistance Stage adaptation lasts for as many years as the body's resources and reserves will allow, while the body continues its attempts to repair itself. Depending upon individual genetic makeup, as well as factors such as nutritional deficiencies, traumas, illnesses, medications, and surgeries which have been acquired in life, the ability to continue to adapt and resist will vary significantly from person to person. This explains why two people faced with apparently identical challenges will respond quite differently. One might meet the challenge with no sign of difficulty, while the other might collapse into serious ill-health.

Most people will display the collection of minor symptoms which seem to have become the norm of Dr. Bland's "vertically ill" as they cope with life's stresses, whether these be structural, biochemical, or emotional. It is at the end of the Resistance Stage, when a person's adaptive mechanisms begin to fail, that the final stage of GAS results, known as the Exhaustion Stage. At this point, the person's ability to cope with repetitive, and often multiple, stress factors will inevitably lead into actual disease, usually of a chronic nature.

Returning to the example of the overworked muscle, one can clearly see how each of these stages would progress. When a muscle is first overworked, the Alarm Stage reaction manifests as pain, stiffness, and perhaps inflammation. If this stress of overwork becomes chronic, during the Resistance Stage the muscle would become increasingly less elastic and more fibrous, placing stress on the points where it is anchored into bone. This creates additional problems of pain, coordination difficulties, and stress on the joints. Left untreated, the muscle will eventually enter into the Exhaustion Stage, with the fibrousness and inflammation possibly degenerating into fibrositis (muscular rheumatism), and the joints, due to the uneven wear and tear caused by muscular imbalances, would show signs of arthritis.

It is the interaction between what is being adapted to and the individual's reserves and resources which decides when, and at what level, ill-health will result. To use another example, treating high blood pressure by prescribing a drug could possibly be effective in momentarily lowering blood pressure, but if it is being caused by emotional stress or improper diet, the underlying causes would be unaffected and could soon result in additional problems elsewhere in the body. Helping the person learn to better deal with his or her emotions, or instructing him or her in the role proper diet and nutrition plays in overall health, would be far more effective long-term approaches.

"The same principles apply to all health problems," states Dr. Chaitow. "If we can remove the cause of the problem, increase the powers of adaptation and resistance, or, ideally, do both of these, we restore the opportunity for the self-regulating mechanisms of homeostasis to operate again and healing can begin."

Other Factors Contributing to Illness

As a growing number of patients struggle with illnesses involving depressed immune function and overstressed hormonal and nervous systems, physicians must cope with the fact that these illnesses simply do not respond to the types of treatments being offered by conventional medicine today. To better understand this situation, we must first look at some of the factors influencing our health.

Genetics—From our parents we receive our genetic inheritance, and are born with constitutional strengths and weaknesses over which we have no control. External factors provide additional layers of influence which act on our genetically acquired ability to adapt and cope.

Diet—Emmanuel Cheraskin, M.D., D.M.D., of Birmingham, Alabama, pictures the sick individual as a layered "onion" whose signs and symptoms serve as the onion's outer layers, with layers of biochemical imbalance lying underneath. At the core of the onion, according to Dr. Cheraskin's research, lies poor diet.

That diet is so essential to health is not surprising. The foods and liquids we consume, along with the air that we breathe, have a fundamental effect on our well-being. A healthy diet of pesticide-free fruits and vegetables, whole grains, seeds, and nuts, along with organically raised, free-range poultry and certain types of fish, can supply us with all of the essential nutrients our bodies require for optimum efficiency, energy, and freedom from disease. Such a diet is rare today, however, having been replaced by foods high in unhealthy levels of fat, preservatives, chemical additives, and, in the case of most of the meat available in the United States, antibiotics and hormones, due to the way our livestock is raised. These factors alone can contribute to much of the chronic ill-health conditions besetting people today.

Mental and Emotional Stress—Research in the field of mind/body medicine has revealed that there is a direct link between mental and emotional distress and the body's ability to resist illness. It has also been discovered that unresolved or unexpressed thoughts and feelings are translated in the body as neurochemicals. These chemicals communicate with other systems of the body, particularly the autonomic nervous system, causing the body to react in a manner similar to when physical stress is present. Fear, for example, arouses the nervous system and triggers a flood of adrenal hormones, causing an accelerated heart rate and intensified breathing. Under healthy conditions, such reactions soon subside, but chronic fear, anger, grief, and other powerful emotions can keep the nervous system in a constant state of arousal. This allows stress to build up in the body, eventually attacking the body's organs and resulting in depressed immunity.

Environmental Pollution—Pollutants in the air, water, soil, and the foods we eat can contribute to illnesses ranging from birth defects and cancer to Alzheimer's disease. They also can create a severe toll on the immune system, leading to many other chronic conditions, such as allergies.

Dental Factors—The relationship between common dental silver amalgam fillings and chronic illness is now becoming recognized by a growing number of dentists, physicians, and researchers. The problem lies with the fact that calling the fillings "silver" is a misnomer because they are actually composed of 50% mercury, one of the metals most toxic to the human body. Over time, the mercury can slowly leech out of the fillings. When this happens, damage may occur to the nervous system, leading to symptoms resembling multiple sclerosis, chronic fatigue syndrome, and senile dementia. Infections in the gums can also diminish health by suppressing immune function and increasing the susceptibility of disease elsewhere in the body. The misalignment between the skull and jaw caused by temporomandibular joint syndrome can also create various types of stress that can result in depression, insomnia, headaches, fatigue, chronic pain, and low back pain.

The Inappropriate Use of Antibiotics—Antibiotics are valuable drugs when they are used appropriately. But the evidence today points to massive overuse. Antibiotics are often prescribed for medical conditions that do not warrant them. For instance, they are routinely given for colds, but many colds are the result of viral infections, and while antibiotics kill bacteria, they have no effect on the viruses.

The use of antibiotics can also result in a variety of side effects due to the way their powerful actions can interfere with the delicate balance of the body's systems. This can result in the destruction of the friendly bacteria in the body, leading to yeast overgrowth, both locally, such as in vaginal infections, and systemically, in the form of candidiasis, interference of nutrient absorption, the development of food allergies, recurrent ear infections, and immune suppression, as evidenced by the large percentage of adults suffering from chronic fatigue syndrome who have histories of recurrent antibiotic treatment as children or adolescents.

Electromagnetic Fields—Electromagnetic fields (EMFs) are invisible yet active forces produced by electrical appliances (including computers, microwave ovens, and even electric razors), power lines, and wiring. Researchers have only recently begun to realize the effects EMFs can have on health. Recently, the Special Epidemiology Studies Program of the California Department of Health Services noted that EMFs can, in fact, change biological tissue, although the full range of their health effects remain unknown. Additional studies by the United States Environmental Protection Agency have found that, in the last twenty years, possible associations have been found between EMFs and miscarriages, birth defects, leukemia, brain cancers, and lymphomas.

Geopathic Stress—Geopathic refers to illnesses that are caused, or contributed to, by areas of harmful radiation from the earth itself. That such a possibility exists has been known to traditional cultures for thousands of years. The Chinese art of feng shui (the study of subtle earth energies and their relation to human life), for instance, takes into account the effects of harmful radiation from the earth to safeguard against building over the locations from which they emanate. According to Anthony Scott-Morley, D.Sc., Ph.D., M.D. (alt. med.), of Dorset, England, as many as 30% to 50% of the chronically ill exhibit some signs of geopathic stress. These include excessive sleeping, cold extremities, respiratory difficulties, and unexplained mood changes and depression. "While geopathic stress may not be the cause of these conditions, it certainly seems likely that it is a contributing factor," Dr. Scott-Morley says.

All of these factors can contribute to a decline in organ and body system function, resulting in illness. Even so, the pathway back to health does exist.

The Return to Health

The vast majority of illnesses are self-limiting, meaning that they get better all on their own. Alternative medicine recognizes this fact, realizing that health will usually arise spontaneously when the conditions for health exist. Therefore, once you are ill, getting healthy again requires the very same inputs that were needed to keep you healthy in the first place.

This may seem obvious but it's a message worth restating. As Dr. Chaitow says, "To regain health once it has been lost we need to begin to reverse some, and ideally all, of those processes which may be negatively impacting us and over which we have some degree of control. This includes taking responsibility for stopping those lifestyle choices which we know are harmful, whether this be smoking, excessive alcohol intake, or using drugs. In addition, we need to start to positively address the real needs that such behavior masks."

Depending on the nature of our health problems, this might involve starting to eat more nutritiously, sleeping and exercising in a more regular and balanced way, and making sure of receiving reasonable exposure to fresh air and sunlight. It may also include hygienic considerations, detoxifying and cleansing our bodies, addressing any structural or mechanical imbalances, as well as learning how to properly cope with stress, and deal with our mental and emotional needs.

"That sounds like a vast prescription," Dr. Chaitow says. "However, even if only some of it can be addressed, such as diet and relaxation, a remarkable phenomenon occurs as homeostasis begins to function more efficiently and health begins to return."

In beginning the journey back to health, we may require help, especially if our bodies have been overloaded and compromised for some time. According to Dr. Chaitow, the help should come from the treatment that is most appropriate for the individual. "This might involve alternative treatments aimed at helping restore nutritional balance or treatments geared toward the removal of toxic burdens in the body. Or it might involve restoring normal nerve and circulatory supply by addressing structural imbalances. One of the advantages of alternative medicine is that it affords the individual the broadest range of health treatment options. Of course, preventive care is always a better choice than waiting to restore health once it has been lost."

Our bodies are not designed to become ill, they are designed to heal and become healthy. "Even if conventional medicine tells you that your condition is incurable or that your only option is to live a life dependent on drugs with troublesome side effects, there is hope for improving or reversing your condition," Dr. Chaitow says.

Treatment

When, for any of a variety of reasons, our homeostatic potential is limited, or when we are more vulnerable and susceptible because of a decline in immune system efficiency, it is time to seek treatment to encourage the recovery processes. The treatment chosen should ideally seek to eliminate causes, remove the obstacles to recovery, or encourage normal homeostasis.

"All alternative healing methods focus on one or more of these key elements," says Dr. Chaitow, "which explains why there are so many different forms of treatment in the field of alternative medicine. The treatments themselves do not 'cure' the condition, they simply restore the body's self-healing ability. Some treatments focus on biochemistry, others address structural imbalances, while some deal with a person's energetic or emotional requirements. Whatever treatment approach works will effectively help homeostasis to function more efficiently and will not have added to the body's burden by increasing toxicity or weakening any element of the body's ability to function."

Selecting the Appropriate Treatment: Many Roads to Rome

Alternative medicine offers a wide variety of treatment options. Some of these, such as chiropractic, osteopathy, craniosacral therapy, and the various systems of bodywork, address structural imbalances within the body. Others focus on maintaining the body's biochemical balance of hormones, enzymes, and nutrients, in order to maintain proper cellular function. These include diet, nutritional supplements, herbal medicine, and enzyme therapy. Still others seek to restore mental and emotional balance, including mind/body medicine, biofeedback training, meditation, hypnotherapy, guided imagery, and neuro-linguistic programming. Finally, systems such as acupuncture, homeopathy, energy medicine, magnetic field therapy, and neural therapy address the energetic levels of the body.

Some systems of alternative medicine, such as Ayurvedic medicine, naturopathic medicine, and traditional Chinese medicine, incorporate a wide range of these methods to offer complete systems of healthcare.

While the treatment methods of alternative medicine may vary in their approach, all of them are linked by a common philosophy that:

■ Focuses on empowering the individual to accept responsibility for at least a part of the task of recovery and future health maintenance

■ Emphasizes sound nutrition as a core requirement for health

■ Recommends a balanced lifestyle, adequate and appropriate exercise, rest, sleep, and emotional tranquillity as prerequisites for a state of health

■ Attempts to ensure detoxification and the efficiency of the organs and systems of the body

■ Recognizes the importance of the musculoskeletal system as a potential source of interference with nerve transmission and the body's energy pathways, and as a reflection of the individual's internal physical and emotional state

■ Most importantly, treats the individual instead of his or her symptoms

Individuality

The late Roger Williams, Ph.D., of the University of Texas, showed that in any group of fifteen to twenty people there can be a range of nutritional requirements from person to person that varies by as much as 700 percent.

"Your actual need for a particular vitamin is almost certain to be different from mine," says Dr. Chaitow, "and our requirements for this vitamin will also vary depending upon our age and any emotional, biochemical, or physical stresses which we may be coping with. What this illustrates is that there is no uniform prescription as to what any of us require nutritionally. Our bodies know what we need, however, and as long as they remain healthy and we supply them with the benefits of a healthy diet, in their own innate wisdom they will automatically take what they need from the food we eat."

Since, even in terms of nutritional requirements, each person is unique, it follows that what is required to return to health also can vary drastically from individual to individual. It is with this in mind that alternative physicians begin their diagnosis and subsequent treatments. Understanding all of the factors that play a role in both health and illness, their focus is on meeting the specific needs of each of their patients, rather than attempting to superimpose any one particular model or approach to health as the answer for every person.

"All too often, this understanding is lacking in conventional medicine, however," Dr. Chaitow says. "For example, the conventional doctor who has twelve patients with asthma will often provide each of them with the same recommendations and prescription drugs, in effect treating the condition and not the patients themselves.

"An alternative practitioner, on the other hand, will realize that asthma has numerous causes. Some of his patients might be experiencing an allergic reaction to foods or something in their environment, others might have succumbed to a viral infection, while still others might be asthmatic because of diminished nerve supply due to a misaligned spine. Such a practitioner will therefore seek to determine the underlying cause for his patients' conditions, and treat each of them differently, using the method that will best stimulate their bodies to heal themselves. This distinction between approaches is a cornerstone of alternative medicine."

The return to health, therefore, is a road which each person must walk according to his or her own unique individuality. It is also a road that needs to address one's entire being, taking into account one's mental, emotional, and physical aspects, as well as the structural, biochemical, and energetic components that shape each of us. It is precisely because alternative medicine honors and understands these concepts, that it is now positioned to become a valuable and necessary pathway for meeting the medical crisis we, as a planet, are currently facing.

Medical Freedom Act

Freedom is at the heart of American society. We have freedom of speech, freedom of worship, and freedom of the press. But Americans lack one freedom which seems increasingly more vital for a truly free society. The freedom to choose the health care of their choice. This basic freedom is being suppressed by state and federal agencies, as well as the vested financial interests of the "medical/pharmaceutical complex," comprised of the conventional medical establishment and the multinational pharmaceutical companies. Despite the fact that conventional treatments are often ineffective, simply mask symptoms, and are subject to troubling side effects, Americans who seek better and more effective medicine must struggle to win the right to open access to alternative practitioners and treatments.

In the last decade:

■ There has been a concerted effort on the part of government regulatory agencies to punish and harass medical professionals who recommend or practice nutritional and herbal medicine and other alternative therapies to maintain health and prevent and treat illness.

■ State medical boards have censured and revoked the licenses of conscientious physicians who practice alternative medicine simply because their treatments are not conventional and do not conform to accepted "standards of care." These actions are taken despite the fact that many of these treatments work.

■ Insurance companies have routinely refused to pay for alternative treatments such as acupuncture, chiropractic, homeopathy, and nutritional medicine, labeling them unapproved therapies, regardless of the benefit received by the patients. This stance denies tens of millions of Americans their basic right to the health care of their choice.

■ The general public has been denied free access to information concerning the documented health benefits of nutritional supplements and herbs by restrictive labeling regulations established by the Food and Drug Administration (FDA). This restriction of information flow comes despite the fact that large scale independent studies have shown that many Americans, especially the elderly, are suffering from nutritional deficits which could be corrected by dietary supplementation.

■ Manufacturers of nutritional supplements and herbs, as well as health food stores, have been the target of FDA seizures in an attempt to block the manufacture and sale of numerous natural substances such as coenzyme Q10 and evening primrose oil, whose therapeutic effects have been scientifically validated.

These strong-arm tactics are being used despite the estimate of former Surgeon General C. Everett Koop that, out of 2.1 million deaths a year in the United States, 1.6 million are related to poor nutrition.

The bias against alternative medicine on both the state and federal level has become clearly established and has links to the campaign of the medical establishment to squelch the emergence of alternative medicine in the United States.

The Food and Drug Administration: Medical Establishment Cops

The FDA's suppression of alternative medicine, and especially of nutritional supplements, constitutes a war for power with billions of dollars and the health of Americans, according to Julian Whitaker, M.D., President of the American Preventive Medical Association and editor of the successful alternative newsletter *Health and Healing*. "This is not a reasonable debate on public safety or honesty in labeling," says Dr. Whitaker. "It is an ugly struggle for power by FDA Commissioner David Kessler, and those who support giving the FDA more power over the nutritional supplement industry, that smacks of the tactics of Joe McCarthy in the 1950s. Whereas Joe McCarthy's witch hunt was based on the theory that communists were everywhere, today's persecution of innocent people by the FDA is based on the premise that nutritional supplements are a menace."

The FDA is a branch of the Department of Health and Human Services. It is funded annually through the United States Congress and has the authority to regulate foods, drugs, cosmetics, and medical devices that are sold between states or imported. The FDA is also responsible for ensuring that products are pure and unadulterated, and not misrepresented through false labeling, declarations of ingredients, or net weight statements. The FDA also regulates certain manufacturing processes, holding jurisdiction over a product from the initial shipment of its raw materials across state lines to the shipment of the finished product from a manufacturing distribution facility outside the state. In addition, some drugs, medical devices, food additives, and food coloring require premarketing FDA approval. If someone markets a product without such approval the FDA can take regulatory action.

"The FDA has very wide-ranging regulatory powers that are restricted only by the courts. However, the FDA is rarely restricted by the courts because it is considered to be an agency of experts dealing with expert issues," notes attorney Jay Geller of Santa Monica, California, an authority on FDA law and former employee in the general counsel's office of the FDA. This lack of restriction allows the FDA to persecute alternative medicine practitioners with a relative lack of accountability. "There are two ways that the FDA is able to harass alternative physicians," says Alan R. Gaby, M.D., of Baltimore, Maryland, of the American Holistic Health Association. "They can raid their clinics or restrict the availability of effective medicinal substances. Whether or not the FDA has overstepped their legal boundary is unclear, but I do believe that what they are doing is improper. If there were unbiased individuals running the FDA this would not be happening, as I think it has much to do with their own bias and attitudes."

Konrad Kail, N.D., past president of the American Association of Naturopathic Physicians, holds a similar view. "The FDA's plan right now is to remove the agents used by alternative physicians, such as supplements and herbs, since they cannot remove the physicians," he says. "They are using the brute force of their power to unfairly police a specific group of individuals who tend to practice alternative medicine. As far as I am concerned this is a politically motivated move by conventional medicine in order to remove the competition from the marketplace. They are using the FDA to accomplish their own political motivations."

The FDA's bias in favor of conventional medicine may stem from the informal but very real connection it has with the pharmaceutical industry. One study, for instance, found that half of the high-ranking FDA officials have been formerly employed as key executives in pharmaceutical companies immediately prior to joining the FDA. In addition, the study found that half of these officials would then serve in an executive capacity in a pharmaceutical company immediately upon leaving the FDA.

The FDA's bias is further shown by its selective implementation of policy directives. Its duty, by law, is to set standards for drug advertisements. Yet, according to a study done last year at the University of California and published in the *Wall Street Journal*, 60% of the pharmaceutical ads from medical journals violated FDA guidelines. But the FDA, to this day, has done nothing about these violations.

Another connection between the FDA and the pharmaceutical industry is through the Pharmaceutical Advertising Council. In 1985, the Pharmaceutical Advertising Council teamed up with the FDA to solicit funds from the pharmaceutical industry for the purpose of combatting medical quackery. "The Pharmaceutical Advertising Council and the FDA also issued a joint statement addressed to the presidents of advertising and PR agencies nationwide asking them to cooperate with a joint venture antifraud and quackery campaign," according to Mark Blumenthal, Executive Director of the American Botanical Council. "The letter has joint letterhead from the FDA and the Pharmaceutical Advertising Council, and is signed by the directors of both organizations. On the surface it appears to be patently illegal. The FDA is supposed to regulate the pharmaceutical industry, but instead they are teaming up to work on an antifraud campaign against an industry that some could construe to be an economic competitor."

Further evidence of the FDA's bias toward drugs as opposed to nutritional supplements is demonstrated by the FDA's Dietary Supplements Task Force Final Report, which reads in part, "The Task Force considered various issues in its deliberations, including…what steps are necessary to ensure that the existence of dietary supplements on the market does not act as a disincentive for drug development.

Freedom of Information and FDA Regulation of the Manufacture and Sale of Nutritional Supplements and Herbs

"The FDA has always had a perceived bias against dietary supplements and has historically looked on them with a jaundiced eye," says Geller. "The agency has expressed virtually no interest in trying to find a balance between the requirements necessary to approve prescription drugs and those appropriate to allow preventive health claims for naturally occurring substances such as vitamins, minerals, enzymes, amino acids, and herbs. Even with the studies that have come out on the potential benefits of vitamin E for preventing heart disease, the FDA's position is that there are not going to be any claims allowed to be made for dietary supplements that do not meet the standards applied to prescription drugs."

The FDA has also seized safe and effective natural remedies such as coenzyme Q10 and evening primrose oil from health food stores and distributors because they did not approve of the statements being made about these supplements, according to Dr. Gaby. "This, despite the fact that extensive scientific literature supports their use. Coenzyme Q10 has been shown to be valuable in treating congestive heart failure, cardiomyopathy [a disease of the heart muscle], and high blood pressure; and evening primrose oil has proven effective in the treatment of eczema, high blood pressure, and arthritis," he notes.

Dr. Gaby also finds that the policies of the FDA make it extremely difficult for consumers to learn about the health benefits of any natural substance, including nutritional supplements and herbs. "According to the FDA's interpretation of the law," he says, "any substance for which a health claim is made becomes a drug, subject to the same strict rules and regulations as prescription pharmaceuticals."

Dr. Kail feels that such rules are unnecessary. "We don't need to have more restrictions on supplements and herbs," he says. "This will only act to benefit the pharmaceutical companies and doctors who are already making enormous profits in this field and make it more expensive for people to take care of themselves. Health care will be taken out of the hands of the people and put back into the hands of institutions. People can do a lot to take care of themselves if they are taught how to do it."

One such example of FDA bias and its damaging effect on national health concerns the use of saw palmetto berries for prostate disease. "The extract of the saw palmetto berry has been shown by scientific studies to be about three times more effective than the Merck prostate drug, Proscar, for alleviating symptoms of prostate enlargement, such as poor urinary stream, urinary retention, and nightime urination," reports Dr. Whitaker. "Furthermore, saw palmetto extract has no toxicity."

On the other hand, Proscar causes impotence, ejaculation dysfunction, decreased libido, and is teratogenic (birth defect-causing), according to the Physician's Desk Reference.

Yet, the FDA has recommended that saw palmetto berry be removed from the market while allowing Proscar to remain available. "As a result," says Dr. Whitaker, "ten million men have been robbed of a safer, more effective therapy."

The bias against natural cures is alarming. For example, according to summaries from the nation's poison control centers, one death was associated with the use of a nutritional supplement from 1983 to 1990, and that was due to regular overuse of niacin by a mentally disturbed individual,. On the other hand, drug use causes fatal reactions in 0.44% of hospitalized patients. This translates to about 130,000 deaths a year, or roughly 356 deaths every day.

"So as not to alarm the public or hurt the pharmaceutical industry, the FDA looks the other way when prescription drugs kill hundreds of thousands and harm millions," says Dr. Whitaker. "But if someone drinking Sleepytime tea has a restless night, the agency raids the health food stores, confiscates the tea, and dupes the TV networks into airing biased exposés on the dangers of nutritional supplements."

The Persecution of Dr. Jonathan Wright

One of the most outspoken critics of FDA policy has been Jonathan Wright, M.D. A widely publicized incident involving Dr. Wright and the FDA illustrates how ruthless the agency's regulatory action can be when directed against physicians practicing alternative medicine. On the morning of May 6, 1992, FDA agents, accompanied by ten officers from the King's County Police Department, broke down the door of Dr. Wright's Tahoma Clinic in Kent, Washington, wearing flak jackets and with guns drawn.

Prior to this raid, the clinic had never been subject to an official FDA inspection nor received a request for an inspection. Yet during the subsequent 14-hour raid, FDA agents confiscated a truckload of items, including patient and employee records; banking statements; payroll data; injectable, preservative-free vitamins, mineral and glandular extracts; noninvasive allergy and sensitivity testing equipment; instruction and training manuals; the entire printed contents of the hard drive on the clinic's central computer system; and even the clinic's supply of postage stamps.

One of the items confiscated in the armed raid was a vitamin B12 complex manufactured in Germany. Though the FDA claims that the sale of these vitamins is against the law, Dr. Wright argues that vitamins, minerals, and other nutrients are not drugs, but natural substances over which the FDA should not have jurisdiction. Because he treats many patients with allergies, Dr. Wright uses the German form of vitamin B12 because it is the only injectable vitamin he has found that does not contain preservatives or additives, both of which can cause adverse reactions in some of his patients.

In addition, the German form of vitamin B12 is in use around the country, and stronger doses of the vitamin made in America are also available in numerous pharmacies.

FDA harassment of Dr. Wright, a former columnist for *Prevention* magazine who is considered one of the world's experts in nutritional biochemistry, began in 1991 when agents confiscated from his clinic a dispensary stock of L-tryptophan that had previously been verified as being uncontaminated.

In August 1991, Dr. Wright sued for recovery of the L-tryptophan. Within three weeks, FDA investigators started systematic searches of the trash bin located in the parking lot of the office complex housing the Tahoma Clinic. Between December and March of the following year, they also visited the clinic posing as patients, leading up to the May raid.

Doctors and alternative care advocates say Dr. Wright was singled out because he has been outspoken about treatment methods that traditional practitioners deem unorthodox. Dr. Wright speculates the action is tied to a lawsuit he has pending with the FDA over the seizure of his stock of L-tryptophan. He also reports that when he and his wife have traveled abroad since the incident, they have been singled out in customs lines and their belongings meticulously searched, something that had never happened previously during his many foreign travels. Upon returning from a recent trip, his wife was even taken to a room and strip-searched. Dr. Wright, a prominent physician with over twenty years of experience in family practice and an international reputation for the safety and effectiveness of his practice, is being treated like a common criminal—simply because he stood up for his right to practice alternative medicine.

The Harassment of Dr. Stephen Levine & NutriCology

Critics of the FDA have long asserted that the agency has unjustly waged health fraud campaigns against alternative treatments, products, or practitioners, while at the same time ignoring gross health violations by major pharmaceutical companies. For instance, when it was discovered that Pfizer, Inc., produced and sold a defective heart valve which resulted in 310 deaths, the heart valve was removed from the market but no fraud charges were filed. And when Bristol-Myers was caught selling unapproved cancer drugs through illegal promotions, they too escaped criminal charges. On May 9, 1991, however, Stephen A. Levine, Ph.D., learned of the FDA's selective practices firsthand.

Holding a temporary restraining order secured by the Department of Justice, U.S. Attorney's Office, and Attorney General on behalf of the FDA, a dozen FDA agents burst into the headquarters of Dr. Levine's small company, NutriCology, in San Leandro, California. To complete their exhaustive search of his offices and warehouse, they effectively shut the company's operations down for two full days. Although the FDA had not warned Dr. Levine of any serious noncompliance for three years prior to the raid, he was now accused of selling "unapproved new drugs" and slapped with a temporary restraining order on nine products. These products were coenzyme Q10, flaxseed oil, geranium, borage oil, OxyNutrients™, citrus seed extract, *Artemesia annua*, Ovalectin™ (an extract of hen egg yolks), and a natural antioxidant called pycnogenol. Dr. Levine maintained that the products were to be classified as foods and not "drugs," because they are reputable supplements that can be found in most health food stores in the United States.

In addition, in the government's memorandum, Dr. Levine was compared to a "snake oil salesman" and the products in question termed "at best worthless." He was also threatened with criminal charges associated with the mail fraud act. Under this act the government can seize property, assets, records, and other belongings of the accused; thus the court was asked to also freeze Dr. Levine's company and personal assets.

Later, depositions of the FDA's two leading experts revealed that they had not read any of the scientific literature substantiating NutriCology's products, and that neither, in fact, had conducted any research personally. Their action was based solely on the hearsay statements of others.

Perhaps one of the reasons the FDA targeted NutriCology, a small company with no history of customer complaints, was because of its leading scientific role in developing new products.

Furthermore, Dr. Levine has played a key role in successfully educating physicians regarding antioxidant therapies through his book, *Antioxidant Adaptation: Its Role in Free Radical Pathology*.

In response to this unprovoked attack, NutriCology submitted evidence from several expert witnesses, affidavits from sixty physicians, and a 12-inch stack of scientific papers supporting the products under FDA attack.

On May 23, 1991, Federal Judge F. Lowell Jenson denied the government's request for a preliminary injunction on the nine products. In a 20-page opinion, Judge Jenson held that the FDA had failed to provide evidence necessary to support its charges against NutriCology. The court even went so far as to state in its decision that to prevent the sale of products the FDA was targeting would "clearly threaten the viability of the business [NutriCology] itself, which, in light of the attestations of numerous physicians, health officials, and other experts, would constitute a real and potentially unnecessary loss to the health needs of the general public."

But the FDA filed for reconsideration and was again denied the motion for the same reasons. In December 1992, the FDA petitioned the 9th

Circuit Court of Appeals for a fourth injunction. When the FDA was questioned as to why it was bringing the case to the appellate level after it had already been denied previous injunctions, it responded by saying that NutriCology was dangerous to the public. The court responded by citing that in the past ten years there were no complaints or injuries arising from NutriCology products, the majority of which cater to medical doctors and health care professionals. The injunction was again denied.

The Medical Establishment and the Suppression of Unorthodox Research

The FDA is not the only force that practitioners of alternative medicine must contend with. In order to receive grants for medical research and be published in the major medical and scientific journals, physicians and researchers are compelled not to stray far from conventional views. Otherwise they run the risk of being shut out of the mainstream and find themselves without the funding they need to carry on their work. The American Society for Clinical Nutrition, for example, publishers of the *American Journal of Clinical Nutrition*, acknowledge at the front of each issue of their journal the "generous support" of certain organizations for selected educational activities of the society. Among the companies that provide this support are the Coca-Cola Company, General Foods Corporation, General Mills Foundation, Gerber Products Company, the Nutra-Sweet® Group, the Pillsbury Company, and numerous pharmaceutical companies. "Would these organizations support research about the damaging effects of the processed foods they are selling?" Dr. Gaby asks, pointing out the unlikelihood of such a scenario.

Furthermore, physicians who abide by a conventional Western medical perspective are more likely to publish papers and end up being on editorial boards of scientific journals than are their peers who hold to different philosophies. "There is kind of a self-selection process where physicians who are against alternative medicine end up being on the editorial boards of the journals," Dr. Gaby says. It's important to bear in mind, too, that a large percentage of medical journals receive a substantial amount of their revenue from the advertising dollars they get from the pharmaceutical industry, whose interests would not be served by articles and studies that recommended the use of alternative medicine over drugs and surgery.

The Case of Dr. Peter Duesberg

The bias against unorthodox medicine has never been more clear than in the case of Peter Duesberg, Ph.D., of the University of California at Berkeley, a specialist in the field of microbiology with impeccable credentials who is recognized internationally as an expert in retroviruses, an area of research he helped to pioneer. Due to the quality of his research work, Dr. Duesberg was awarded a $250,000 federal research grant as an independent investigator, meaning he could choose his own area of research. But when Dr. Duesberg went against conventional wisdom to assert that HIV (human immunodeficiency virus) was not the cause of AIDS, as is commonly believed, but possibly only an incidental factor, the government took away his grant and his views were dismissed out of hand. Now, however, some four thousand cases of AIDS have been discovered where no trace of the HIV virus exists, giving weight to Dr. Duesberg's position. In addition, research from the renowned Pasteur Institute in Paris, France, which was responsible for the discovery of HIV, has also shown that HIV is not the sole cause of AIDS and, in fact, requires co-factors for the disease to develop. Despite this, Dr. Duesberg continues to be discounted, and even vilified, by the medical establishment.

Repression of a Cancer Drug That Works:
Dr. Joe Gold and Hydrazine Sulfate

In the area of cancer, the National Cancer Institute (NCI) has shown an equal bias against alternative practitioners. Despite the apparent failure of the costly "war on cancer," NCI continues to wage a campaign against nutritionally-based cancer treatments that may be one of the keys to halting, and even reversing, cancerous growths. An example of this can be found in the case of Joe Gold, M.D., of Syracuse, New York.

A veteran of NASA's medical corps, Dr. Gold discovered that an easily synthesized substance called hydrazine sulfate could help cancer patients reverse their disease by preventing the wasting-away process that accompanies cancer and which inhibits the body's normal processing of nutrients. In fact, a significant percentage of cancer victims die of the malnutrition caused by this inhibition, rather than the cancer itself.

Hydrazine sulfate is inexpensive, and was first developed by Dr. Gold at the Syracuse Cancer Research Institute in the early 1970s. It has subsequently undergone more than 20 years of controlled testing at both UCLA Harbor Hospital and the Petrov Research Institute in St. Petersburg, Russia. Results showing that hydrazine sulfate is able to stop, and even reverse, tumor growth in many cancer patients have been published in leading medical journals, including *The Lancet*, *Cancer*, and the *Journal of Clinical Oncology*. And in a 1991 multi-institutional study, a team of scientists from the Petrov Institute reported that hydrazine sulfate stopped tumors in roughly half their patients, including those tumors which attack the breast, ovaries, cervix, endometrium, and vulva. A smaller but significant number of patients had even more profound results, with their tumors disappearing altogether.

The NCI has not followed up on the Russian study, which American cancer officials have dismissed as "poorly done work...not up to our standards." Compounding the NCI's omission is the fact that U.S. clinical trials conducted in 1992 and 1993 were allowed to occur without heeding Dr. Gold's warnings that hydrazine sulfate is not effective when used in conjunction with incompatible substances such as alcohol, sleeping pills, and tranquilizers. Patients were allowed to ingest these substances, in effect scuttling the test results, which were inconclusive. Instead of initiating further tests and conducting them according to Dr. Gold's established protocol, NCI officials continue to reject hydrazine sulfate as a viable cancer treatment, informing physicians that its use is little more than "quackery."

State Medical Boards:
Does Conformity Equal Competence?

In 1847, the American Medical Association (AMA) was formed, ostensibly to protect the public from charlatans, since, at that time, anyone could offer medical services and drugs uncontested. For the remainder of the nineteenth century, the AMA successfully lobbied states to require licensing of all physicians. Eventually, the AMA set up a Council on Medical Education to oversee all medical schools. The AMA was so successful that the number of medical schools in the United States actually decreased by half between the early 1900s and 1944, from 160 in 1904 to just 77 in 1940. Today, the AMA is able to prevent doctors who do not subscribe to its views from serving on hospital staffs and it also controls medical boards on the state level.

The purpose of such medical boards is to protect the public against incompetent and unscrupulous doctors. But, as Dr. Gaby notes, "they often inappropriately extend that function to eliminating doctors that deviate from the arbitrary standards of care that are based on what they understand. The excuse for censuring a doctor or revoking his license is that he is incompetent, and the proof is that he deviates from the standards of care. Therefore, by definition, if you deviate, you are incompetent."

The Persecution of Dr. Warren Levin

A telling example of the power of state medical boards to censure and harass competent physicians who deviate from conventional therapies is the case of Warren Levin, M.D., of New York City. The medical establishment so strenuously objected to Dr. Levin's effective use of chelation therapy, vitamin supplements, exercise, and counseling that it waged a 16-year campaign against him, at a cost of approximately $1 million.

Despite its efforts, the Office of Professional Medical Conduct of the New York State Health Department was unable to come up with a single allegation of patient injury attributed to Dr. Levin. Nevertheless, the state medical board's hearing officers managed to ignore and insult a parade of highly respected physicians and scientists who came to Dr. Levin's defense, including two-time Nobel Prize–winner Linus Pauling.

At the same time, the hearing officers did accept and honor the testimony of a doctor who denounced chelation therapy as useless. And although the prosecution witness in question admitted under cross-examination that he had never read anything about chelation therapy, met a doctor who used it, or even seen a patient who received it, the panel found him to be a "credible and authoritative witness." The panel, therefore, recommended that Dr. Levin be stripped of his license to practice.

It is ironic that at the same time the government is searching for highly effective, lower-cost approaches to the nation's health care needs, a physician like Dr. Levin, who for years was providing his patients with exactly such an approach and achieving impressive results, could be prevented from practicing his profession.

Positive Developments in Protecting Your Medical Freedom of Choice

Since 1990, nine states (New York, North Carolina, Georgia, Alaska, Colorado, Oregon, Oklahoma, South Dakota, and Washington) have passed freedom of practice statutes, allowing physicians to practice alternative forms of medicine without fear of retribution from their state medical boards. The statutes state that failure to conform to standards of care shall not by itself be considered incompetence unless patients are harmed or exposed to unreasonable risk.

These new laws are paving the way for medical freedom in the United States, providing citizens with a true choice in their medical treatment. The United States Congress is also beginning to recognize the validity of alternative medicine. In 1992, Congress established the Office of Alternative Medicine at the National Institutes of Health (NIH), with an annual budget of $2 million to be used to investigate the potential of promising alternative therapies. Although this is hardly adequate funding for such an important task, it is clearly a step in the right direction.

Both developments are in the spirit of the World Health Organization's call for the integration of the various forms of "traditional medicine," such as homeopathy, naturopathic medicine, traditional Chinese medicine, Ayurvedic medicine, and herbal medicine, with conventional modern medicine in order to help meet the global health care needs of the twenty-first century.

In order for change to take place in the practice of medicine in America, it is important to have alternative physicians on state medical boards. In fact, certain laws already on the books may help to put this into action. Vincent

Speckhart, M.D., of Norfolk, Virginia, reports, for instance, that in dealing with the State Medical Board of Virginia, he discovered a 100-year-old state law that required that two homeopaths always sit on the board, a law that had been ignored for over 20 years.

The state of Alaska, meanwhile, is taking the lead in this area. On July 23, 1992, Alaska Governor Walter J. Hickel, appointed Robert Jay Rowen, M.D., to the State Medical Board. Dr. Rowen is an alternative physician from Anchorage, Alaska, whose dedicated effort led to the passage of landmark legislation on freedom of practice, making Alaska the first state to adopt such a measure. Governor Hickel announced his bold move in the following press release:

"I am putting Dr. Rowen on the Medical Board not to be controversial but to be helpful. He is a strong advocate of prevention as the first line of defense. And as the costs of traditional medical care continue to go up, it will be those who care for themselves through prevention who will live better lives. He believes prevention simply costs society less."

The governor went on to proclaim, "Dr. Rowen has a sound medical background, yet he is open minded about new ideas that can help heal. I think we need that now more than ever. I believe a balanced perspective in this seven-member board is best for Alaskans, and best for the future of health care."

Actions We Can Take to Restore Our Medical Freedom

A combination of grassroots activity, market forces, and public awareness about the full benefits of alternative medicine will do much to restore medical freedom in America. Because people can feel powerless in the face of large, influential institutions such as the FDA or Congress, it is essential that they are able to find a common vehicle through which they can empower themselves and affect change.

Alexander Schauss, Ph.D., executive director of the non-profit health care advocacy groups Citizens for Health and the American Preventive Medical Association (APMA), cites the effect grassroots movements can have on legislation: "A United States senator was trying to introduce an amendment that would delay restrictive labeling laws for dietary supplements. It was predicted to be defeated. Through our network, we were able to initiate a series of 1,800 phone calls through our national phone tree, and we reached an additional 15,000 people through a fax network. Within 48 hours, the United States Senate was receiving approximately 10,000 phone calls per hour. That helped the bill to be easily passed by a margin of 94 to one, and shows that people really can make a difference."

In North Carolina, grassroots forces also demonstrated their ability to effect change. Doctors statewide were losing their licenses as a result of alternative health care modalities which they incorporated into their standard practices. The movement started out as 12 people fed up with government interference in their freedom to make health choices, but soon grew to a core group of 3,000 people. The group ended up having a dramatic impact on state legislators.

As Dr. Schauss points out, people often underestimate the power of grassroots organizations. "The average congressional district has around 200,000 people and only about 10% or 15% of those people vote," he says. "So you only need half of those voters to keep a person in Congress."

Therefore, one of the most practical ways citizens can hasten the acceptance of alternative medicine is to organize letter-writing campaigns to Congress and the President demanding that research into these methods be conducted, and that persecution of practitioners, manufacturers, and researchers of alternative medicine cease.

It is important to note that this is not to imply that all new medicines should be approved without proper testing, as reasonable safeguards are always desirable. But in a time when some legislators are proposing that it be illegal to purchase vitamins without a prescription, it is essential to promote freedom of choice in both gaining access to information on new treatments as well as access to the treatments themselves once they are established as viable alternatives.

"If everyone in this country wrote a truthful and honest letter to all their congressmen and senators at both state and federal levels expressing their feelings about the medical industry and demanding a choice in health care, we could see a big change," states Dr. Kail. "Tell them that you want to be able to choose your health practitioners—an acupuncturist, a chiropractor, a naturopath, or an M.D.—who can practice alternative therapies without fear of losing their licenses."

As alternative medicine continues to wage its battle against the seemingly unyielding forces of government and conventional medicine, grassroots organizations will play perhaps the most important role in raising public awareness and in initiating both legislative and societal change. If alternative medicine is to gain its proper place in preventing and alleviating health problems, citizens must organize, mobilize, and act.

ACUPUNCTURE

Acupuncture uses needles to penetrate and stimulate specific points in the body to restore normal function and energetic balance. It is a recognized form of treatment and prevention that is practiced in hospitals and in private practice throughout the world.

Nationwide

Chesapeake Electromedical
3 Church Circle Ste 165
Annapolis MD.................................800/872-0399

Alabama

Birmingham

Chen Gregory Shu
3245 Lorna Rd 205/979-4079

Fairhope

Stump John L DC OMD P
401 N Section St...........................334/928-5058

Alaska

Anchorage

Jade Acupuncture & Behavioral Medicine
8437 Jade St..................................907/243-3031
Manuel F Russell MD
4141 B St Ste 209........................907/562-7070
Rowen Robert MD
615 E 82nd Ave Ste 300..............907/344-7745

Wasilla

Martin Robert MD
PO Box 870710.............................907/376-5284

Arizona

Lake Havasu City

Kuhns Bradely OMD PHD
1641-25 McCulloch Blvd 602/453-6245

Phoenix

Abromovitz Alan M
1725 E Osborn Rd 602/274-9302
Addesso Anthony DC
2525 W Greenway #214 ....602/843-9249
Donatello Lance A
4315 E Thunderbird Rd Ste 2 ....602/996-6745
Highhouse Susan
4419 N 46th Pl 602/952-8959
Kail Konrad ND
13832 N 32nd St Ste 2-4 ....602/493-2273
Kimata Lori G ND
13832 N 32nd St Ste 2-4 ....602/493-2273
Lee Tom S ND
13832 N 32nd St Ste 2-4 ....602/493-2273
Lee Terry J DDS
4210 N 32nd St 602/956-4807

Nassan Susan H
4419 N 46th Pl 602/952-8959

Prescott

Cocilovo Anna M
PO Box 10602 ....602/445-1643

Scottsdale

Feingold Jeffrey H NMD
5743 E Thomas Rd Ste 1 ....602/945-8773
Wadsworth Chloe F
9270 E Mission Ln Unit 207 ....602/391-0615

Sedona

Binswanger Carole Ida
PO Box 10207 ....602/282-1206
Boericke Keith
315 Capitol Butte Dr 602/282-1342
Butterfield Carol
PO Box 1429 ....602/282-0585
Evie Kay M DAC
2756 West Hwy 89A 602/204-1347

Tucson

Deloe Paul NMD
6161 E Speedway Blvd 602/886-9988
Harrell-Stokes Sunana
3232 N Little Creek Pl 602/881-8848
Jaffrey David M
1735 E Fort Lowell Rd Ste 12 ......602/323-8940
Kimbrell L Caitlin RN MS MA
2542 E La Madera Dr 602/327-1134
Morris Lance J
1001 N Swan Rd 602/323-7133
Parker Margo Jordan
4725 E Sunrise Dr # 154 ....602/529-0433
Stumpf Susan Mac ACP
4007 Flowing Wells Road 602/887-7699

Arkansas

Harrison

Sinclair John H Dds
702 N Main 501/741-2254

Hot Springs

Ranft Michael Edward
239 Hobson Ave 501/623-5433

Leslie

Taliaferro Melissa
PO Box 400 ....501/447-2599
Vigh Janice
PO Box 465 ....501/447-6166

California

Agoura Hills

Gentile Teresa PHD ND
28247 Agoura Rd........................ 818/707-3126

Alameda

Lam Harvey M

2303 Buena Vista Ave 510/522-8482
Weber Margaret
   2236 Buena Vista Ave 510/769-7139

Albany
Liao Richard Y T
   1033 Solano Ave 510/524-8148

Aptos
Singer Charles R
   8065 Aptos St 408/685-1800

Arcadia
Hs Ouyang Donald
   1742 Vista Del Valle Dr 818/355-6744
Hsi Eric Y
   600 Walnut Ave 818/576-7528

Arcata
Yamas John S
   48 Sunnybrae Ctr 707/822-7400

Aromas
Breslin Joseph
   1560 Cannon Rd 408/726-3212

Artesia
Soon Cho Kyu
   11742 E Artesia Blvd 310/924-0723

Bakersfield
Sook Kim In
   8812 Ginger Oak Ln 805/665-8689

Balboa Island
Murray Ann L
   209 Crystal Ave Ste A....................714/673-9504

Belmont
Sheehan Timothy Walter
   2704 Barclay Way 415/570-5991

Berkeley
Carter Joseph BS LAC
   2291 Eunice St 510/524-4151
Chasin Gilbert E LM
   816 Contra Costa Ave 510/843-7492
Cutler Karen B
   2006 Dwight Way Ste 204-205 ....510/654-3873
Dierauf Benjamin Edward LM
   2510 Grant 510/652-6667
Douthwaite Tisha
   3099 Telegraph Ave Ste 108 ....510/486-0988
Guenther Tamminen Ann LM
   1420 Hearst Ave 510/845-2094
Helms Joseph Moll
   2520 Milvia St 510/841-7600
Kalfus Frances OMD LAC
   2615 Ashby Ave 510/841-1753
Kitts David B LAC
   1720 Bancroft Way 510/486-1682
Lewis Roberta A
   Bancroft Center of Chinese Medicine

   1834 Dwight Way 510/540-8528
Lourie Carol MD LAC
   1442 A Walnut St #410 ....510/526-2028
Macnair Barbra E LAC
   3021 Telegraph Ave #B 510/649-8054
Marcus Alon LAC DOM
   1650 Alcatraz Ave 510/652-5834
McElyea Mink Katie
   Bancroft Center of Chinese Medicine
   1720 Bancroft Way 510/849-1809
Mink Jeffrey S
   267 Arlington Ave 510/528-0134
Partridge Elizabeth LM
   2130 Derby St 510/845-8081
Peler Eva Marie
   2929 Martin Luther King Jr Way ...510/848-5951
Sordean John R OMD LAC LM
   3021 Telegraph Ave #C 510/849-1176
Tamminen Ann Guenther
   1502 Walnut St 510/845-2094
Wong Henry Ks
   2728 Webster St 510/845-5345
Zieger Robert B
   3031 Telegraph Ave Ste 106.........510/843-7397

Beverly Hills
Afifi Simin G LM
   300 S Beverly Dr Ste 310 ....310/551-0828
Holmes Mark OMD LAC
   Center for Regeneration
   9730 Wilshire Blvd Ste 108..........310/706-2540
Ishikawa Keiko LAC DAC
   Ishikawa Acupuncture & Shiatsu Clinic
   441 S Beverly Dr Ste 4 ....310/203-8548
Lippman Cathie A MD
   2915 La Cienega Blvd Ste 207 ...213/653-0486
Nagaser Tom Y
   PO Box 1177 ....213/550-0179
Waterhouse Michael H
   9730 Wilshire Blvd Ste 215 ....310/859-0444

Bolinas
Angel Patricia
   PO Box 599 ....415/868-1486

Buena Park
Nambudripad Devi S
   6714 Beach Blvd 714/523-0800

Burbank
Livingstone Patricia M LM
   1117 N Niagara St 818/843-3496

Burlingame
Orlinsky Walter A
   1118 Majilla Ave 415/579-3743

Calabasas
Depew Karole M
   23540 Calabasas Rd 818/347-7236

Mann Laura OMD CA
  Calabasas Center for Healing
  5000 Calabasas Parkway #105 ...818/222-8031

Calistoga
Fennen Brian C
  2436 Foothill Blvd Ste D 707/942-9380

Camarillo
Cooper Carol LAC LCSW
  425 Mariposa Dr 405/388-7663

Campbell
Viet Ta Hoang
  138 Gilman Ave 408/374-2959
Wilson Mark R
  116 E Campbell Ave Ste 7 ....408/378-2424

Canoga Park
Zhang Xiao Xing
  21050 Community St 818/407-0514

Cardiff By The Sea
Levitt Steven D
  PO Box 355 ....619/436-6004

Carlsbad
Levee Sandra Jean
  800 Grand Ave Ste C-1 ....619/434-1832
Maxwell John K
  4891 Sevilla Way 619/729-4498
Tsai Rujun
  800 Grand Ave Ste B-1 ....619/434-7832

Carmel
Lerner Melanie Grace
  26621 Carmel Center Pl Ste 201 408/625-6161

Carmel Valley
ARANA EDWARD M DDS
  PO Box 856 ....408/659-5385
Kirby Pauline
  PO Box 138 ....408/659-1733

Carmichael
Hee Do-Yoo Young
  6735 Fair Oaks Blvd Ste 11......... 916/485-2624
Kauffman Jeffrey D MD LAC
  6241 Fair Oaks Blvd 916/485-8158

Carpinteria
Wolfe Melissa J
  3802 Via Real 805/684-7795

Chico
Lerner James RN LAC
  5 Governors Ln Ste B 916/343-8932

Chino
Wu Lily Li-Hsia
  13041 Detroit Ct 213/388-8968

Concord
Crist Richard LAC
  2342 Almond Ave..........................510/602-0582
Hellmuth Karen Summers

  1106 Ridge Park Dr 510/930-6115
Shpak Michael Simeon
  4094 Hamlet Dr 510/682-2275

Copperopolis
Derock J Lauren DVM
  United Equine - IVAS Certified
  PO Box 312 ....209/785-4100

Corralitos
Fresco Rachel
  144 Pioneer Rd 408/724-4140

Corte Madera
Shima Miki
  21 Tamal Vista Blvd Ste 110 ....415/924-2910

Costa Mesa
Said Sepideh Z
  3420 Bristol St Ste 305 ....714/557-1010
Tseng Woo Henry
  1491 Baker St Ste 1 ....714/545-3181

Cotati
Stuart Mary P LAC
  429 E Cotati Ave 707/795-4399

Covina
Chi Hung Cheng
  672 E Rowland St 818/966-2596
Chuan Liang Kin
  130 E Cypress St 818/331-1541
Goodkin Valarie D
  237 S 3rd Ave 818/452-9231

Cupertino
Wen Thomas Sintan
  20445 Pacifica Dr 408/446-2007

Daly City
Lai Kim Man CA DCM D
  50 Skyline Plz Ste E 415/994-6020

Dana Point
Tomanjan Jeanne
  24843 Del Prado #515 ....714/661-5646

Danville
Chen Paula L
  919 San Ramon Valley Blvd Ste ..415/820-8451
Keng Shyan-Chyi
  1044 La Gonda Way 510/831-9717
Romanow Candice
  161 Morninghome Rd 415/584-7803

Davis
Utter Johanna Lunn
  622 E 8th St 916/757-2064

Del Mar
Del Mar Astrid E
  13983 Mango Dr Ste 103 ....619/481-3500
Kuster Kristen M
  1155 Camino Del Mar #445 ....619/436-5296
McCusker April Janet
  1155 Camino Del Mar Ste 445 ...619/792-8981

Morris Rhonda Terry
  1011 Camino Del Mar Ste 214 ...619/431-7919
Nathan Pamela S LAC
  13983 Mango Dr Ste 206 ....619/755-3340
Roland Melinda
  1349 Camino Del Mar Ste A 619/259-1553

Desert Hot Springs
Chang Stanley 66565 12th St 619/251-3098

Downey
Bang Lee Joo
  8200 Firestone Blvd 310/923-1111

Dublin
Karami Manouchehr Mike
  7990 Amador Valley Blvd 510/828-3333

El Cajon
Lee Benshiuann
  1027 Greenfield Dr Ste 1A 619/444-3166

El Cerrito
Brody Laurel A 6931 Stockton Ave...510/524-5995
Lollis Patricia Rose
6822 Lincoln Ave...............................415/528-8210
Wallace Susan L 8614 Arbor Dr 510/559-9103

El Monte
Chen Hong-Ping 4432 Shasta Pl 818/575-0663

El Sobrante
Tamaki Yoshimasa
  3755 Ramsey Ct 510/758-5644

El Toro
Gahn Holly A
  23704 El Toro Rd Ste 5422 ....714/364-4434
Quinto Michael 22471 Eloise Dr 714/768-0601

Elk
Marks David B 3900 Cameron Rd ..707/877-3543

Encinitas
Davidson Robin K
  102 Neptune Ave 619/632-7026
Kovida Fisher Roswitha
  874 Eugenie Ave 619/436-5877
Laine Sheri 271 A Hillcrest Dr 619/436-6959
Mann Davis Lisa 121 W E St 619/584-7670
Meister Pamela R 465 1st St 619/942-5995
Merkle Gordon Lyle
  2127 Summerhill Dr 619/298-8548
Parry William L
  454-B N Hwy 101 ....619/753-4283
Rundle John F
  454-B N Hwy 101 ....619/753-4283
St Diane D RN AA
  1152 Devonshire Dr 619/436-7541
Szymczak Matthew J
  1048 Hermes Ave 619/942-8646
Weber Shelly A
  317 N El Camino Real Ste 101 ... 619/944-6874

Encino
Abraham Iona MD
  17815 Ventura Blvd 818/345-8721
Haykin Gary A
  4808 Densmore Ave 818/784-6676
Wells David DC
  5363 Balboa Blvd Ste 234 .... 818/789-6077
Yedvab Miriam
  4263 Mooncrest Pl 818/784-4451

Escondido
Almquist Tama Jo
  7841 Harmony Grove Rd Ste 18 . 619/744-6523
Embry Eden K
  2034 Sleepy Hollow Rd 619/745-7059

Eureka
Downey Denise D
  350 E St Ste 507 ....707/445-0583

Fair Oaks
Gantt Roc H
  9915 Fair Oaks Blvd Ste D 916/961-4268

Fairfax
Jurzykowski Yolande L LAC
  4 Sherman Ave 415/457-6951
Odom Marvin J
  98 Porteous Ave 415/453-6786

Forestville
Chan Norbu L PO Box 98 ....707/887-1859
Kenner Daniel C 7455 Poplar Dr 707/887-9018

Foster City
Minami Hideshiro
  820 Sea Spray Ln Apt 307 .... 415/361-1341

Fountain Valley
Asai Shinji
  18367 Mount Kristina St 714/962-2418
Broadwell Robert J ND DMD
  18837 Brookhurst St Ste 205 .....714/965-9266
Firooz David RPT LAC
  PO Box 8969 ....714/966-2008
Le Thanh V 16138 Challis St 714/775-0838
Tarng Chaur-Yang
  10382 La Tortola Cir 714/962-5978
Yen Emilio
  9624 Gardenia Ave 714/531-5310

Frazier Park
Linero Jeannie PO Box 6081 ....805/242-0149
McLoughlin Donald Ross
  3400 Mt Pinos Way 805/245-3456

Fresno
Moore Tim LAC DAC
  5066 N Fresno St #104 ....209/229-8202
Muzychenko John LAC RN
  Acupuncture Healing Arts Center
  726 W Barstow Ave Ste 103 ....209/233-5554

Nickel Ruth L LAC
  2651 N Hughes Ave 209/498-3309
Fullerton
Kim James 2107 W Seaview Dr 714/526-3961
Minh Lam Khanh
  2201 W Olive Ave 714/680-5410
Muldoon Constance Mary
  Traditional Chinese Medical Center
  336 W Brookdale Pl 714/497-4963
Rho Bong Ho 1716 Chantilly Ln 714/526-7503

Garden Grove
Chi Phan James
  1352 Yockey St 714/892-8268
Chinh Nguyen Duc (David)
  10701 Beacon Ave 714/839-3912
Hwa Lee Ha Soon
  8810 Hewitt Pl Apt 6 ....714/898-7061
Hyun Baik Seong
  12162 Jentges Ave Apt 7 ....714/530-3050
J Nam Kyung
  9928 Garden Grove Blvd 714/530-9907
Jun Kuon Wuh
  12724 Pinehurst Ct 714/534-5143
Keun Ha Jeong
  8810 Hewitt Pl Apt 6 ....714/898-7061
Nguyen Hai N T
  13878 Brookhurst St 714/636-8166
Opran Ionela LAC
  12751 Brookhurst Way 714/636-2441
Pao Phong Lan 8791 Treva Cir 714/893-3578
Se Shin Young
  9928 Garden Grove Blvd...............714/530-3560
Sugato Thien Y
  12292 Magnolia St 714/530-9641
Thuong Nguyen Phuc
  10701 Beacon Ave 714/839-3912
Truong Van-Hung
  13262 Greentree Ave 714/750-1438
Truong Thomas S
  10701 Beacon Ave 714/839-3912
Van Bui Hoai 13182 Hilton Ln 714/748-1749
W Kim Jang 6561 Killarney Ave 714/891-1347
Yuan Xia Yuan 8521 Boyd Ave 714/891-8893

Gardena
Min Kim Jung
  16229 S Western Ave Ste 10 ....310/329-5558

Glendale
Hentoff Karen E
  1066 Thompson Ave 818/507-5778
Hirano Tatsuo
  125 E Glenoaks Blvd Ste 101 .....818/244-2287
Ja Ohm Kwee
  2724 E Chevy Chase Dr 818/956-6920
Kwang Ohm Han
  2724 E Chevy Chase Dr 818/956-6920
Tsai Ta-Ko

  125 E Glenoaks Blvd Ste 106 .....818/956-2172
Glendora
Yu Sam 217 N Vermont Ave 818/335-4658
Goleta
Robertson Mary P 131 Carlo Dr 805/967-7283
Granada Hills
Won Yoon Chi
  16236 Devonshire St #20 .... 818/846-5438
Zung Lee Hwa
  17916 Mayerling St 818/363-7160
Grass Valley
Sharp Gregory Alan
  PO Box 3572 ....916/274-8505
Hacienda Heights
Chi Lai Kuang
  15058 Wedgeworth Dr 818/333-8318
Chung Yu Francis
  15584 Gale Ave 818/330-6028
Eiko Yano Jean
  3040 Rio Lempa Dr 818/330-0846
Lieu Fong-Yi
  1668 Clayhill Ave 818/330-6192
Healdsburg
Jackson Jessica LAC
  513 Center St 310/433-7714
Helena
Frame Kay T
  1336 D Oak Ave St 707/963-2022
Landry Cara
  1336 D Oak Ave St 707/963-2022
Hemet
Sup Lee Yong
  911 E Florida Ave 714/925-0548
Hermosa Beach
Lowry Kathleen R LAC DAC
  1322 Hermosa Ave Ste 9 ....310/379-0559
Hillsborough
S Hsu Kuei
  20 Summerholme Pl 415/697-2888
Huntington Beach
Brizendine William E
  21521 Brookhurst St 714/964-3111
Fang Li Jing 6542 Esta Cir 714/848-4865
Kato Ray M PO Box 3603 ....714/887-7280
Wagner Lucille Marie
  17456 Beach Blvd 714/841-2688
Huntington Park
K Na Soon
  7902 California Ave 213/588-7442
Imperial Beach
Eckert Starr Jeanann
  229 Elkwood Ave 619/575-8191
Irvine

Nguyen Minh V
5101 Yearling Ave 714/559-5429
Pham Quyet K 51 Castillo 714/730-3624
Wang Wen-Jing 21 Alaris Aisle 818/548-0937
Yen-Sun Kao Nancy 19 Toscany 714/250-1989
Yoon Byung H
17502 Jordan Ave Apt 11D 714/733-2194

Jamul
Alwa Allyn C
2084 Honey Springs Rd 619/468-3054

Jenner
Bonas Anna Marie PO Box 95 ....707/632-5038

Kensington
Dreyfuss Robert N CA OMD D
267 Arlington Ave 415/528-0132

Kentfield
Slonetsky Michael Bohdan
43 Briar Rd 415/461-8399

La Jolla
Keefe Donna LAC MTOM
8950 Villa La Jolla Dr Ste 112 .....619/450-0620
Moss Charles A MD
8950 Villa La Jolla Dr Ste 216..... 619/457-1314
Odegaard Martha
8950 Villa La Jolla Dr Ste 121..... 619/558-1204
Warren Ii Richard E
8457-38 Via Mallorca 619/587-0161

La Mesa
Bieg Greg C LAC
8240 Pkwy Dr 619/698-8688
Riley David R OMD LAC
4711 4th St 619/462-7890

La Palma
Hae Ye Jung 5052 Cottonwood Ln ..714/739-5578

La Puente
Shih Nancy Mc 2428 Brisa Ln 818/598-3595
Tong Chen Jeih
18720 Alderbury St 818/913-9683
Yuan-Da Chen Alex LAC OMD
1124 N Hacienda Blvd 818/917-2121

Laguna Hills
Hamedi-Tabari Fereshteh
25411 Gallup Cir 714/831-6975

Lake Forest
Grossman Michael J MD
24432 Muirlands Blvd...................714/770-7301
Steenblock David A DO
22706 Aspen Ste 500 ....714/770-9616

Lakeport
Baker Deborah S 320 1st St 707/263-1100

Lakewood
Chen Mark Lakewood Doctors Building
5220 Clark Ave Ste 460 ....213/915-1131

Elser Martha
5840 Adenmoore Ave 310/925-6948
Fang Chen Mei
4826 Conquista Ave 310/596-6306
Ich Chiem Sanh
2816 Del Amo Blvd 213/418-8437
Yun Aesuton
12232 Centralia St 310/865-2221

Larkspur
Selandia Elizabeth PO Box 827 ....415/457-1674

Lemon Grove
Ann Lisa
2239 Camino De Las Palmas 619/698-7844
Felicetta Geralynn Ann
2239 Camino De Las Palmas 619/698-7844

Leucadia
Aplington Barbara P PO Box 2811 ..619/436-6592

Lompoc
Walsh Mary Angell
East West Health Center
601 E Ocean Ave Ste 22 ....805/736-0051

Long Beach
Born Chhay Hor
2212 N Long Beach Blvd 310/490-9508

Los Altos
Black Margaret K
80 Main St 510/486-0316

Los Angeles
Belenyessy Laszio MD
12732 Washington Blvd #D 213/822-4614
Albalas Moses
12732 W Washington Blvd Ste A ..213/306-3737
Aldridge Alita D
5358 Sanchez Dr 213/298-1961
Allen Linda Jean
1562 S Spaulding Ave 213/965-9144
Alvino Denis Michael
124 N LaBrea Ave Ste D 213/965-8246
Arnstein Novack Sarah
1033 Gayley Ave Ste 117 ....310/208-1567
Baik Chun Choo
425 Southwestern Ave Ste 1 ....213/388-1516
Baptie Bruce T
1414 Westwood Blvd Apt A 310/474-0872
Benedict Steven Ludlow
12579 Venice Blvd 310/390-3561
Berger Lisa Lynn
4325 Coolidge Ave 310/397-8939
Berkheim Lila
1035 N Edinburgh Ave 213/650-7344
Bienenfeld Linda PHD OMD
2211 Corinth Ave Ste 204 ....310/477-8151
Bresler David E PHD LAC
2211 Corinth Ave #204 ....310/477-8151

Caraco Jack A 2194 Ponet Dr 213/462-7602

Chan Pedro 5266 Pomona Blvd 213/721-0774

Charno Sara

   11850 Wilshire Blvd #102 ....213/312-0717

Chen Paul Tm

   920 S Robertson Blvd Ste 3 .... 310/659-7455

Cheng Esther S

   1109 Magnolia Ave 213/385-4713

Chi Hung Wai

   1011 N Broadway Ste 203 ....213/222-5090

Choe Choel M

   310 N Heliotrope Dr Apt 201 .... 818/249-8010

Cohen David M

   6404 Wilshire Blvd Ste 701 ....213/852-9704

Coleman Beverly E

   6111 Homer St 213/939-3255

Crow David

   12217 Santa Monica Blvd Ste 20 310/826-7793

Eberstein Jocelyne LAC DMD The Eberstein Center

   10780 Santa Monica Blvd #210. 310/446-1968

Eyring Thomas MSAC LAC

   944 1/2 N Croft Ave 213/654-4141

Fridman Efim

   217 N Carondelet St 818/342-5732

Galitzer Michael

   12381 Wilshire Blvd 213/820-6042

Goldberg Kate

   1033 Gayley Ave Ste 117 ....310/472-0100

Green Elliott Saul

   10120 Hollow Glen Cir 310/271-4474

Hee Lee Min

   959 S Gramercy Pl Apt 106 ....909/861-8506

Heller Beverly G LAC D

   1033 Gayley Ave Ste 117 ....310/208-2923

Hong Chung Jae

   737 S Oxford Ave Apt 2 ....213/487-3346

Hoon Kim Yong

   2528 W Olympic Blvd Ste 11 ......213/389-2183

Hwan Yom Tae

   567 S Western Ave 213/669-1457

Hye Son Min

   549 N Serrano Ave 213/465-0441

Hyong Kwon Paek Paul

   950 S Western Ave 213/733-5975

Hyun Moon Jung

   1125 W 6th St #2 ....213/385-4392

Il Sim Hae

   3150 W Olympic Blvd 310/454-0748

Jahangirl M MD

   2156 S Santa Fe Ave 213/587-3218

Jehn Noh Yum

   866 1/2 S San Andrews Pl 213/739-1279

Kelly Paul A 1824 Burnell Dr 213/222-3144

Kessler Dennis S

   1125 S Beverly Dr Ste 610 ....310/552-0649

Keun Yoon Jong

   1001 S Vermont Ave Ste 209 ......213/380-0074

Khalsa

   1536 S Robertson Blvd 310/274-8291

Kihn E Douglas

   1976 S Sepulveda Blvd 310/473-2971

Kit-Ching Chan Jane

   2827 Avenel St 213/666-4390

Kum Mindy M 3671 W 6th St 213/383-8496

Lazares Ellen J

   3758 Mentone Ave Ste 201..........310/558-8422

Levy Judith S PO Box 241884 ....310/479-0948

Lydick William S

   230 S Coronado St Apt 1 ....213/384-3805

Manrique Norma G

   12577 Venice Blvd 213/815-0266

McCallum Joyce E

   5157 Dahlia Dr 213/258-2475

McNamee Kevin P DC LAC I

   3407 Cabrillo Blvd 818/591-2732

Melchiorre Mark

   6301 Eunice Ave 818/585-8877

Migdali Ilan LAC DAC

   7080 Hollywood Blvd Ste 1012 ..213/962-8586

Miller Harold Jay

   4071 Grand View Blvd Trlr 2 ....310/391-1162

Morgan Scott Eric LAC OMD

   11611 San Vicente Blvd Ste 310/826-8606

Nam Lee Chung

   822 1/2 Crenshaw Blvd 213/389-9640

Naruse Takako

   11941 Wilshire Blvd Ste 3 ....310/473-3499

Ok Chang Jae

   942 S New Hampshire Ave 213/389-1572

Palay Cindy Eileen

   1101 S Orange Grove Ave 310/285-9241

Park Junsik

   1133 S Vermont Ave Ste 17 ....213/365-1585

Reeves-Migdali Lesley J

   7080 Hollywood Blvd Ste 101 .....213/673-9995

Rousek Yancey R

   12021 Wilshire Blvd Ste 802 ....310/478-5301

Ryu Wonchung M

   532 N Westmoreland Ave Apt 1 ...310/327-1386

Sciabbarrasi Joseph MD

   2211 Corinth Ave #204 ....310/477-8151

Seon Chung Il

   737 S Oxford Ave Apt 2 ....213/487-3346

Shahamati Farima

   2180 S Beverly Dr Ste 118 ....310/203-9292

Shik Shin Soon

   950 S St Andrews Pl Apt 307 ...... 213/735-3359

Sick Lee Voo

   3545 Wilshire Blvd Ste 218..........213/385-4392

Soo Han Joon

   3545 Wilshire Blvd Ste 218 ....213/385-4392

Sook Han Jeung

   327 S Western Ave 213/935-8889

Staffa Rosanna

1903 Berkeley Ave 213/353-0216
Steele Jan Kay
1149 S Highland Ave 213/936-3162
Taek Park Ki
3261 W 4th St Suite 202 ....714/871-8750
Tsuzomu Harada Vaughn
PO Box 25457 ....310/457-6379
Uy R MD
6317 Wilshire Blvd Ste 202 ....213/655-5628
Wiggins-Woolf Sandra L
1725 Silver Lake Blvd 213/665-9432
Wilcox Lorraine
12233 W Olympic Blvd Ste 130 ..310/207-3600
Wu Moon-Aung
608 S Citrus Ave 213/931-3203
Y Choi Kenneth
1655 W Olympic Blvd Ste 208 ....818/332-0262
Yong Auh Kwang
906 Crenshaw Blvd 213/934-1749
Yoo Paul K
1300 N Vermont Ave Ste 305 ......213/665-9550
Yoo Sang Soo
4734 Oakwood Ave Apt 101.........213/738-1657
Yung Tsau Chun
4029 Bledsoe Ave 310/397-9583

Los Gatos
Schwaderer Terri Anne
160 Villa Ave 408/354-6719

Malibu
Morgan-Tydings Barbara
28290 Rey De Copas Ln 310/457-5137

Manhattan Beach
Bailey Tracey L LAC MS O
1104 Highland Ave Ste I 310/318-2225

Marina
Kim Chang K
326 Reservation Rd Ste E.............408/384-2313

Martinez
Nachtwey Nancy Jane
704 Sterling Dr 510/372-7971

Mendocino
Bayer Judith Ann PO Box 241 ....707/937-4338
Greensfield Zvika PO Box 143 ....707/935-6851

Menlo Park
Waters Margaret J PO Box 2043 .....415/366-9739

Mill Valley
Beyers Kathryn
295 Miller Ave Ste D 415/383-4443
Prudhomme Lisa LAC
333 Miller Ave 415/383-7224
Gold Iris OMD LAC
131 Camino Alto 415/381-3838
Grace Paul LAC DAC
25 Evergreen Ave Ste 3B 415/389-6003

Graves Paul V
25 Evergreen Ave Ste 3B 415/389-6001
Griffin Maureen LAC
25 Evergreen Ave #3B 415/381-2802
Himmel Raymond
147 Lomita Dr Ste C 415/383-7730
Mathews Lauren PO Box 2603 ....415/383-5326
Reich Gatya LAC
642 Northern Ave 415/927-0776
Rohrwig Reich Renata
12 Patricia Ln 415/381-1160
Rossman Martin L Academy of Guided Imagery
10 Willow St #4 ....415/383-3197
Soleil Alvita PO Box 807 ....415/388-7859

Milpitas
Farkas Robin L
475 Los Coches St 408/946-9332

Mission Hills
Eichelberger Bruce David
15545 Devonshire St 818/785-1922
Wood Mary E
11151 Sharp Ave 818/365-3814

Monrovia
Hung Lin Tzu 2603 Doray Cir 818/447-9091

Monterey
Guiffre-Cook Karen Ann
1000 8th St Ste 101 ....408/375-5117

Monterey Park
Bun Ng Man
415 Mooney Dr Ste A 818/573-2768
Chou Michael
209 Baltimore Ave 818/307-0237
Cuan Shauyuin 218 Ransom Way ...818/573-3708
Gasper Louis
313 W Andrix St 213/722-7353
Gasper Nellie Mabel
313 W Andrix St 213/722-7353
Heng Tu Shiao
512 S Huntington Ave 818/280-2194
Ho Vivian Y
507 Pomelo Ave Ste C 818/307-6908
Li Jiahui 502 N Lincoln Ave Ste A 818/572-9818
Lohrungruang Tiva
216 S McPherrin Ave Ste 2..........818/573-1376
Man Kim Jae
943 S Atlantic Blvd Ste 222 ....818/284-2833
Suon Duan-Tyi
209 Baltimore Ave 818/307-0231

Morro Bay
Brajkovich Wendy R LAC ACP
665 Main St Ste C 805/772-5807

Mount Baldy
Kissner (Hunt) Peggy Sue
PO Box 370 ....714/949-2294

Napa

Wright Robert C
1020 Clinton St Ste 208 ....707/255-5124

National City

Uda Georgiana N
1635 Sweetwater Rd Ste G 619/477-4111

Nevada City

Flower Essence Service
PO Box 1769 ....800/548-0075
Hill Turiya 707 Zion St Ste B 916/265-4141
Tucker Dennis PHD LAC
127 Argall Way 916/265-8202

Newport Beach

Kunze Maret Irene Long Life Medical Clinic Inc
3355 Via Lido Ste 235 ....714/675-2729
Mae King Melanie
3700 Newport Blvd Ste 303A 714/723-0423

Nipomo

Kandel Herb J 776 Inga Rd 805/929-3609

North Hollywood

Cardenas-Rios Rodolfo F
6862 Vanscoy Ave 818/765-5337
Hearn Karen G
6160 Whitsett Ave Apt 2 ....818/506-7477
Katz David OMD LAC
10628 Riverside Dr #5 ....818/508-6188
Ottaviano John
5316 Lankershim Blvd N...............818/506-4701
Penner Joel OMD LAC
5223 Corteen Pl Apt 8 ....818/344-1983

Norwalk

Ok Joo Sun
13805 Graystone Ave 310/868-5068
Roc Doo Young-Ming
16203 Jersey Ave 310/921-5233

Oakland

Barlay Brian A
461 43rd St 510/654-4925
Bauer Ulrike M
2888 Delaware St 510/839-8430
Cai Lai Fu
1830 Lakeshore Ave Apt 408........510/893-6230
Chapman Jeanne E
6391 Heather Ridge Way 510/339-3720
Chee Ho Pui 2048 7th Ave 415/834-2048
Chung Frank LIAC OMD
5664 Broadway 510/655-0668
Cronin Connie M 574 Forest St 510/655-4650
Curry Mary V
3837 Huntington St 510/530-8886
Donner Daniel
3927 Piedmont Ave 510/655-0555
Dorsett Robert J
832 Erie St Apt 3 ....415/893-7922
Fong Byron B LAC DOM

220 Grand Ave 510/451-8244
Gandy Michael W
2109 Macarthur Blvd 510/531-4325
Ginsberg Steven P
280 Lee St 510/763-8304
Jackson Franchesca
5349 College Av 510/653-6029
Keenan Patricia Ann
465 Stow Ave 510/835-2758
Liang Victoria P
2544 E 16th St 510/534-8473
Louie Choi-Sing C
3901 Vale Ave 415/482-3660
Lui Danny 706 Hillgirt Cir 510/832-8322
Morris Kenneth 5459 Shafter Ave ...510/658-6857
Qiu Wang Ying
2709 Grande Vista 415/967-5797
Ross Gregory W
3521 Laguna Ave 510/531-0530
Roth Gloria L
3641 Dimond Ave 415/530-0244
Strang Joann
5349 College Ave 510/655-7776
Wei-Tzu Chung Frank
5664 Broadway 510/655-0668
Woodcox Larry H
2647 E 14th St 510/436-0336
Zhe Huang Zhou Xiao
2136 E 15th St 510/534-3341

Ojai

Edgcomb Laurie E
PO Box 1162 ....805/646-1360

Orange

Ai Au Chau
2027 W Sycamore Ave 714/978-9823

Pacific Grove

Gill Jason M
164 Forest Ave 408/373-0373

Pacific Palisades

Ivanhoe Eliot R
16009 Northfield St 310/828-5220
Kalina Leonard E
15324 De Pauw St 310/454-8678

Pacifica

Doecke Robyn
1015 Rio Vista Dr 415/285-4512

Palm Desert

Lee Vivian Y K
74-090 El Paseo 619/340-3838

Palm Springs

Degnan Sean MD
2825 E Tahquitz McCallum Way .. 619/320-4292
Fitzpatrick Alice P
1815 Sandcliff Rd 619/323-2842

Palo Alto

Loman Scott J DDS
416 Waverley St Ste A 415/326-3290
Neustaedter Randall OMD LAC
360 Bryant St 415/324-8420

Paradise
Struthers John E
1278 Storybook Ln 916/872-5746

Pasadena
Cao Thanh Dong
529 E Washington Blvd #6 ....818/794-8165
Fleming Kerry A
1848 N Michigan Ave 818/791-4570
Hilsdale Karen
Acupuncture Association of Pasadena
301 S Fair Oaks Ave #102............ 818/585-8877
Hui Hsieh Hong
290 Anita Dr 818/793-5698
Mainferme Nic D
427 Virginia Ave 818/795-6758
Melchiorre Mark
301 S Fair Oaks Ave #102 ....818/585-8877

Paso Robles
Lee Pamela LAC PHD
939 Oak St 805/237-1011
Cahoon Laurie 411 B St Ste 8 ....707/763-7683
Fannin William J 519 Upham St 707/778-1929
Prange William LAC OMD
245 Kentucky St #A 707/778-3171

Placentia
Babcock Henry George
219 Demmer Pl 213/828-1942

Pleasanton
Ming-Sun Shen Mason LAC PHD
5150 Case Ave Apt N112 ....510/449-4327
Shen Mason M
1393 Santa Rita Rd #A 415/820-8451
Wei-Zhu Tan Joe
2235 Delucchi Dr 415/846-7036

Pomona
Hehn Kim S
42 Stagecoach Dr 714/622-9543
Tao Yi-Yuann
42 Stagecoach Dr 714/622-9543

Poway
Malik Dianne Grace
17124 St Andrews Dr 619/486-1718

Rancho Cucamonga
Kuo-Hui Lee Joanna
7365 Carnelian St Ste 126 ....714/948-8418

Redding
Campanale Frank Joseph
4692 Bear Mountain Rd 916/275-5375

Redlands

Minjares Therese Anne
316 E Olive Ave 909/793-9573
Vanornum Theresa E
1528 Clay St 714/335-1505

Redondo Beach
Boone Karen
2323 Huntington Ln #A 310/417-8485
Leigh Snelson Connie
615 Esplanade St Apt 412 .... 310/316-7669
Liu Marina M
3007 Blossom Ln 310/379-9275

Redway
Medoff Linda S PO Box 1538 ....707/913-4610

Redwood City
Cold Sandra E
1170 Chesterton Ave 415/363-0630
Deaton Kathleen
1510 Jefferson Ave 415/363-2020
Soo Han Jong
133 Arch St Ste 3 ....415/364-2828

Reseda
Light Daniel
Victory Tampa Medical Square
19231 Victory Blvd Ste 151 .... 818/344-9973
Milch Ruth Marion
6212 Hesperia Ave 818/881-6849
Preston Dunn Jan
6548 Balcom Ave 818/342-1764

Richmond
Cross Christina G
622 36th St 510/234-6566
Krestan Sandy
1500 Aqua Vista Rd 510/236-4669

Riverside
Lovell Phyllis D
392 5th St 714/683-1694

Rolling Hills Estate
Su Chin-Lang
715 Silver Spur Rd Ste 208......... 310/541-4379

Rosemead
Chen Quincy C & H Acupuncture & Herbs Clinic
3135 San Gabriel Blvd 818/288-1233
Chiu Daryl T
2511 Pamala St 818/573-9241
Phung Chi N
7833 La Merced Rd 818/288-1525

Roseville
Brown Gregory C
1751 E Roseville Pky Apt 1435 ...415/571-6464

Rowland Heights
Jan Shiow-Lih
19268 Tranbarger St 818/913-9806

Sacramento

Ertel Aeriel 2410 K St Ste A 916/443-8107
Phillips Stephen B
   3301 Alta Arden Expy Ste 6 ....916/483-4657
Reuben Carolyn LAC
   3825 Marconi Ave 916/483-2359
Wang Hu-Shen
   5316 57th St 916/457-9612
Yamazaki Daichachi S Japan Institute of Acupuncture
   3430 Balmoral Dr Ste 3 ....916/486-8122

San Anselmo

Broffman Annapurna G
   124 Pine St 415/485-0484
Kutchins Stuart OMD DAC
   32 City Hall Ave 415/459-1868
Martin Rita
   PO Box 901 ....415/457-0602
McCulloch Michael F
   114 Pine St 415/485-0484
Mini John W
   761 Sir Francis Drake Blvd 415/454-4574
Weissbuch Brian Kie
   165 Tunstead Ave 415/459-4066

San Clemente

Fu Yuan Zhi 155 Ave Del Mar 714/361-2046

San Diego

Disch Barry LAC 435 Rosemont.......619/551-8284
Mouna Peaceful Earth
   Black Kim....................................619/474-4050
Black Vince 619/584-7670
Broadwell Robert J
   18837 Brookhurst St #205 ....714/965-9266
Burke Susan Ann
   4015 Park Blvd Ste 200 ....619/297-3100
Castro Carmencita G Asian American University
   2043 El Cajon Blvd 619/299-0030
Derin Gail 619/233-5484
Douat Joseph A
   5325 Penny Pl 619/583-1910
Elliott Carol R LAC Acupuncture Institute
   4015 Park Blvd #200 ....619/297-3100
Foley Susan
   841 Turquoise St Ste G 619/488-0357
Frieder Glenn DC..............................619/574-1874
Fusco Henry LAC OMD Mission Bay Acupuncture
   2611 Denver St 619/276-4188
Gold Richard M PHD LAC
   3446 Cromwell Pl 619/624-0623
Hoover Kimberly DAC Acu-Care Health Center
   3660 Clairemont Dr Ste 4 .... 619/270-2371
Hung Marguerite M LAC OMD
   3963 Broadlawn St 619/277-4989
Ivey Martha OMD LAC 619/291-1655
   4254 5th Ave 619/543-9904
Kastner Mark Albert
   1042 Devonshire Dr 619/222-3818

Keller Loisanne OMD LAC
   3737 Moraga Ave Ste A5 ....619/272-8215
Lichterman Daniel M
   3634 Engle St 619/294-6990
Merkle Gordon LAC DAC
   4565 Ruffner St Ste 100 ....619/560-4366
Montano Victor E
   6011 Schuyler St 619/472-1133
Mortensen Richard A
   4765 Voltaire St 619/224-1387
Mouna 3718 Vermont St 619/574-6669
Nagel Jeffrey R
   3833 Eagle St 619/542-1903
Narins Toni
   3644 Front St 619/291-5908
Obata Claudia L
   4640 Jewell St Ste 102-A 619/274-1341
Parker Linda MS LAC
   2422 San Diego Ave 619/295-3006
Raskin Erin MS LAC
   5333 Mission Center Rd Ste 100 619/542-0884
Riggs Cathy D Pacific Center of Health Acupuncture
   4545 Campus Ave Apt 6 ....619/297-6705
Rosenberg Z'ev DOM LAC
   6667 Fisk Ave 619/546-8309
Sekito June Chiropractic & Pain Clinic
   7878 Clairemont Mesa Blvd Ste.. 619/576-7337
Tan Richard T
   4550 Kearny Villa Rd Ste 107 .....619/277-1070
Tang Shengying
   9248 Regents Rd 619/452-3560
Timmons Colleen M
   1648 32nd St 619/233-3957
Tom Celia Maria
   3652 Clairemont Dr #A 619/581-6953
Wang Tai-Nan
   4295 Gesner St Apt 1A 619/483-7795
Wexler Marly Beth
   215 Spruce St Ste A 619/295-7121

San Fernando

Rehwalt Sybil S
   1500 Glenoaks Blvd Ste A 818/365-0653

San Francisco

Abrams Sally N
   138 Cortland Ave 415/824-6216
Angus Liane
   3819 23rd St 415/641-4268
Balles Thomas John LAC Traditional Acupuncture Clinic
   1863 Union St 415/921-4808
Beinfield Harriet Chinese Medicine Works
   1201 Anderson St 415/285-0931
Berkelhammer Lisa Ann
   1380 Filbert St 415/474-0540
Chan Henry P
   2943 Balboa St 415/386-2024

Chang Cynthia M L
2118 Hayes St 415/386-4619
Chau Eva M
2038 16th Ave 415/731-3169
Chen Susan C
738 40th Ave 415/386-6273
Chen Kuei-Fa
4223 Geary Blvd 415/752-0170
Chen Rong-Wen
4223 Geary Blvd 415/752-0170
Chow Effie P Y
450 Sutter St Rm 916 ....415/788-2227
Chun Su Chin
4223 Geary Blvd 415/771-0170
Clemente Susan
109 Bradford St 415/285-1312
Cohen Misha R 30 Albion St 415/861-1101
Corbett Kelly
214 Connecticut St 415/431-1825
Coupez Therese Ann
3933 25th St 415/821-1405
Currie Donald H 4006 25th St 415/285-6595
Dunphy Daniel J
343 Lombard St 415/391-7102
Dunphy Gerard R RN LAC
2216 Jones St 415/775-1972
Espinoza Sandy M
306 Delano Ave 415/584-6539
Feichtmeir Janis
689A 4th Ave 415/221-1387
Fen-Kue C Hang Fanny
4223 Geary Blvd 415/752-0170
Forsberg Larry C
1201 Noe St 415/648-8084
Germain Robin E
336 San Jose Ave 415/647-3795
Graham John F
650 Parker Ave 415/666-6473
Hamako Fujimura Sue
127 Fair Oaks St 415/826-6241
Hangee-Bauer Carl ND LAC
Soma Acupuncture & Natural Health
862 Folsom St 415/974-5596
Heyob Robert M
3552 23rd St 415/641-1418
Hoon Lee Dong
1610 Post St Ste 201 ....415/929-1007
Horn Anne M
203 Prospect Ave 510/208-5135
Hotoyama Jun R
150 Glenbrook Ave 415/665-5890
Hsu Hsieh Yun
2714 Noriega St 415/665-6782
Inn Martin Cs
143 Rippley St 415/285-9408
Jane Tang Bick 1943 31st Ave 415/564-0147

Jiao Daniel 455 Arkansas St 415/282-9603
Jin Zhen 227 14th Ave 415/221-4822
Kai Tak Chan Peter
1184 Capitol Ave 415/333-7257
Kan Tsao Henry 1109 Powell St 415/391-3691
Kaplan Susan
519 Castro St Ste M17 ....415/641-7436
Kernan Adrienne
890 Carolina St 415/550-7251
Keung Lau Yin
1181 Clay St Ste 6 ....415/771-7038
Khalighi Khosrow
1863 Union St 415/921-4808
Kolenda John A 1335 Ulloa St 415/566-8865
Korngold Efrem Victo Chinese Medicine Works
1201 Noe St 415/285-0931
Kwee Su Chen Daniel
85 Duncan St 415/282-7672
La Forgia Brian
1532 Union St 415/474-6195
Li Jing 584 San Jose Ave 415/282-1880
Liane Strecker Karen
159 Vicksburg St 916/641-5811
Loh Chee-Chang
1663 30th Ave 415/759-9003
London Eugene R
816 Waller St 415/864-1121
Mark Denise R MD
345 W Portal Ave 415/566-1000
Martin Joel
311 11th Ave Ste 4 ....415/752-4478
Marx Emmett D
1863 Union St 415/911-4808
McMullen Sally A
120 27th St 415/550-7732
Ming Coo Hang
775 7th Ave 415/386-0184
Moffet Howard Hugh
60 Sharon St 415/861-5994
Newman Milton Lewis
149 Arkansas St 415/863-2449
Newmark Irene E
181 Noe St 415/552-3813
Ng Daniel W
4444 Geary Blvd Ste 102 ....415/386-7169
Oh Faith M
404 Balboa St 415/221-8751
Pao-Chih Liu Doris
1646 43rd Ave 415/681-9818
Pomianowski Mark Steven
1250 48th Av 415/267-1873
Poy Yew Chow Effie
450 Sutter St Rm 916 ....415/788-2227
Pretot Urs 450 Connecticut St 415/285-3749
Prongos Jennifer Lee
1686 Union St Ste 209 ....415/921-8505

Robert Evelyn M
  3131 Kirkham St 415/566-5447
Sanders Patricia L
  1883 Vallejo St 415/821-4264
Shaw Stephen S 17 Ross Aly 415/397-1798
Sinclair Thomas M LAC MS
  4219 21st St 415/824-3649
Singh Nam
  1289 43rd St 415/661-7160
Sorkin Zhanna
  660 Sloat Blvd 415/759-7644
Spear Loraine M
  380 Ivy St 415/626-7326
Stepto Steven G
  774 7th Ave 415/668-6218
Tong S Scott
  1200 Gough St 415/563-4567
Wang Li-Kuo 531 12th Ave 415/751-7337
Wang Yei-Jan 4 Jakey Ct 415/824-1617
Woon Ng Shek
  710 Grant Ave Apt 203 ....415/421-8435
Wu Angela C F
  703 Clement St 415/752-0170
Yat-Fai Lee Jeffrey
  973 Greenwich St 415/673-6765
Yee John S
  4448 California St 415/752-9518
Young Michael Glenn
  3450 16th St 415/252-8711
Zhen Jin 3147 Geary Blvd 415/751-0128
Zhu Ming Qing 1523 Irving St 415/566-0822

San Gabriel

Bin Mok May
  2005 Redding Ave S 818/280-8568
Lee Christina
  1304 S Del Mar Ave 818/307-0433
Tien Huang Kuang
  1405 Prospect Ave Apt C 818/457-8669

San Jose

Bhu Song Minn
  100 O'Connor Dr 408/286-9237
Chen Daren LAC OMD
  167 N Bascom Ave 408/998-1838
Devlin Grace Marla
  1081 Avondale St 408/378-2424
Fisher Mary G
  482 Tuscarora Dr 408/281-8389
Hsu Denise D
  1521 Greensboro Ct 408/436-1762
Kim Nam H
  259 Meridian Ave Ste 19 ....408/293-0461
Nei King Yu 3034 Crater Ln 408/263-7700
Soo Kang Jin 1820 Lencar Way 408/264-1038
Tarvin Mary Louise
  3320 Cherry Ave 408/723-7336
Tran Trang T

  2857 Senter Rd Ste M 408/226-6115
Tu Jason
  10787 South Blaney Ave 408/257-4146
Van Tran Nhien
  5015 Page Mill Dr 408/262-8336

San Leandro

Gee Steven H MD
  595 Estudillo Ave 510/483-5881
Wan Kim Jong
  15287 Hesperian Blvd Ste 11..... 510/278-3250

San Luis Obispo

Doyle Laurel E
  2103 Broad St 805/541-6242
Kavanagh Kimberly OMD DAC
  2103 Broad St 805/541-6242
Cadwallader Claudia LAC
  891 Pismo St 850/541-2563

San Marcos

Kubitschek William C DO
  1194 Calle Maria 619/744-6991

San Marino

Hui-Yee Chu Herrick
  1941 Wellesley Rd 818/285-0063

San Mateo

Cho Jiyon A
  19 W 39th Ave Ste 2 ....415/570-5531
Wuji Huang Albert
  220 E 3rd Ave Ste 1 ....415/343-2112

San Pedro

Dewey Nancy N CAC
  2020 S Western Ave Unit 8 ....310/833-3294

San Rafael

Fairfield Peter
  134 Villa Ave 707/935-7072
The Atma Group
  185 N Redwood Dr Suite 220 .....415/499-3319
Preventive Medical Center of Marin
  25 Mitchell Blvd Ste 8 ....415/472-2343
Hobson Laura
  84 Scenic Ave 415/454-4576
Luon Stephanie
  369 3rd St #D 415/459-2245
Stuetzer Paul H
  710 C St Ste 10 ....415/381-1604
Tavily Farangis
  PO Box 2775 ....415/257-5256

Santa Ana

Azizi Amir S
  1125 E 17th St Ste W239 ....714/558-0844
Boling Mark Alan ACT
  13122 Prospect Ave 714/532-9532
Cooper Wan-Tzy
  1506 W Cleghorn Way 714/751-8131
Kim Ronald R
  11171 Arroyo Ave 714/832-1475

Le Joseph T 707 S Mascine St 714/839-1963

Minh Doan King
2525 Huckleberry Rd 714/554-7936

Ngoc Tran Thuat
1813 W Glenwood Pl 714/241-0274

Thanh Tran Bao
1813 W Glenwood Pl 714/241-0274

Wempen Ronald MD
3620 S Bristol St Ste 306 ....714/546-4325

You Yu 1618 E Avalon Ave 714/647-0227

Santa Barbara

Wu M Lonnie RN LAC
4046 Foothill Rd 805/682-2153

Arcudi Melanie M
PO Box 2423 ....805/682-0381

Davis Deborah LAC 805/969-1992

Diamond Daniel
1625 State St 805/569-1771

Fadden Jan Scott 912 Olive St 805/569-2153

Francis Katharine Shell
385 N La Cumbre Rd 805/563-2272

Jahnke Roger OMD Health Action
243 Pebble Beach........................ 805/682-3230

Merryweather Bambi OMD PHD
PO Box 5573 ....805/684-7099

Pinnick Mary Kay
PO Box 92008 ....805/964-9254

Riskin Ronald M
206 W Anapamu St 805/963-9429

Salazar Sylvia
226 E Canon Perdido St Ste C 805/966-6963

Scaran Mary T
122 Skyline Cir 805/965-0448

Silvestri Thomas A
521 E Arrellaga St Ste 5 .... 805/963-1637

Silvestri Tony
521 E Arrellaga St #5 ....805/963-1637

Smith Sheelah R
38 S La Cumbre Rd Ste 2 ....805/964-0333

Sorgman Joann
1919 State St 805/569-1541

St Denis Aliki
1919 State St Ste 204 ....805/961-3757

Thiessen Patricia C
27 E Victoria St Ste L 805/963-8181

Weinheimer Laurel E
522 De La Vista Ave 805/687-6115

Wu M Lonnie RN LAC OMD
4046 Foothill Rd 805/682-2153

Santa Clara

Bum Yoon Mun
1490 Kiely Blvd 408/985-0895

Gih Hu Lucy
2041 Bowers Ave 408/773-8790

Nah Ho 4768 Gillmor St 415/794-5520

Sook Kim Young
1088 Kiely Blvd 408/244-6143

Sun Yoon Tea
1490 Kiely Blvd 408/985-0895

Valerie Ryan M
Modern Acupuncture & OM Clinic
3669 Eastwood Cir 408/737-2873

Yuanpu Jiang Yutao
PO Box 3075 ....408/247-8116

Santa Clarita

Morris-Devine Leitia OMD LAC
Santa Clarita Pain Treatment Center
18285 Soledad Canyon Rd 805/250-9010

Santa Cruz

Atkinson Carolyn LAC DAC
Meridian Acupuncture
626 Frederick St 408/423-3818

Beck Susan Leslie
100-B West Ave 408/425-8052

Benedict Martha S
427 Locust St 408/425-5977

Bernstein Marilyn Mariposa
Po Box 1015 ....408/458-3110

Bourland Glenn A
3710 Gross Rd Lot 27 ....408/662-1334

Brott-Atkinson Carolyn A
116 Yosemite St 408/427-3440

Carr Craig I
Center For Int'l Healing Arts...........408/457-2076

Chenping Chao Joanna
200 7th Ave 408/476-8211

Elias Felice Ann
550 Water St Ste F-4 ....408/423-6413

Gunsaulus-Tierra Lesley H
208 Locust St 408/429-8066

Haber Cally E
709 Frederick St 408/458-0809

Johnson Susan LAC
550 Water St Bldg C......................408/425-5037

Klapman Gary
260 Meadow Rd 408/426-5660

Lewis Sally 408/425-7707

Lewis Sally Ann
132 6th Ave Apt 1 ....408/475-1885

Lindaro Tala
115 Maple St 408/425-4691

Lynn Raqib
3528 Mission Dr 708/479-9228

Murphy Shayne Kristen
2870 Chesterfield Dr 408/479-3242

Nadborny Ina
212 Ocean View Ave 408/426-4306

Pouls Kathleen Marie
820 Capitola Rd 408/475-8885

Seeger Sandra

111 Alamo Av 408/429-1243
Smyth Edward M
740 Front St Ste 330 ....408/267-5578
Strawhacker Dale
740 Front St Ste 330 ....408/423-8344
Tierra Michael LAC OMD
912 Center St 408/429-8066

Santa Maria
Tadashi Kaneko Robert
406 S Pine St 805/434-4623

Santa Monica
Agarwal Seema
825 Grant St #1 ....310/652-1076
Apollo Richard M
2926 Santa Monica Blvd 310/828-6994
Armijo Richard
2309 Main St 310/396-2130
Avery Judith
1544 6th St Ste 104 ....310/458-9662
Benoit Lebel Marc
821 3rd St Apt 106 ....310/394-2783
Birch Patricia OMD LAC
1150 Yale St Ste 7 ....310/828-5588
Chilkov Nalini OMD LAC
530 Wilshire Blvd Ste 206 ....310/395-4133
Dal Kim Bong
1807 Wilshire Blvd Ste B 310/453-8833
Deorio Keith MD OMD
2901 Wilshire Blvd Ste 435 ....310/828-4480
Fay Monique Bodymind Systems Medical Center
2450 Wilshire Blvd #1 ....213/273-5270
Griggs R Leroy
PO Box 5673 ....213/399-4272
Grossman Richard D
1250 Franklin St Apt A 310/828-0767
Gumenick Neil R
2926 Santa Monica Blvd 310/453-2235
Harrie Shashi M
1438 10th St #7 ....310/395-4650
Hirsh Roger OMD LAC
1247 7th St Ste #201 ....310/319-9478
Hutson-Lange Susan E
1411 5th St Ste 405 ....310/395-9525
Jacob Lauren
1411 5th St Ste 405 ....310/815-0266
Kandel Herb
225 E Mill St 805/922-4490
Kearney David P
1821 Wilshire Blvd Ste 610 ....310/455-2037
Klee Mary Ellen
2926 Santa Monica Blvd 310/454-7570
Lakshmi Lambert F
1227 Euclid St Apt 2 ....310/393-0961
Lehrer Danise LAC OMD HMD
1411 5th St Ste 405 ....310/395-9525
Mackinnon Lesley J

1002 Grant St Apt C 310/452-1194
Meyer Susan R
1502 Montana Ave Ste 207 ....310/455-3380
Ni Maoshing LAC OMD
1314 2nd St Ste 101 ....310/917-2200
Obey Frederick C
918 9th St Apt E 310/458-2901
Ray Timothy
1740 Sunset Blvd 310/396-5472
Thompson Laura
429 Santa Monica Blvd Ste 3 ..... 310/451-4419
Weinstein Michael
612 Santa Monica Blvd 310/395-6014
Zand Janet LAC OMD
1437 7th St Ste 301 ....310/458-8020

Santa Rosa
Chung Vicki Lynn
3033 Coffey Ln 707/579-4371
Every Janet F
736 McConnell Ave 707/528-0335
Su Terri MD 1038 4th St # 3 ....707/571-7560
Walker David B 917 Deturk Ave 707/578-9233

Sausalito
Freiberg Julie W 11 Marie St 415/332-1912
Smith Nicki Melanie
13 Tomales St #B 415/331-0552

Seal Beach
Green Allen Md
909 Electric Ave Ste 212 ....714/851-1550

Sebastopol
Crist Richard
11933 Barnett Valley Rd 707/823-7741

Sepulveda
Do Min Byung
8927 Swinton Ave 818/895-7489
Steeh (Engel) Kathleen Ann
16350 Labrador St 818/894-1594

Shasta
Hsu Shen 500 McCloud Ave 916/926-5007

Sherman Oaks
George-Rydberg Susan RN LAC
4910 Van Nuys Blvd Ste 104 ......818/981-3440
Miller Neal Stuart
12926 Riverside Dr 818/789-2468

Simi Valley
Dimopoulos Stephanie A
1750 Wexford Cir 805/527-4272
Niederman Stephanie Acupuncture Pain Relief Center
1834 Cochran St 805/527-2759

Sonoma
Hoke George G 158 W Napa St 707/996-4511
Hong Cecilia LAC LMT Sonoma Holistic Center
164 W Napa St 707/996-7358

Sonora

Alpern Steven CA
103 S Shepherd St 209/533-9226

Soquel
Carter-Hinson Julie 2955 Park Ave ...408/476-1886
Shwery Richard A
630 Aurora Rd 408/479-3760

South Lake Tahoe
Sult Thomas A
2070 Lake Tahoe Blvd 916/542-4181

Spring Valley
Duerrstein Allen R
695 Sweetwater Rd Ste 250 ....619/579-1236

Stanton
Jitae Kim Edwin
11849 Beach Blvd 714/373-5450
Thi Le Tran Quyen
8376 Chanticleer Rd 714/821-8339

Studio City
Blake Claudia
11432 Canton Dr 213/654-9165
Bleicher Nancy C
4212 Rhodes Ave 818/508-1327
Law Jr Charles E MD
3959 Laurel Canyon Blvd Ste 1 ... 818/761-1661
Miller Neal S
12940 Moorpark St 818/981-2468

Sunland
Honjio Steven M
10630 Johanna Ave 818/353-4826

Sunnyvale
Abel Karen
1055 Sunnyvale-Saratoga Rd 408/739-3777

Sylmar
Varela Federico M
13856 Baddock St 818/362-5503

Tahoe City
Barr Stephen E PO Box 7696 ....916/583-9407

Tarzana
Nixon Terri L
5132 Garden Grove Ave 818/881-3126
Tucker Rand S
5132 Garden Grove Ave 818/881-3126

Temple City
Cheng Tsao Jenny
8825 Elm Ave 818/285-7536
Young Hua Ming
10634 Daines Dr 818/350-9387

Thousand Oaks
Lu Lawrence Y
166N N Moorpark Rd Ste 203 .....805/373-0699
Nielsen Erik OMD LAC
1864 Orinda Ct..............................805/492-1811
Rose Johanne

5707 Corsa Ave Ste 105 ....818/889-1421
Ryf Hope
223 E Thousand Oaks Blvd Ste 3 805/497-4074
Shaul Ofira
264 Larcom St 818/989-1008
Sik Park Chang
100 E Thousand Oaks Blvd Ste 2 805/495-0360
Wang Shui-Lan
166 N Moorpark Rd Ste 203 ....805/373-0699

Toluca Lake
Miko Robert W 10153 1/2 Riverside Dr Ste 417
....818/609-8656

Topanga
Clarke Murray C 20485 Callon Dr ...310/393-5949
Keeler Deloris 23333 Valdez Rd 818/592-6816
McLean Bonnie S
19711 Valleyview Dr 310/455-3276

Torrance
Barnett Nancy A
4010 W Sepulveda Blvd 310/791-2624
Halverson Oda S
3655 Lomita Blvd Ste 412 .... 310/373-4462
Karsten Yuki
23441 Madison St 310/373-0368
Klein Maxine LAC DAC
4015 Pacific Coast Hwy Ste 101 .310/791-7080
Lin Anna
1835 W 175th St 310/318-5288
Quang Vu Thuc
17213 Atkinson Ave 310/324-5126
Sakamoto Jenny OMD LAC
Acupuncture Associates
23441 Madison St Ste 215 ....310/373-0368
Sakamoto Mary
23441 Madison St Ste 215 .... 310/373-0368
Skinner Suzanne M PHD ND DSC HHD
2204 W Torrance Blvd....................310/518-4555

Tustin
Cu Luong
17021 Kenyon Dr #B 714/731-4980
Dang Hao T
2032 Fallen Leaf Pl 714/832-7764
Hue Phan Phi
2032 Fallen Leaf Pl 714/832-7764
McGinnis Jerry Lee
1291 Olwyn Dr 714/730-9474
Moore Marjorie
1034 Irvine Blvd 714/528-0216
Talebi Fatima
1101 Bryan Ave Ste E 714/544-1080

Upland
Wang Mei-Chih
2274 O'Malley Ave 714/982-5226

Vallejo

Cole John Alfred
535 Whitecliff Dr 707/552-4738
Sunbeam Alan LAC
721 Marin St 707/644-4325

Van Nuys

Hu Yu - Chinese Medical Academy
14435 Sherman Way # 104 ....818/901-7889

Venice

Dermont Celia
1802 Washington Way 310/821-1659
Krech Douglas K
13900 Fiji Way 310/395-3626

Ventura

Bergman Elizabeth Gail
1168 Cornwall Ln 805/653-0603

Walnut

Wang Andrea S Y
1259 Athena Dr 714/598-4179

Walnut Creek

Charles Alan S MD
1414 Maria Ln 510/937-3331
Tu Angela Y
1563 Palos Verdes Mall 510/932-4002
Ying Tu Angela
1563 Palos Verdes Mall 510/932-4002

Watsonville

Mark Maryellen
600 Corralitos Ridge Rd 408/462-2838
Marra Sarah 277 Sundance Ln 408/724-1313

West Covina

Hangi Fung Henry
1414 S Azusa Ave Ste 16 ....818/919-0415
Van Dao Duc 1229 W Ituni St 818/338-2392
Yu Sam 1507 E Vine Ave 818/308-9882

Westminster

Dang Paul M
6072 Apache Rd 714/984-9787
Han William C
5262 Shrewsbury Ave 714/897-9225
Mui (Diane) A Ly
15822 Monroe St 714/897-7315
Tran Hoang M
10491-A Bolsa Ave 714/775-6664
Truong Tho V
14024 Magnolia St Ste 200 ....714/892-6133
Van Dao Kiem
14461 Castle St 714/895-3286
Van Phan Du
15650 Brookhurst St Apt C 714/839-3666

Whittier

Lui Ming 6740 Bright Ave 310/698-3056

Woodland Hills

Farahmand Salar
5649 Rawlings Ave 818/348-0246

Hui Tiao Winnie
22563 Flamingo St 818/888-9697
Jordan Linda S
5353 Topanga Canyon Blvd Ste 8.818/704-9736
Kwan Abel S
22949 Califa St 818/702-0198
Li-Chen Kwan Santina
22949 Califa St 818/702-0198
Meisinger Susan B
22020 Clarendon St Ste 305 ......818/883-1245
Wong Perez Janis
22554 Ventura Blvd Ste 205 ....818/716-8330

Yountville

Rose David J PO Box 2685 ....415/454-7768

Colorado

Aspen

Aspen Health Works
3010 Glenwood Spring..................303/920-8753
Cargile William M BS DC FIA CA
3010 Glenwood Spring..................303/945-2693
Goodrich Mary C PO Box 2245........303/927-9617
Roberts Brendan PO Box 44 ....303/925-6035

Aurora

Sun Fan-Shin 10722 E Cliff Ave 303/752-1782

Boulder

Storrie Scott
3065 Center Green Dr Ste 100 ...303/440-8010
Alper Johanna
1435 Hawthorn Ave 303/444-3319
Bellows Warren E
944 Grant Pl 303/444-8527
Binder Timothy A DC ND
2321 Mapleton Ave 303/786-8116
Burnell Suzanne S
1800 30th St Ste 307 ....303/442-5441
Denman Katheryne C
1404 Wonderview Ct 303/442-4031
Flaws Robert S CMT DAC
Iris Acupuncture Associates
3405 Penrose Pl Ste 107 ....303/442-0796
Frank Douglas Charles
3011 Broadway Ste 32 ....303/449-3114
Gingrich Alan R
2922 Glenwood Dr 303/939-9405
Gottlieb William Jia
1120 Alpine Ave Ste F 303/444-2425
Henderson Andrew
1705 14th St Ste 227 ....303/444-0412
Hendryx Jan Do
2575 Spruce St Ste A 303/444-8844
Huang Pao-Chin Ruseto
2900 Valmont Rd Ste E-1 ....303/449-1686
Liu Yong
1531 Lodge Ln 303/939-9732
Macritchie James Acupuncture Center of Boulder

2730 29th St 303/442-2250

Metke Mary E
2111 30th St Suite D 303/442-2545

Oakley Stephen D
584 Peakview Rd 303/447-8481

Rao Nancy A ND RAC
Goose Creek Plaza
2880 Folsom St # 210A 303/449-8581

Reaves Whitfield PO Box 2039 ....303/442-6399

Socolov Leonard Jay
2769 Iris Ave Ste 109 ....303/444-5202

Temple Lisa M 4931 Carter Ct 303/530-4130

Terres Lora Stephanie
2919 Belmont Av 303/449-9800

Wolfe Honora Lee
1775 Linden Ave 303/447-0740

Zhou Mingying
735 Mohawk Dr 303/499-1691

Colorado Springs

Cooper Stevan R
3608 Windsor Ave 719/528-6952

Juetersonke George DO
5455 N Union Blvd Ste 200 ....719/528-1960

Liu Jian Wei
6485 Nanette Way 719/598-1897

Tucci Jill Adrian
3113 N Prospect St 719/596-9148

Denver

Grogan Colleen DAC Cherry Creek Acupuncture
3665 Cherry Ck Dr N 303/320-1240

Hill Laurelle L
9045 E Girard Ave Ste 54 ....303/751-5143

Kelley Robert T
1100 E Evans Ave 303/789-2330

Kitchie George H OMD LAC Acupuncture Wellness Ctr
2121 S Oneida St Ste 250 ....303/757-7016

Moore Dennis R DA Moore Acupuncture
2121 S Oneida St Ste 250 ....303/757-7016

Silver Eric M
3329 E Bayaud Ave Apt 7-H 303/355-2010

Tao Eric H Y 3200 E Mexico Ave 303/758-7045

Tichy Robert J 905 S Gilpin St 303/733-2564

Truong Van
1860 Larimer St Ste 330 ....303/298-8602

Dillon

O'Brien Carol E PO Box 2741 ....303/567-4397

Durango

Albright Mary Ellen
2320 County Rd 303/259-6347

Edwards Louise N
929 E 3rd Ave 303/247-2043

Levens Geoffrey D
PO Box 3794 ....805/682-2126

Vandover Nancy Gae
831 E Animas Rd 303/247-0719

Englewood

McCain Sally Arent
5885 S Monaco St 303/779-1109

Evergreen

Carlee Adrienne L
16391 Wolverine Trail 303/670-9419

Carmer PO Box 2156 ....303/674-8595

Hayes Donn William
28257 Lupine Dr 303/674-4790

Fort Collins

Coseo Marc C
4109 Trowbridge Dr 303/532-3024

Helenschild Margaret
638 Endicott St 303/224-4787

Glenwood Springs

Cargile William M DC LAC
1322 Grand Ave 303/945-2693

Lee Bing Fay
214 8th St Ste 303 ....303/945-2802

Menten Kathleen M
Rocky Mountain Acupuncture
826 1/2 Grand Ave 303/945-2768

Golden

Fisher-Rosenberg Lee A
33 Conifer Rd 303/526-1051

Greeley

Liscum Gary A
1028 8th St 303/356-9803

Lafayette

Fratkin Jake Paul
204 W Brome Ave 303/541-9055

Lakewood

Nowinski Gary M
1213 S Gray St 303/922-2309

Littleton

Bonde Jean D 4 Catamount Ln 303/972-3323

Longmont

Elliott Diane Kay
15168 County Road 7 ....303/922-4878

Lyons

Padilla Patricia Ann PO Box 146 ......303/823-6318

Pagosa Springs

Norman Edward Nils PO Box 1751 .303/264-4772

Paonia

Brooks Dennis R PO Box 1071 ....303/527-6652

Pueblo

Skonieczka Don
Golden Flower Health Center
251 S Santa Fe Ave 719/542-9210

Steamboat Springs

Simcoe Mark A
PO Box 770926 ....303/879-7544

Telluride
Clifton Nikki Jo PO Box 611 ....303/728-6660

Connecticut

Bethel
McKnight William R
74 Sunset Hill Rd 203/778-8292

Danbury
Shih Deying
73-3 Great Plain Rd 203/748-8107

East Hartford
Greenberg Stephen R
52 Oakland Ave 203/528-7111

Greenwich
Assadi-Baiki Abdoreza
48 Ritch Ave 212/722-6248
Harris Marie A
22 Lafayette Place 203/869-9340
Meade E Babs   DIPL AC
523 E Putnam Ave 203/661-2933

Mansfield Center
Thompson Peter Guy LAC
Japanese Body Balance Shoppe
452 Storrs Rd 203/456-3010

Middletown
Reneson Joseph PHD
148 College St 203/347-8894

Milford
Fleischman Gary Franklin Milford Acupuncture Center
26 Lafayette St 203/878-0061

Mystic
Poole Kathleen T Mystic River Acupuncture
PO Box 249 ....203/536-3362

New Haven
Davis Paul S DAC Microcurrent Research Inc
1440 Whalley Ave Ste 224   ....800/872-6789
Ritterman Robin B
2558 Whitney Ave 203/230-2200

Norwalk
Lok Kai-Yee
29 Granite Dr 914/946-7704
Schweitzer Marvin P
71 E Ave Ste F 203/853-6285

Orange
Sica-Cohen Robban MD
325 Post Rd 203/799-7733

Redding
Wiegaard Ingri Boe
43 Wood Rd 203/938-8693

Salem
Browne-Carey Bonnie Lee
400 Round Hill Rd 203/859-3844

Southport

Zimmerman Jeffrey C
22 Rockview Dr 203/221-9877

Stamford
Carpenter Corrine C
Acu-Therapy
1360 Bedford St 203/964-4725
Haase Corrine C
Acupuncture & Acupressure Therapy
1360 Bedford St 203/964-4725
Karn Eileen M DAC
Acupuncture Health Services
37 Glenbrook Rd 203/353-8811
Semel Abbey
93 Riverbank Rd 203/322-4977
Shen John Hf
50 Strawberry Patch Ln 203/324-1982

Washington Depot
Loreto Conrad C
39 Hifield Dr 203/746-5030

Wilton
Strasmore Kassandra
197 Old Kings Hwy 203/834-0413

District of Columbia

Washington
Gao Jingyun
4520 Natashsa Bl Suite 108....... 202/338-5490
Heaton-Levering Sarah
1712 Kilbourne Pl NW 202/234-2329
Jackson Deng
4000 Albemarle St NW Ste 206...202/237-0197
Na Hong-Do DAC
1244 5th St NE 202/544-2929
Ross John Nathan
2914 33rd Pl NW 202/333-3170
Shu Mengda
2141 Wisconsin Ave NW D-1 ....202/625-1603
Stang Sarah E
Acupuncture Associates
2019 Park Rd NW 202/328-6591
Taylor Julie E
5524 MacArthur Blvd NW 202/363-2455
Wu Shi-Hua MD
1505 6th St NW 202/789-2094
Wu Jing Nuan
5524 Macarthur Blvd Nw 202/363-2455

Florida

Boca Raton
Gottesman Simm
8904-F SW 22nd St 407/488-4887
Hedendal Bruce DC
Hedendal Chiropractic & Nutrition Center
301 Crawford Blvd 407/391-4600
Iannelli Michael PO Box 3611 ....305/480-4540

Lee Yao Wu
875 Meadows Rd #321 ....407/368-6502
Marshall Michael L
5642 Santiago Cir 407/278-1513
Zoll Stuart Joel 7301 W Palmetto Pk Rd Ste 103C
....407/395-2667

Boynton Beach

Burstein Rosalyn Acupuncture Plus
2828 S Seacrest Blvd #207 ....407/369-8900

Bradenton

Fee Wang Peng
4816 Dundee Dr 813/792-6872

Bradenton Beach

Nussbaum Irma
3701 E Bay Dr Apt 5 ....813/778-9367

Casselberry

Huang William
2905 Lakeview Dr 407/830-0012

Coral Springs

Landy Leslie AP
9465 W Sample Ste 201 ....305/345-7571
D'Costa Harriet M MD DAC
1481 Belleair Rd 813/584-7246
O'Neill John E 1700 McMullen Booth Rd Ste D2
....813/726-7333

Cocoa

Patrignani Victoria
1314 Clearlake Rd Ste 3...............407/633-4363

Deerfield Beach

Pennell David J 418 N River Dr 305/481-2285

Fort Lauderdale

Chen Chao CA MD
1930 E Sunrise Blvd......................305/761-7115
Chu Yen Johanna
Yen's Acupuncture Center
1051 SE 17th St 954/522-6405
Lumbert Jeffrey
1050 NE 5th Ter 305/525-5069

Gainesville

Barry Juanita
10231 SW 75th Way 904/885-4406
Bole David N
6425 NW 54th Way 904/378-2669
Smith Pamela J
1833 NW 6th St 904/376-3975

Hallandale

Abdurr Jata Muhamud
517 SW 10th St Ste 2 ....305/454-0795

Hialeah

Chin Linda Whei-Lin DAC
Multi-Rehab Health Institute
166 E 49th St 305/825-3035

Hollywood

Chen Chao CA MD
800 S Federal Hwy 305/923-8500
Dolinsky Jerome
6670 Taft St 305/961-6400

Jacksonville

Kowalski Michael B AP DAC
Acupuncture & Holistic Health Center
4237 Salisbury Rd Ste 107 ....904/296-9545
Lim Chang Dong
3653 Riveredge Dr 904/744-5597
Murphy Joyce
1 San Jose Pl Ste 28 ....904/292-1048

Jupiter

Hollifield Steven C
Calm Spirit Health Care Inc
725 N A-1a 407/575-6800

Kissimmee

Iida Takatoshi
1900 Boggy Creek Rd 407/933-4878

Lady Lake

De Meo Vincent J PO Box 520 ....904/753-4289

Lake Mary

Holistic Options
3895 Lake Emma Rd 407/333-2603

Lake Worth

Lee Samuel K
6118 Seven Springs Blvd 407/966-8677

Lakeland

Hong-Sun Ou Henry
1604 E Gary Rd 813/644-6152
Ou Henry H
1604 E Gary Rd 813/687-9480
Ying Ou Susan Y
1604 E Gary Rd 813/644-6152

Largo

Johansen Roger L DC
918 W Bay Dr 813/581-2774

Lauderdale Lakes

Yen Francis E
4297 N State Rd 7.......................954/485-9188

Leesburg

Demeo Vincent
734 N 3rd St Ste 215 ....904/787-8882

Lynn Haven

Eckhaus Muhammad
1301 Ohio Ave 904/265-1204

Melbourne

McAlhster Wendy A
905 E New Haven Ave Ste 204 ....407/728-4463

Merritt Island

Burleson Marie
215 Lucas Rd 407/453-5466

Miami

Chen Agnes
3800 Collins Ave Apt 814 .... 305/534-2518
Colangelo Marleen AP
Myotascial Therapy & Acupuncture
7550 S Red Rd Ste 209 ....305/669-1351
Duwat Michael M
239 E Enid Dr 305/856-5629
Font Ruben
300 SW 107th Ave Ste 212 ....305/551-3147
Grossbard Harvey Jay
17435 NE 12th Ct 305/652-5336
Holder Jay DC MD PHD
5990 Bird Rd 305/661-3474
Kocica Bodhi F LMT
814 Ponce De Leon Ste 417 ....305/444-9984
Konefal Janet PHD LAC
3478 Royal Palm Ave 305/548-4751
Korotkin Lois LAC
6001 Riviera Dr 305/667-1314
Lan Xu Zong
8475 SW 94th St Apt 126-E 305/279-8180
Lo Sophie
7125 SW 95th St 305/666-7510
Nhat Yuan Van
3430 SW 87th Ave 305/220-8637
Pagani Luis
1720 79th St Causeway Ste 118 305/868-6801
Ruggiero Enrico
2944 NW 10th Ave 813/327-0180
Russell Robert V
7522 SW 62nd St 305/667-8787
Sachi 330 W 58th St 305/861-1070
Sanchez Camilo
Acupressure Acupuncture Institute
9835 Sunset Dr #206 ....305/595-9500
Schweizer David Jon
5790 SW 54th Ter 305/663-1578
Trinh Binh Ngoc
Happy Healthy
3430 SW 87th Ave 305/220-8637

North Miami Beach

Chiu Aidan Y MD
Chinese Health & Cultural Center
360 NE 167th St 305/949-2228
Holder Jay M DC PHD DAAPM
975 Arthur Godfrey Rd (41st)........305/534-3635
Larsen Terre G
1545 NE 167th St 305/940-7763

Naples

Caccamesi Charles
PO Box 9723 ....813/353-7063
Hubbard Stanley J Acupuncture Center of Naples
231 9th St S 813/263-2322
Nair Dan PHD AP
2500 Tamiami Trl N Ste 220 ....813/261-6601

New Port Richey

Raney Joann C
7113 US Hwy 19 ....813/846-7266
Pierson Rebecca
7113 US Hwy 19...........................813/846-7266

Okeechobee

Douglas Edward DC
Douglas Health Center
916 W N Park St 813/763-4320

Orange Park

Chin Robert
350 Eldridge Ave Ste 5 ....904/264-3069

Orlando

Hou Joseph P 2224 E Concord 407/896-3005
Wong Peter K 3708 E Grant St 407/894-4972

Oviedo

Yong Shou Dong 425 Geneva Dr 407/366-3183

Palm Bay

Chen Hsiu S 201 Eldron Blvd SE 407/951-3764

Palm Beach

Regard Pierre G 250 Ocean Ter 407/848-8770

Palm Beach Gardens

Carianna Ember
11211 Prosperity Farms Rd #22 .407/622-4706

Pompano Beach

Landy Leslie RN AP
9465 W Sample Rd Ste 201 .... 305/345-7571

Punta Gorda

D'Aprile Delores
740 Taimimi Trail 813/743-7500
Moffatt Vincent
2195 Gulfview Rd 813/635-2033

Saint Augustine

Smith John W 43 Cincinnati Ave 904/829-1487

Saint Petersburg

Liang Ku Su 5473 66th St N 813/541-2666
Sommers Frank 5735 31st Ave S ...813/381-4925

Sarasota

Center for Trad Chinese Medicine
RJ Zhao OMD PHD Clinic Director
1299 S Tamiami Trail #1209 ....813/365-8008
Allen Marilyn B
7717 Holiday Dr 813/924-1346
Donaldson Kimberly Jeanne
RR 10 Box 331A 813/371-2862
Kaltsas Harvey J DAC
The Healing Center
505 S Orange Ave......................... 813/955-4456
Miller Terese M
2831 Ringling Blvd Ste 203B 813/365-1283
Reese James T
4724 Sloan Ave 813/921-2770

Tallahassee

Kresge Carol A RR 7 Box MLC...........904/878-1598
Trescott Carol 501 E College Ave 904/224-1964

Tampa

Celpa Luis O Celpa Health Center
2707 W Tampa Bay Blvd 813/875-4444
Eubanks Charles R
1704 N Lincoln Ave 813/875-2187
Heigh Gregory AP MD PHD DNBHE
13014 N Dale Mabry #352 ....813/968-6260
Lee Eugene H MD
1804 W Kennedy Blvd #A 813/251-3089
Zhang Lin
1602 W Sligh Ave 813/935-4744
Zuby William L
4302 Menderson Blvd 813/251-3866

Tarpon Springs

Geier Larry S
1006 Lake Avoca Ct 813/934-2002
Sullivan Patrick Enite Crane Center
9 Hibiscus St 813/942-4249

Tequesta

Groll Edwin H 4 Shady Ln 407/747-8197

Vero Beach

Quaranto Danny BS DAC
Acupuncture Center of Vero Beach
1717 20th St 407/778-8877

West Palm Beach

Auger Nicole CA Health & Beauty Acupuncture Center
11 Waltham 407/471-2917
Carianna Ember AP
2601 N Flagler Dr Ste #212 .... 407/835-6821

Georgia

Doraville

Ho Kiin Sung
5269 Buford Hwy NE 404/455-6511
Yeol Yoo Han
5312 Buford Hwy NE 404/457-9516

Fayetteville

Kim Tae Chong
590 Hawthorne Dr 404/461-5922

Norcross

Lee Samuel
4418 John Dr 404/279-2254

Roswell

Anderson Seneca Anderson Health Center
1265 Minhinnette Dr 404/642-4646

Hawaii

Ewa Beach

Tanji John Tsuguo Nak
91-1364 Kaihuopalaai St 808/677-3777

Haleiwa

Himmelmann Richard T
59-525 Akanoho Pl 808/638-8061

Hanalei

Amdur Carol Latifa Acupuncture & Natural Healing Ctr
PO Box 1232 ....808/826-1163

Hilo

West Sarah
90 Kamehameha Ave Ste 2 ....808/935-8088

Holualoa

Lawrence Felicitas G PO Box 763 ....808/322-1663

Honolulu

Burke Jack 615 Piikoi St 808/537-4345
Chang Stewart St
609 Coolidge St Apt 3 ....808/946-8597
Chang Henry J
2222-A Young St 808/955-6175
Cheng Cecilia Sy
1212 Nuuanh Ave 808/524-2402
Horowitz Geraldine S
321 N Kuakini St Ste 712 .... 808/537-9413
Hwang Min-Der
181 S Kukui St Ste 206 ....808/536-3611
Kwon Bong Ahn
1704 Anapuni St Apt 3B 808/947-6896
Lee Lucy Ling H Hawaii Acupuncture Associates
181 S Kukui St Ste 206 ....808/536-3611
Lin Henry
305 Royal Hawaiian Ave #208 .....808/923-6939
Loo Cyrus W
2727 Kolonahe Pl 808/536-6383
Mercer Fielding L
2160 St Louis Drive 808/737-9564
Monasch Eugene
1750 Kalakaua Ave #3-519 ....808/949-8966
Monasch Ruby E
1750 Kalakaua Ave Ste 3-529 ....808/949-8966
Ono Eric
99-433 Ulune Street 808/488-1535
Pham Khahn Thuy
Acupuncture Center
90 N King St Ste 217 ....808/599-3743
Siou Lily
1073 Hind Iuka Dr 808/373-2849
Siou Shih C
111 N Beretania St #D206 ....808/545-1287
Vani Kyong
PO Box 23152 ....808/947-4799
Watanabe Ted S
2065 N King St Rm 311 ....808/941-9074
Xiao Shi-Zhong
1655 Makaloa St Apt 2003 ....808/536-6807
Yee Suen Hang
1016 Maunakea St 808/531-6680
Yiu Heung H
1314 S King St Ste 1264 ....808/524-8297

Yoo Byung Rae
35 N Kukui St Apt 1602 ....808/521-8434
Young Jon
206 Kapalu St 808/536-7437

Kahuliu

Anand Kabba
444 Hana Hwy Ste 213 ....808/572-2562
Chung Susan RN
The Acupuncture Herbal Clinic of TCM
417 Uluniu St 808/263-0333
Davison Kevin J ND LAC
Maui East West Clinic Ltd
444 Hana Hwy #211 ....808/871-4722
Kroll Joni LAC DAC
Kailua Acupuncture Center
320 Uluniu St #2 ....808/262-4550
Kruger Daniel DAC
140 Hoohana St Ste 301 ....808/871-8777
Pitman Shelley DAC
Acupuncture & Herbal Clinic
417 Uluniu St 808/263-0333

Kailua Kona

Maekawa Chieko Joyce DAC
Knoa Clinic of Acupuncture
72-3996 Hawaii Belt Rd 808/325-7778
Mallon Tisha M
Village Professional Plaza
75-5759 Kuakini Hwy Ste 200 ....808/326-5688

Kamuela

Toubman Karl Jeremy LAC MT
Waimea Natural Health Center
PO Box 1739 ....808/885-9661

Kaneohe

Clough Babette L
47-591 Puapoo Pl 808/239-9849

Kapaa

Stuinpf Ii Edwin E
129 Aleo St 808/822-0838

Kealakekua

Gannon Joan
PO Box 1786 ....808/328-8040

Kekauoha

Jacinta Dana
PO Box 2143 ....808/329-8108

Kihei

Fitzgerald Susan
107 Luluka Place 808/879-4327

Kihei Maui

Christman J Randol LMT DAC............808/879-4341

Kilauea

Wright Victoria
PO Box 933 General Delivery 808/828-1198

Kula

Howden Michael S LAC

PO Box 667 ....808/878-3922

Lahaina

Biancardi Marco Lahaina Health Center
180 Dickenson St 808/878-2717

Makawao

Cotter Makik
PO Box 843 ....808/572-6091

Idaho

Boise

Burden John C
916 E Washington St 208/343-5155

Ketchum

Blair Margret Jane PO Box 3591 .....208/726-2761

Lewiston

Klein Elwin C 1130 11th Ave 208/743-1168

Nampa

Thornburgh Stephen DO
824 17th Ave S 208/466-3517

Sandpoint

Goldblum Arthur
219-B Church St 208/263-9687

Illinois

Arlington Heights

Connell Louella M
1048 N Carlyle Ln 708/394-4225
Sukel Phillip P DDS
1640 N Arlington Heights Rd 708/253-0240

Bensenville

Yates Betty V 238 Marshall Rd 312/641-0151

Champaign

Song Keychun 2509 W William St ...217/356-6488

Chicago

Anderson William James Chicago Acupuncture Clinic
3723 N Southport Ave 312/871-0342
Browne Patrick J DIP LAC (NCCA)
2740 N Pine Grove Ste 12G 312/935-4775
Cubacub Daniel V
2100 W Bradley Pl 2nd Fl 312/281-5530
Fen Xin-Xiang
3138 S Morgan St 312/421-7661
Guo Zhengang 327A W 23rd St 312/842-2775
Howard Martha H
706 W Junior Ter 312/935-0029
Jenkins Hugh A ND
2148 W 95th St 312/445-6800
Komen Julie E DAC
509 W Aldine Ave 312/477-6353
Kreuser Maureen Frances
639 W Diversey Pky #211.............312/525-7469
Lee Mary Helen BS DAC
1309 W Albion Ave 1st Fl 312/743-5229
Luban Michael

55 E Washington St Ste 164........ 312/553-2020
Lynch Linda G
  1823 N Fairfield Ave 312/929-7916
Maguire Paul J
  3333 W Peterson Ave 312/478-6870
Marino Mary Ellen
  2400 N Ashland Ave 2nd Fl 312/296-6700
Marino Mary Ellen DIPL LAC
  Chicago Holistic Center
  5353 N Virginia Ave 312/728-2025
Markowski Nadrien T
  3719 N Sacramento Ave 312/539-1989
Marks Brenda
  100 E Walton St #41-7 ....312/787-1180
Morland Clifford E
  2156 W Giddings St 312/878-9310
Northage-Orr Althea
  1522 W Nelson St 312/975-1655
Perry Robert F
  1421 North Hoyne 312/342-4572
Pirog John E
  3541 W 61st St 312/434-2792
Plovanich Dan Chicago Holistic Clinic
  2400 N Ashland Ave 2nd Fl 312/296-6700
Pomeroy Justin
  1350 W Schubert Ave 312/281-4450
Qi Rebecca Chicago Holistic Center
  2400 N Ashland Ave 2nd Fl 312/296-6700
Qian Mei Ling MD Harmony Herb Company
  3210 S Halsted St 312/791-0025
Rogel Mary I
  10 W 35th St #14E3-1 ....312/955-9643
Speckman Jodine Ann
  3047 N Lincoln Ave Ste 430 ....312/281-3341
Suddeth Toy Frances DC CA D
  Lincoln Park Chiropractic
  2202 N Lincoln Ave 312/248-2790
Tong Rosa Yeu-Fen
  6151 N Maplewood Ave 312/975-1295
Uretz Allen
  2400 N Ashland Ave 2nd Fl 312/296-6700
Wallach Pamela Chicago Holistic Center
  2400 N Ashland Ave 2nd Fl 312/296-6700
Wilson Wardell
  PO Box 19701 ....312/468-4083
Yurasek Frank Chicago Holistic Center
  2400 N Ashland Ave 2nd Fl 312/296-6700
Zheng Jin Quan
  3420 S Paulina St 312/225-1854

Dekalb
Faivre Patricia Ann
  2309 W Fairview 815/756-5039

Des Plaines
Oiso Akio MD CA
  1455 E Golf Rd Ste 114 ....708/296-5437

Elgin
Sabanis John V
  1124 Leawood Dr 708/888-4839

Evanston
Baker Claudette TM DAC
  527 Forest Ave 708/866-8116
North Mitzi
  1215 Cleveland St Apt 2 ....708/869-2462

Highland Park
Chow Chi DAC LAC Chinese Healing Art
  1854 Clavey Rd 708/831-1609

Lake Bluff
Lambrecht Sarah E
  243 W Blodgett Ave 708/234-0842

Naperville
Cullen Olivia CA LAC D
  845 Edgewater Dr 708/357-3320

Niles
Chen Raymond
  7356 W Carol St 708/470-1026

Oak Park
Dunn Dale A DC DAC
  Synergy Health Systems
  PO Box 1130 ....312/386-8822
Eckholm Jacquelyn Marie
  200 S Kenilworth Ave Apt 2N....... 708/386-5478
Pattee Jodie DAC
  711 South Blvd #4 ....708/386-5667
Ryan Mary Kay
  1033 S Highland Ave 708/386-7802
Yurasek Frank - The AcuCenter
  816 S Oak Park Ave 708/445-0455
Yurosek Frank MA ACT O
  816 S Oak Park Ave 708/319-0192

Richmond
Dunbar Irene Helen
  7801 Barnard Mill Rd 815/728-8015

Skokie
Zhou Qi 8414 McCormick Blvd 708/674-1951

Tinley Park
Dieska Daniel R DDS
  17726A Oak Park Ave 708/429-4700

West Chicago
Slater Martin A
  27 W 570 Ridgeview St 708/293-1345

Westmont
Pai Maria Chia
  18W 066 71st Street 708/969-6091

Wheeling
Romano Augusto DAC
  500 W Palatine Rd #106 ....708/459-5950

Wilmette

Friedman Andrea J
2936 Central Ave 312/251-4420

Indiana

Bloomington
Jia Ying BTCM
400 E 3rd St 812/336-6216

Crown Point
Howey James A
4207 W 121st Ave 219/662-9800

Evansville
Sparks Harold T DO
3001 Washington Ave 812/479-8228

Gary
Nabors Joh PO Box 6117 ....219/949-7544

Valparaiso
Trowbridge Myrna D DO
850-C Marsh St 219/462-3377

Iowa

Des Moines
Roberts John T
6536 University Ave 515/279-9120

Iowa City
East-West Center 424 Highland Ct...319/354-1866

Sioux City
Coulter Diane Kay
1520 Whitcher Ave........................712/233-1398

Kansas

Kansas City
Baker Steven W
5435 Turner Rd 913/287-7171
Thompson-Rentscaler Anne
1039 S 53rd St 913/287-7066

Wichita
Beyrle Stanley NMD
Kansas Clinic of Traditional Medicine
2708 E Central Ave 316/687-0035
Gao Qizhi CA
550 N Hillside #203......................316/688-7154

Kentucky

Louisville
Odell James Paul OMD
Traditional Chinese Health Arts Institute
305 N Lyndon Ln 502/429-8835

Louisiana

Baton Rouge
Lee Tu-Kung
9201 Airline Hwy 504/924-1331

Breaux Bridge

Churchill Heather M OMD CA
513 Grant Ave 318/269-0444

New Orleans
Nguyen Theresa Hong
14452 Peltier St 504/254-9228

Roseville
Brown Gregory Channel LAC
901 Sunrise Ave 916/782-6683

Maine

Bangor
Atwood Donna Lm
109 State St 2nd Fl 207/945-5586
Myerowitz Zev J
1570 Broadway 207/947-3333
Roseberry Mary M
115 Franklin St Ste 1B 207/942-0494

Blue Hill
Evans Howard M LA PO Box 838 ....207/374-9963
Pollard Vicki C PO Box 838 ....207/374-9963

Camden
Brand Katherine
13 Grove St 207/236-2794
Rockett Jolinda CA
29 Mountain St 207/236-3601

Falmouth
Marland Miranda ND LAC
4 Fundy Rd 207/781-7600

Hallowell
Klobas Russell A
220 Water St #2 ....207/621-0985

Kittery
Gansecki Meattey Alice
Pepperrell Green 74 State Rd St ..207/439-5809
Hart Netta Acupuncture Health Service Inc
72 Rte 236 N Kittery Business 207/439-6627

Portland
Connolly Colleen RN
48 Deering St 207/828-0059
Ganberg Sheldon RF DAC Acupuncture Health Care
278 State St 207/775-5020
Hopkins Devereux
145 Newbury St 207/775-0058
Jonas Coleen Ellen
PO Box 8463 ....207/828-0059
Riesenberg Anne R 43 Macy St 207/775-0058

Smyrna Mills
White Casey RN FNP PO Box 42 .....207/757-8994

Yarmouth
Marks Paul R 78 Main St 207/846-6464
Marland Miranda J
8 Farnell Dr 207/781-7600
Tsao Fern S PO Box 798 ....207/846-4433

Maryland

Annapolis

Chesapeake Electromedical
  3 Church Circle Ste 165 .... 800/872-0399
  168 West St Ste 201 .... 410/280-6488
Mullins Margaret M
  1182 River Bay Rd 301/757-3613

Baltimore

Brown Robert B LAC
  711 W 40th St Ste 316 .... 410/235-2998
Clarke Penny R
  1200 E Joppa Rd 410/339-7820
Cost Denise
  4801 Yellowwood Ave 410/367-0606
Daniel Jack M
  51 River Oaks Cir 410/486-3406
Dorst Heather
  4801 Yellowwood Ave 410/367-0606
Drechsler Dorothy R RN
  3410 University Pl 410/467-2175
Dunn Katherine E
  4540 Keswick Rd 301/366-5761
Gershowitz Susan
  3655 Old Court Rd Ste 10 .... 410/484-3709
Johnson Eric L
  1305 S Hanover St 410/783-1331
Kramer Bruce T RAC
  1777 Reisterstown Rd Ste 290 ... 410/486-9370
Lewis Viola G
  1732 Moreland Ave 410/728-0841
Mahone Patricia L
  Little Patuxent Pkwy 410/997-3770
Nguyen My-Hanh T
  1501 Sul Grade Av 410/367-4900
Phelps Mary A RN RAC
  4803 Yellowwood Ave 410/367-0606
Weng Marisa Y 909 Starbit Rd 410/321-5774

Bethesda

Brenner Zoe Dee
  4733 Bethesda Ave Ste 804 .... 301/718-0953
Durana Carlos MA
  4933 Auburn Ave 301/654-0080
Kari Carol C RN
  5654 Shields Dr 301/897-0806
King Houng Kaung
  8218 Wisconsin Ave Ste 417 .... 301/656-6547
Lee Dominic Duhyong
  7220 Bradley Blvd 301/365-5460
Shapero Leslie Ann
  5654 Shields Dr 301/530-7240
Tsang Grace Wong
  4400 E West Hwy 301/652-2828

Brinklow

Lansdale Johnsen Robin

  20300 New Hampshire Ave 301/779-5860

Chevy Chase

Kopelove David
  4601 Davidson Dr 301/718-1028

College Park

Foster David Karl
  7526 Sweetbriar Dr 301/474-9124

Columbia

Baker Elizabeth M
  10716 Little Patuxent Pky 301/997-7040
Barnes Cyrie L
  10716 Little Patuxent Pky 410/992-0080
Choe Jay Ho
  6507 Sewells Orchard Dr 301/381-4723
Connelly Dianne M
  American City Bldg 301/997-3770
Delong Mary P RAC
  10716 Little Patuxent Pky #21 .... 410/997-7040
Duggan Robert M
  American City Bldg 301/596-6006
Finn-Gilbert Hope M
  9244 Hobnail Ct 410/730-2042
Finn-Gilbert Hope M AC ACQU
  10716 Little Patuxent Pky............. 410/997-7040
Gallagher Deborah
  11360 Tooks Way 410/730-7008
Ignatius Haig PO Box 817 .... 410/730-4224
Kerr Charlotte Rose
  American City Bldg 301/997-3770
Marinakis Peter G
  American City Bldg 410/997-3770
Measures Julia
  American City Bldg #10 .... 301/596-6006
Pescetto Giovanni
  10716 Little Patuxent Pky 410/997-5814
Phillips Michael A
  American City Bldg 410/997-3770
Rhinelander Nanine DAC
  5653 Harpers Farm Rd Unit B 301/694-2383
Rhinelander Nancy C
  5243-I Brook Way 410/997-2414
Smith Sharon M
  10716 Little Patuxent Pky............. 410/997-7040
Spivey Clayton MA RAC
  8342 Old Montgomery Rd 410/799-5883
Talbot Elisabeth J
  10716 Little Patuxent Pky............. 410/992-0080
Umidi Suzanne J
  9743 Summer Park Ct 410/730-2320
Zawacki Judy
  10314 Tailcoat Way 410/740-3288

Easton

Mercier David G
  32 S Washington St 410/820-7545
Reynolds Howard W

32 S Washington St 410/820-7545

Edgewater
Daniel Kathleen M
   224-E Mayo Rd 410/269-6032

Ellicott City
Lao Lixing
   4609 E Leisure Ct 410/281-9008
Marshall Bruce
   3462 Harrington Dr 410/461-4921
Vivino Barbara L
   633 Oella Ave 410/465-5843

Gaithersburg
Perretz Perry RAC
   19 Big Acre Sq 301/924-3834

Hyattsville
Clinic
   5400 Tuxedo Ave 301/341-9595

Kensington
Wong Grace OMD
   9709 Hill St 301/588-7570

Laurel
Brandt Edna M
   9811 Mallard Dr Ste 112 ....301/953-3413
Korbly-Canter Frances
   9811 Mallard Dr #209 ....301/953-3413

Mechanicsville
Barth Phebe J
   1150 Woodburn Hill Rd 301/884-8101

North Potomac
Huang Hui-Hsiung
   14816 Soft Wind Dr 301/762-1659

Owings Mills
Fradkin Mark
   9199 Reisterstown Rd Ste 211C .410/484-8147

Potomac
Han Injon 12212 Devilwood Dr 301/424-2223
Li Gui Fu
   11 Maidens Bower Ct 301/590-1055

Rockville
Chan Yeh Chong
   11125 Rockville Pike #G4 ....301/881-7866
Debarros Daniel M
   16 Maxim Ln 301/340-3077
Health Management Institute
   11140 Rockville Pike Ste 550 ......301/816-3000
Rossoff Michael LAC DIPL LAC (NCCA)
   5901 Montrose Rd Ste S-208 ....301/881-6400
Rukus Monika L 5014 Macon Rd ...301/881-6754
Shapero Robert C
   2272 Dunster Ln 301/340-6073
Su Shin Shin 5814 Hubbard Dr 301/881-0363
Yu Rong S
   11125 Rockville Pike Ste G4 ....301/881-7866

Silver Spring
Andreae Kristen M RN CMT
   3944 Rickover Rd 301/942-2146
Beatty Margaret M RAC
   722 Ritchie Ave 301/587-3874
Duncan Alaine D
   8830 Cameron St #501 ....301/565-2700
Goodman Harold DO
   8609 2nd Ave Ste 405B 301/565-2494
Grissmer Jane A
   2405 Eccleston St 301/229-2453
Kang Paul Myungsup
   12503 New Hampshire Ave 301/622-6660
Koppelman Joan
   523 Ashford Rd 301/585-1084
Lee Koo
   11905 New Hampshire Ave 301/622-3610
Lewis Joan
   8830 Cameron St #501 ....301/565-2700
Li Nianzu
   817 Silver Spring Ave Ste 100 .....301/495-0058
Ngoc Phan Han
   10407 New Hampshire Ave 301/431-0279
Wang Huai Ken 12804 Ruxton Rd ..410/566-1982
Wang Chin-Hua
   2354 Deckman Ln 703/871-3878

Takoma Park
Hecker Arnold 6631 Eastern Ave 301/270-0095
Norton Reggi 13 Sherman Ave 301/270-5511
Soldinger Eve C
   6935 Laurel Ave Ste 203 ....301/270-2117
Tepper Lawrence
   6935 Laurel Ave 301/891-2737
Van Tran Sen MD
   8108 Hammond Ave 301/439-6476

Timonium
Patz Nelson
   22 W Padonia Rd #C-245 ....410/560-1960

Westminster
Cross Deborah
   112 E Main St 410/857-1614
Hartman Alison LAC MAC
   218 E Main St Ste 2 ....410/857-1614

Woodstock
Fishman Jed E
   10117 Davis Ave 410/750-2090

Massachusetts

Acton
Hanson John Sanger
   532 Great Rd 508/263-0110

Amherst
Grossman Nancy ACUP DIP Commonwealth Acupuncture
   150 Fearing St Ste 23 ....413/549-5855
Huang Jingfei
   616 North Village 413/546-2166

King Dedie S LAC Traditional Acupuncture Office
592 Main St 413/253-9761
King Helen S
592 Main St 413/253-9761
Klate Jonathan Shaw
48 N Pleasant St Ste 201 .... 413/253-9558
O'Rourke Ellen S LAC Acuhealth of Amherst
502 Main St 413/256-8558
Smith Verena J RAC DAC
19 Cosby Ave 413/549-2830

Ashby

Caiander Richard M PO Box 325 ....508/386-5696

Baldwinville

Stuart Charles L 2 Chestnut St 508/939-8544

Belchertown

Ehret Joanne G 13 Maple St 413/323-9310
Moran James D Belchertown Wellness Center
21 Everett Ave 413/323-7212

Beverly

Legault Mariane E First Choice Health Center
266 Cabot St 508/922-0831

Boston

Barton Shivanatha
1152 Beacon St 617/277-4150
Cargill Marie LAC
25 Huntington Ave Ste 422 ....617/247-1446
Lee Susan 15 Kenwood St 617/625-8840
McCabe Mary M 77 Holland St 617/776-2020
Naeser Margaret A LAC DAC Boston Chinese Medicine
8 Whittier Pl Apt 19-D 617/723-9487
Shaw Karen J RN LAC
63 Dunboy St 617/254-1114

Boxboro

McMahon-King Cynthia Lynn
25 Stow Rd 508/263-4026

Brighton

Gerard Marianne
1505 Commonwealth Ave Ste 37 ....617/782-0267

Brookline

Ammen Jonathan B
385 Harvard St 617/738-7499
Boltax Jay David
22 Bowker St 617/131-0219
Delaney Carol C
1152 Beacon St 617/277-4150
Ginsberg Alan M
209 Harvard St Ste 302 ....617/738-9144
Holroyde Nancy Joan
6 Perry St Ste 5 ....617/731-4859
Kung Ching Ling
126 Harvard St 617/566-3603
Mandell Richard LAC
52 Lanark Rd 617/566-9766
Sempert Martha A

16 Davis Ave 617/566-2354
Sollars David LAC
1093 Beacon St 617/734-0928

Burlington

Hurley Judi A
171 Cambridge St 617/270-9555
Weinstein Judith Ann
171 Cambridge St 617/270-9555

Cambridge

Barney Heather Baird
32 Speridakis Ter 617/354-1060
Clarke Savitri The Health Alliance
2166 Massachusetts Ave 617/492-8300
Courtney Terry S Central Square Acupuncture
6 Bigelow St 617/661-2010
Cruichshank Ronald E
5A Lancaster St 617/547-4133
Gamble Andrew
4 Greenough Ave 617/926-4271
Kaptchuk Ted
27 Bay St 617/926-1788
Kay Joseph
400 Broadway 617/547-7119
Maguire Karen A
114 Willow St #4 ....617/863-9565
McCormick James S
335 Broadway 617/354-8360
Mueller William Henry
335 Broadway 617/354-8360
Pak Won Kyung
10 Pleasant St 617/864-4600
Pepper Anne L
6 Garden Ct Ste 5 ....617/491-6619
Quinn Dana Rae
6 Agassiz St Apt 5 ....617/354-7613
Singer Joyce LAC 617/868-8885
Zucker Michael
7 Arlington St 617/661-4070

Canton

Harris Susan Kay
9 Hillsview St 617/828-8308
Wernick Jeffrey S
197 Turnpike St 617/828-6636

Chelmsford

Halley Beverly
59 Boston Rd 508/256-1903

Chestnut Hill

Burstein Joseph S Reservoir Medical Associates
824 Boylston St Ste 101 ....617/739-1001
Dumont Patrick J Reservoir Medical Associates
824 Boylston St Ste 101 ....617/739-1001
Wallace Richard LAC REGD Brookline-Newton Health
850 Boylston St Ste 400 ....617/731-3399

Colrain

Evans Gail A PO Box 155 ....802/368-2929

Concord
Gerzon Robert E
  77 Bolton St 508/369-3539
Paino Sarah E
  252 Shadyside Ave 508/371-2355
Umphress Catherine M LAC
  42 Thoreau St 508/371-1228
Weinstein Kerry Community Health Resources
  1260 Main St 508/369-1131

Cummington
Ginzberg Jonathan N
  PO Box 300 ....413/634-5575

Dennis Port
Taloumis Louis PO Box 398 ....508/385-7280

Fairhaven
Waclawik Laurice Hall BS CLS DAC
  Accupoint Family Care
  888 Sconticut Neck Rd 508/991-5911

Fitchburg
Stuart Charles
  Options for Health
  910 Main St 508/354-6424

Framingham
Nie Qiangde MD
  16 Blackthorne Rd 508/872-7077

Georgetown
Gaudet Madeline
  24 Bradford Loop 508/352-8292

Gloucester
Jacobe Eliha LAC DAC
  2 Magnolia Ave 508/546-7170

Gloucester
Ventresca James W
  457 Washington St 508/283-0401

Great Barrington
Bunn Maribeth 113 Division St 413/499-3459
Goldberg Peter PO Box 10 ....413/528-5055

Greenfield
Edwards Nancy H 474 Main St 413/774-6611
Sachs Daniel A 278 Main St 413/774-3487

Hanover
Cohen Richard MD
  51 Mill St Ste 1 ....617/829-9281
Vanrenen Louis John American Acupuncture
  171 Rockland St 617/826-7606

Haverhill
Kane Susan E
  3rd Floor One Pkwy 508/372-7403

Hingham
Lane Genevieve P
  160 Old Derby St #12 ....617/740-1320

Holbrook
Black Karen LAC LSW
  Center for Wellness
  97 Belcher St 617/767-2336

Jamaica Plain
Kelter Ronald Alan
  29 Lakeville Rd 617/524-2220

Leeds
Mager Amy E
  481 Kennedy Rd 413/586-1577

Leverett
Shamey James N
  128 Shutesbury Rd 413/548-9757

Lexington
Blake Brigitte U 36 Shirley St 617/862-5729

Lowell
Kaufman Svetlana MD
  24 Merrimack St #323 ....508/453-5181

Malden
Bellini Joshua 452 Pleasant St 617/321-8293

Manchester
Siegelman-Nathan Diane Joan
  25 Harbor St 508/526-8334

Mendon
McSweeney Sandra M
  37 Cape Rd 508/473-5574

Methuen
Choi Young C Oriental Acupuncture
  11 Constitution Way 508/683-7779

Natick
Wendel Renato 16 Pinewood Ave 617/522-1493

New Bedford
Schwartz Daniel R
  123 Alva St 508/997-4158
Skaliotis Dionysios A
  203 Hawthorn St 508/994-9400

Newbury
Valaskatgis Peter E 19 High Rd 508/465-5080
Valaskatgis Pauline W
  New England Center for Holistic Medicine
  65 Newburyport Tpke 508/465-9770
Watson Pauline LAC DAC
  65 Newburyport Tpke 508/465-9770

Newburyport
Davis Susan P 552 Merrimac St 508/465-8674

Newton
Chen Wen Juan
  1424 Center St 617/331-6630
Doyle James Comprehensive Medical Services
  555 Commonwealth Ave 617/965-3306
Highfield Ellen S
  11 Chesley Rd 617/497-1185
Leydon Patricia

44 Grove Hill Park 617/527-8365

Newton Center

Pomerantz Wendy Sue
11 Chesley Rd 617/776-6578
Shapiro Maxine M
53 Marshall St 617/964-7191
So Isabel Yee
236 Spiers Rd 617/332-8502

Northampton

Ehret Joanne LAC DAC
53 Gothic St 413/586-9594
Fukushima Elizabeth
245 Main St Ste 206 ....413/586-3325
Kolchin Marjorie J
16 Center St Ste 518 ....413/584-0421
Mascaro Lisa M
16 Center St Ste 523 ....413/584-7949
Robinson-Hidas Linda
53 Gothic St 413/253-2900

Norwood

Levine Barry 10 Hillshire Ln 617/769-7363

Paxton

Chen Yvonne Szh 17 Lincoln Cir 617/757-2859

Pittsfield

Reynolds Donna B
246 North St Ste 315 ....413/499-0940

Provincetown

Spiegel Mary Jude PO Box 1747 ....508/487-9027

Quincy

Karp Daniel S LAC
12 Dimmock St 617/471-5577
Ryan Sandra E 59 Warren Ave 617/328-7237

Revere

Ellis Candice C 142 Kimball Ave 617/286-8755

Roslindale

Kantor Jerry M 623 South St 617/327-3227

Sandwich

Myers Arlene G 8 Pine Tree Cir 508/428-3922

Seekonk

Woo Chong K 1563 Fall River Ave ...508/336-6870

Sharon

Sternick Susan R 5 Mark Rd 617/784-5430

Somerville

Blake Valerie 15 Kenwood St 617/625-8840
Chan Lai Chun
15 Beacon St Apt 15 ....617/547-0139
Chen Ci 9 Myrtle St 617/524-8165
Cunningham Patrick M
186 Willow Ave 617/666-1798
Kay Joseph A
322 Beacon St 617/492-4822
Kung Ching Ling

77 Albion St 617/776-5910
Sarah Rebecca
69 Berkeley St 617/628-4448
Schultz Brian T
341 Washington St 617/666-9811
Whittington Jeanne Ann
46A Spring St 617/629-2251

South Lancaster

Liao Joseph PO Box 1464 ....508/368-1007

Springfield

Chou David St 517 Boston Rd 413/783-5355
Suen Yu Van LAC 308 Maple St 413/733-0007

Still River

Townsend Kathleen PO Box 163 .....508/456-6970

Stockbridge

Jarrett Lonny S PO Box 1093 ....413/298-4221

Stoneham

Stern Fred Franklin St Medical Assoc
139 Franklin St 617/438-6132

Stow

Howard Stephen H LAC
150 Harvard Rd 508/897-5979

Vineyard Haven

Lau Mebie Majorie H MASTER DAC
PO Box 2225 ....508/693-2776

Wakefield

Ferro Barbara D 28 Morrison Ave 617/245-0678

Watertown

Birch Stephen
30 Common St 617/926-4271
Brumson April L LAC DAC
30 Common St 617/926-4271
Feldman Martin
30 Common St 617/926-4271
Grodsky Ora Aqua Retreat Center
30 Common St 617/787-2143
Heeb Dolores Turning Point
26 Sunnybank Rd 617/923-4601
Kinneavy Mary B 30 Common St 617/924-9102
Zhang Yao 30 Common St 617/926-4271

Wellesley Hills

Cole Stephen
267 Washington St 617/431-7137

Wellfleet

McCarthy Maryann PO Box 744 ......508/349-7592

West Harwich

Taloumis Louis G
115 Main St 508/432-4140

West Roxbury

Dearborn Lindas CA.........................617/323-3343

Woburn

Seagrave Sandra Lee

414 Main St 617/938-1779

Worcester

Tamilio Kathleen LAC DAC
465 Park Ave 508/754-0211

Michigan

Ann Arbor

Lincoln Charles J Complementary Care
2345 S Huron Pky 313/973-1012

Battle Creek

Crapo Mark
107 Old Wentworth Pl 616/962-2836
Hubbs Renee
551 Michigan Ave E 616/962-2836

Bloomfield Hills

Rousseau Robert D DDS
6405 Telegraph Rd #J-3 ....313/642-5460

Bloomfield Township

Lielais John DDS
6405 Telegraph Rd #J-3 ....810/642-5460

East Lansing

Zhang Yu Qin
361 Rampart Way 517/355-9908

Farmington

Vincent Michael Andrew DAC
27650 Farmington Rd Ste 101.....810/489-1313

Grand Rapids

Wang Rujil
3441 Newcastle Dr SE 616/241-0515

Okemos

Lincoln-Midlam Deborah
4655 Dobie Rd Ste 270 ....517/349-6430

Paw Paw

Bayha Carl DS DIPLAC
27231 38th Avenue 616/668-4730
Wechter Elizabeth Sloco
34654 32nd St 616/657-3479

Redford

Wang Qian 17702 Fox St 313/532-2563

Richland

Krofcheck David
7622 Gull Creek Dr...................... 616/962-3283

Minnesota

Albert Lea

Winegar Wallace A
222 Fast Main 507/373-2919

Bemidji

Fors Gregory C
310 Minnesota Ave NW 218/759-2117

Bird Island

Neubauer David B
PO Box 169 ....612/365-4635

Neubauer Thomas J
210 Hwy Ave 612/365-4635

Bloomington

Jung Hee Wook
8100 Penn Ave S Ste 124 ....612/888-3454

Edina

Dong Yan-Ping
7225 Comelia Dr 612/832-9328
Durand Frank J
6457 McCauley Trl S 612/476-6612
Durand Cheryl Solange
6135 Kellogg Ave #226 ....612/925-9516
Haywood Rosemary A
5124 France Ave S 612/928-0802

Forest Lake

Kari Gerald W
967 Lake St S 612/464-1113

Fridley

Peng Shu-Dian
7300 Van Buren St NE 612/780-8324

Maple Plain

Conroy Patrick D DAC
1750 Deer Creek Rd 612/472-8642

Maplewood

Wagner James Richard BS
Family Physical Therapy Assoc Inc
1812 N St Paul Rd 612/779-8550

Minneapolis

Acupuncture Association
of Minnesota 612/641-0467
Cong Hung Nguyen
2342 Ferrant Pl 612/521-4973
Culliton Patricia Dawn DAC
825 S 8th St Ste 206 ....612/347-6238
Davis Edith R DAC
4421 4th Ave S 612/825-4362
Gross Diana J Dac
1111 W 22nd St 612/879-0191
Haynes Albert Z S
4235 5th Ave S 612/824-4247
Helffrich Michael
1935 Arthur St NE 612/789-9671
Holle Ned A DAC
4854 Park Ave 612/822-8207
Hung Nguyen Cong
2342 Ferrant Pl 612/374-2162
Kieu Duc DIPL & CER
3721 Chandler Dr NE Apt 202 .....612/572-1305
Klucas Patricia Ann
3653 Bloomington Ave 612/724-8374
Lucking Andrew J ND
3546 Grand Ave 612/924-8112
Mielke Debra K
1111 W 22nd St Ste 110 ....612/377-7107
Nguyen Hung Cong

2342 Ferrant Pl 612/521-4973

Peters Christopher Jay
  3255 Hennepin Ave #227 ....612/827-1226

Radel Vicky Lynn RN DAC
  Group Health Inc
  2701 University Ave SE 612/627-3525

Ragir Judity S
  4146 Pillsbury Ave 612/827-7721

Ross Scott M MD
  2545 Chicago Ave S 612/863-4700

Wu Jiny
  840 18th Ave SE 612/378-0885

Youcha Victor J
  6200 Excelsior Blvd Ste 204 .... 612/925-4639

Minnetonka

Crawford Les H
  15830 Lake St 612/935-2737

Park Rapids

Smart Arthur G
  PO Box 208 ....218/732-5295

Plymouth

Vitalis Nancy J
  2225 Urbandale Ln N 612/473-4773

Saint Paul

Desmarais Russell C
  569 Selby Ave 612/291-7772

Hays Sandra Ann
  105 Milton St S 612/222-8517

Liu Hong
  2024 Commonwealth Ave #A-32 .612/623-4881

Stowell Thomas W ND Wellspring Naturopathic Clinic
  1365 Englewood Ave 612/644-4436

Thatcher Robert L
  3673 Lexington Ave N 612/227-2071

Wang Yi-Rou
  2049 Kapp Ave 612/644-3166

Wells Margery A
  1449 Grand Ave 612/699-9876

Ye Zhu-San
  490 Asbury St 612/647-9116

Stewartville

Jensen Robert James
  100 20th St NW 507/533-4777

Mississippi

Ocean Springs

Waddell James H MD
  1520 Government St 601/875-5505

Missouri

Blue Springs

Dewitt Patricia
  1324 N Hwy 7 ....816/229-3210

Boonville

Wright William DC
  PO Box 14 ....816/882-3333

Chesterfield

Li Bo-Ning
  14392 Rainey Lake Dr 314/535-8785

Independence

Dorman Lawrence DO
  9120 E 35th St S 816/358-2712

Runyon Joseph DC PHD
  Christian Clinic Services
  15605 E Hwy 24 ....816/254-1969

Kansas City

Boyle Gregory LAC DAC
  6304 E 102nd St 816/763-1339

Rowland James DO
  8133 Wornall Rd 816/361-4077

Swickard Kenneth
  2518 NE 43rd St 816/452-0200

Yennie Richard D DC
  4140 Broadway St 816/931-0287

Saint Charles

Kulkarni Satish R
  Building A1 Westbury Sq 314/946-8851

Montana

Bigfork

Beans Donald R RN LAC DAC
  245 Commerce St 406/837-5757

Marie Sara NTS ID
  245 Commerce St 406/837-5757

Bozeman

Kremer Linda W PO Box 1541 ....406/586-0677

Kremer Neil Atkinson
  PO Box 1541 ....406/586-0677

Lee Bahn PO Box 644 ....406/585-5580

Sexton Thomas LAC DAC
  1015 W Mendenhall St 406/587-7177

Butte

Aagenes Nancy
  1820 Harrison Ave 406/723-6609

Emigrant

Wickersham-Kremer Linda Lee
  PO Box 241 ....406/333-4572

Hamilton

Daily Janet Hillary
  173 Blodgett Camp Rd 406/363-4041

Helena

Bergkamp Michael John
  516 Fuller Ave 406/442-2091

Bump Thomas Allan
  816 S Rodney St 406/443-6476

Mazurek Bridgette J DAC
  311 N Jackson St 406/449-4914

Missoula
Haynes Amy G
521 S 2nd St W 406/728-2415

Saint Ignatius
Medicine Tree Clinic
56 Old Hwy 406/726-3000

Nebraska

Omaha
Kim Kihyung
4808 1/2 Dodge St 402/551-5577

Nevada

Las Vegas
Kang Ji-Zhou J MD
5613 S Eastern Ave 702/798-2992
Lee Ju-Cheon
919 E Charleston Blvd 702/382-1335
Lee Duk Joon
6990 Edna Ave 702/871-5524
Lok Peter P
1818 E Desert Inn Rd 702/732-0178
Lok Yee Kung
1818 E Desert Inn Rd 702/732-0178
Milne Robert D MD
2110 Pinto Ln 702/385-1393
Pfau Terry DO
2810 W Charleston Blvd Ste 55 ..702/258-7860
Stefanatos Joanne
1325 Vegas Valley Dr 702/735-7184

Reno
Tsuda Marjory K
PO Box 50185 ....702/323-6400
Wang Jason
4282 Muirwood Cir 702/825-2103

New Hampshire

Keene
Moore Michele C MD 115 Key Rd ...603/357-2180

Portsmouth
Komisar Mitzi M PO Box 6535 ....603/431-3675

Rochester
Meattey Alice Gansecki
20 Hillside Dr 603/335-1425

Rye Beach
Rothermich Lisa Ann PO Box 230 ...603/641-2838

New Jersey

Avenel
Hu Wen-Chou 19 Livingston Ave 201/372-0566

Bricktown
Wu Fu Min 2020 Roule 88 ....908/840-1180

Bridgewater
Berend Eva LAC DAC

97 Bond St 908/707-0152

Cherry Hill
Liu Chien Kuo
125 Saxby Ter 609/261-3256
Xu Yong Hui
303 Cranford Rd 609/427-4464

Collingswood
Keller Robert
702 Park Ave 609/869-9405

Cranford
Decker Norman L
301 North Ave E 908/272-9307

Dover
Chin James Ming
5 Richards Ave 201/989-0907

East Brunswick
Su Chun Lang
215 Hwy 18 ....908/972-7721

Eastontown
Yu Wei-Na
6 Slony Hill Rd 908/544-9317

Edison
Lee C YMD
952 Amboy Ave 908/738-9220
Sy Rodolfo T MD
952 Amboy Ave 908/738-9220

Elizabeth
Locurcio Gennaro MD FAAFP
610 3rd Ave 908/351-1333

Englewood
Mason Sheila Ann CA RAC
8 James St #2E 201/871-8633

Guttenberg
Yanes Naser Jaber
130 69th St 201/869-9512

Hackensack
Federico Vincent David
144 Main St Ste 212 ....201/473-5143

Hackettstown
Alexander Carol J RN CA
490 Schooleys Mountain Rd #3B............908/852-1267

Jersey City
Ali Colette K 53 Crescent Ave 201/435-5556
Lee Jenny 16 Saddlewood Ct 201/659-0275

Lawrenceville
Urich John P
1651 Lawrenceville Rd 609/883-0080

Little Falls
Del Sardo James M 26 3rd Ave 201/256-5181

Maplewood
Cai Peiti
22 Fernwood Rd 201/378-8153

Marlboro

Yun Lu
  3 Crestview Ct 908/780-7824

Neshanic

Dillman-Shaw Kristina
  150A Amwell Rd 908/369-5145

North Brunswick

Xie Fen
  1680 Hudson Ave 908/846-2412

Nutley

Shiuey Su-Jung OMD CA
  331 Bloomfield Ave 201/667-2394
Skelly Marion Louise BS MS MA
  86 Myrtle Ave 201/661-5147

Paramus

Xu Teresa Z 53 Engle Rd 201/261-6038

Parsippany

Chan Seong Leng 60 Hamilton Rd ..201/428-8186

Plainsboro

Liu Kecheng 14 Krebs Rd 609/936-1709

Princeton

Schwartzman Nicolette E
  84 Wheatsheaf Ln 609/921-2874

Rahway

Kinley David 668 Ranton Rd 908/382-4477

Red Bank

Seidman Katzman Sheryl
  65 Mechanic St Ste 103 ....908/758-1801

Runnemede

Belko Kathleen R
  615 W Clements Bridge Rd 609/939-6663

Scotch Plains

Solondz Janet L
  1240 Lenape Way 908/561-0087

Spring Lake

Carmody James E
  111 Warren Ave 908/449-7129

Toms River

Kim Ki Min 555 Lakehurst Rd 201/240-5507

Union City

Lee Chuan Chi
  2113 New York Ave 201/223-0858

New Mexico

Albuquerque

Cao Jiao
  4410 Lomas Blvd NE 505/268-9047
Cook-Wilcox Angelique S
  3924 Carlisle Blvd NE 505/884-3039
Cowan Tony P
  515 Bryn Mawr Dr SE 505/255-2367
De Vries Marijke S DAC

  1819 Carlisle Blvd NE 505/296-7277
Friedman Michael
  3122 Central Ave SE 505/266-1609
Hostetler Nancy J
  4209 Goodrich Ave NE 505/473-2697
Kelly David L DOM
  801 Encino Pl NE #C-14 ....505/265-5185
Laing Christine
  312 Louisiana Blvd SE 505/266-3223
Liu Der S
  1829 San Mateo Blvd NE 505/255-3442
Lockhart Wilcox Glenn
  3924 Carlisle Blvd NE 505/884-3039
Luciani Ralph J DO
  2301 San Pedro Dr NESte G 505/888-5995
Polasky Diane Hilary MA ODM L
  540 Chama St NE Ste 9 ....505/262-0555
Roberts William Norman
  218 Hermosa Dr SE 505/266-8247
Stone Linda A
  3212 Monte Vista Blvd NE 505/888-4847
Taylor John T Do
  6208 Montgomery Blvd Neste D .505/271-4800
Trujillo Alexcia
  120 Amherst Dr NE 505/265-6206
Wilcox Glenn L
  7000 Cutler Ave NE #E5 ....505/884-3039
Wu Jane Lo
  2709 Wyoming Blvd NE 505/299-2944

Bernalillo

Sirwinski Neal
  PO Box 993 ....505/867-3007

Espanola

Zarola John Joseph LAC RN
  PO Box 1231 ....505/753-4466

Las Cruces

Clifton Sidney Catherin
  1120 Burke Rd 505/523-4088
Cooney Jeffrey
  416 W Griggs Ave 505/526-1789

Mesilla

Krueger Theodore Henry
  PO Box 900 ....505/473-4980

Pecos

Bruce Daniel J DOM
  1301 St Francis D #C 505/988-5106

Placitas

Monda Lorena C Omd Dac
  3 Calle Taraddei #B 505/867-1879

Santa Fe

Abbate Anthony
  712 W San Mateo Rd 505/988-3538
Bakken Beverly Ann
  839 Paseo De Peralta Ste D 505/988-4460

Bradley Monika M
  1704 Paseo De La Conquista 505/984-8750
Brandon Catherine L
  1205 Gonzales Ct 505/989-7184
Bruce Daniel J DOM
  1301 St Francis Dr #C...................505/988-5106
Busch Elizabeth Lyn
  2538 Camino San Patricio 505/471-2997
Canzone David J
  1850 Otowi Rd 505/989-7418
Celine Ariana
  PO Box 6044 ....505/984-1722
Creelman Janet M
  615 W Alameda St 505/989-8652
Diaz Maria Dolores LAC DAC
  1502 S St Francis Dr 505/984-0928
Doughty Lisa
  PO Box 5514 ....505/986-8213
Duckworth Thomas K MD LAC
  11 Pueblo Dr 505/983-9570
Easton Jade
  209 McKenzie St 505/983-9133
Ehling Dagmar
  RR 9 Box 15F 505/473-7916
Erdely Maximilian A
  2003 Hopi Rd 505/984-8564
Factor Karen
  1710 Paseo De La Conquista 505/982-3070
Fineberg Leah
  4012 Old Santa Fe Trl 505/983-5529
Flannery Martha Grace
  104 E Faithway St Ste C 505/986-9129
Frenkel Judy Rose
  249T Saw Mill Rd 505/983-2532
Gardner-Abbate Skya LAC OMD
  712 W San Mateo Rd 505/988-3538
Hall Theodore Henry
  1713 Santa Fe River Rd 505/988-8021
Hanna Lucy A
  2300 W Alameda St Apt C-4 ....505/982-5001
Hannah-Rose Allison
  127 Mesa Verde St 505/982-2708
Hasson Randy
  33 Old Arroyo Chamiso Ste A 505/471-7714
Heller Henry J
  PO Box 8654 ....505/982-1153
Jeffs Elizabeth R
  13 Encantado Loop 505/983-8208
Kauffman Mahabba
  RR 9 Box 80 ....505/984-1248
Keefe Gaynl
  1500 5th St Bldg 12 ....505/988-7350
Khalsa Gurusant Singh
  301 E Palace Ave #3 ....505/984-0934
La Badie Carl
  1544 Cerro Gordo Rd 505/986-0638
McLoughlin Dairne

  1331 Cerro Gordo Rd 505/982-5371
Millikin Anne T
  500 N Guadalupe St #G-36 .... 505/982-9561
Mojica Maria I
  PO Box 5888 ....505/986-0647
Moore James M
  1500 5th St Bldg 13 ....505/982-2138
Quanyin West Sarah
  2741 Calle Serena 505/473-2697
Ross John D
  1500 5th St Bldg 12 ....505/989-5777
Santos Daniel L
  RR 10 Box 88D 505/984-1148
Sautter Elke
  PO Box 4096 ....505/989-7022
Schoofs-Torres Elizabeth A
  1117 Don Juan St 505/454-8920
Shankman Roseann
  306 W Gomez Rd 505/989-8609
Skardis Jonas R OMD DRAC
  411 St Michael's Dr 505/988-5551
Spies Sondra K
  547 Franklin Ave 505/983-8250
Story Judith
  108 La Placita Cir 505/988-7117
Tate Michael J
  1043 Don Diego Ave 505/983-1386
Thill-Relyea Jeanne M
  401 1/2 Delgago 505/983-3649
Tunnell Lynsay E
  1500 5th St Bldg 12 ....505/988-7350
West Quanyin
  712 W San Mateo Rd 505/988-3538
Zeng Michael D MD MOD L
  10 Calle Zanate 505/471-5258
Zeng Nancy 10 Calle Zanate 505/471-5258

Taos
French Peggy L PO Box 6559 ....505/758-9462
Hanson Marcia F PO Box 1692 ....505/758-0533
Sowanick Paul J PO Box 448 ....505/758-8230

Taos Ski Valley
Sparks Freeman Vicky LAC DAC
  PO Box 10-C 505/758-2969

Tijeras
Searles Rachel PO Box 1321 ....505/281-2654

New York

Accord
Starrett Ron
  86 Ricci Rd 914/687-9169

Bayside
Yom David J H
  215-36 26th Avenue 718/225-1128

Bearsville
Stone Flower Mountain Health

PO Box 459 ....914/679-4872

Bethpage

Haughney George Joseph
10 Hoover Ln 516/796-6196

Bronx

Iglesias Richard
104 Neptune Lane 718/892-2225

Brooklyn

Biteye Dafina LAC
163 Clifton Pl 718/789-3264
Chester Karen Ruth
201 Eastern Pky Ste 5-0 ....718/783-5333
Clegg Suzanne
348 12th St 1L...............718/788-5924
Fafarman Mona
594 6th St 718/499-8122
Harrison Christopher
345 86th St Apt 106 ....718/921-7264
Lao He Hon
2048 Haring St 718/769-7701

Manhattan

Lee So Young
146th W 29th St 212/268-4300
London Yefim
1285 Delmar Loop Apt 2A 718/642-8357
Pascal Jeffrey B
276 Henry St 718/875-8745
Rondon Selma
290 President St 718/858-4875
Rothman Linda L
414 Prospect Ave 718/965-9879
Wu Lili 6811 Fort Hamilton Pkwy 718/439-8805

Buffalo

Bychkov May
1088 Delaware Ave Apt 11-I 716/885-9414

Canandaigua

Bevin Deanna MAPC
426 S Main St 716/396-0475

East Hampton

Craig Sigler Carol
PO Box 2065 81 Gould St 516/324-7960

Elmhurst

Son Hye Min 87-08 Justice Ave 718/321-7863

Elmont

Keyrouze Frances Eileen
179 Waldorf Ave 516/358-0054

Floral Park

Ringel Shoshana Pinto
PO Box 403 ....516/593-6938

Flushing

Chang Hsin Chi
33-30 Union St 718/359-2703
Chang Shu-Mei

3640 Union St 2nd Floor 718/461-7960
Chen Warner
34-45 Leavitt St 718/461-0369
Chen Shi Ling
36-40 Union St 7th Floor..............718/461-7960
Huang Rong Fang
PO Box 1469 ....718/463-0665
Li James 151-13 33rd Rd 718/961-5605
Lu Cheng-Ih
148-14 61st Rd 718/353-7864
Shelley X. Y. Peng
43-18 Robinson St 718/463-3483
Wu Yuen-Woo
144-44 Sanford Ave 718/359-2307
Yi Jang Yol 139-15 Franklin Ave........718/961-7272

Forest Hills

Abe Hiroyasu
104-60 Queens Blvd 718/830-0223
Crofton Janice M
109-15 Queens Blvd 718/897-8109
Li Tian Cong
71-11 Yellow Stone Blvd 718/575-2866
Tu Henry Sinfui
105-05 69th Ave 718/459-8239

Ft Ewen

Allen Robert S PO Box 1163.............914/338-8846

Great Neck

Feldman Lauretta 51 Bayview Ave ...516/829-9841

Greenlawn

Delney Siobban K
800 Pulaski Rd 516/261-3168

Haupauge

Freidkes Raul 157 Village Dr 516/361-3680

Hillcrest

Gluckstein Rachel RN
77-03 167th St 718/380-2261

Hurleyville

Humphrey Janet PO Box 150 ....914/434-2000

Ithaca

Abrams Judith LAC PAC
342 Dewitt Mall 607/277-7713

Jackson Heights

Xu Jia-Hao
35-50 75th Street 718/672-1367

Kingston

Huang De Ying
264 Smith Ave 914/338-6045

Long Beach

Knell Thomas J
465 Shore Rd 516/432-1646

Long Island City

Kuhnke Christine E............................212/946-1280

Mahopac

Kwon Mi Cha
  3 Fabri Ct 914/628-7262

Millerton

Kisslinger Karen L
  RR 1 Box 72A 518/789-6206

Monticello

Garfinkel Abraham
  15 Hamilton Ave 914/794-8844

Mount Kisco

Kornhaber Eugene 10 W Hyatt Ave ..914/241-0682

Nanuet

Cha Yoon Ok 134 East Rt 59 ....914/623-4187

New City

Xu Yong H 7 Capitol Ct 914/639-9007

New Falls

Elias Jason 3 Paradiws Ln.................914/255-2255

New Hyde Park

Pei Sun F 1 Fairfield Ln 516/775-5285
Zuo Hailiu 54 Edgewood 718/921-2696

New Paltz

Dubitsky Peter LAC DAC
  PO Box 1062 ....914/255-7178

New Rochelle

Lamb Darien S
  140 Lockwood Ave.........................914/633-3799
Song Hui-Jun
  650 Main St #422 ....212/714-0140

New York

Ash Richard N MD
  860 Fifth Ave.................................. 212/628-3133
Atkins Robert C MD
  Atkins Center
  152 E 55th St 212/758-2110
Behr William T
  123 W 79th St #3 ....212/799-4633
Bengston Carolyn Ann
  214 W 16th St Apt 4S 212/989-7279
Bisio Thomas F
  293 Church St 212/226-3140
Bloom Phyllis
  150 5th Ave #804 ....212/675-1164
Bong Mei-Yuen
  39 Bowery Ste 105 ....212/925-7128
Brameier Constance A
  318 W 14th St 212/255-5909
Brown Alan L
  329 E 82nd St 212/288-5930
Call Elizabeth Ann
  50 E 81st St #4B 718/204-8272
Certner Roberta L
  677 W End Ave Ste 4A 212/865-7505
Chen Shin-Yang
  45-48 Union St 718/353-2665

Chen De Ren
  134-27 Maple Ave 718/539-5118
Churchill Margaretha
  377 W 11th St Apt 2B 212/675-2571
Glanzman Gary S
  77 E 12th St Apt 13D 212/420-9534
Gong Kenny
  241 Centre St 212/966-2406
Gorman Pat
  5 E 17th St 212/620-0506
Hadadi Letha G
  310 W 21st St 212/807-1006
Henderson Imetai M
  200 East 11th 212/505-9318
Hurwitz Beverly
  30 W 63rd St Apt 12S 212/262-0027
Janssen Elaine P
  211 W 56th St Apt 18M 212/757-6138
Johnson Rush M
  242 W 76th St 212/496-6611
Khalsa Harigopal Singh
  25 E 10th St Apt 2A 212/228-0869
Kremnetsov Yury G MD
  777 Lexington Ave #800 ....212/888-8877
Lee Catherine Mary
  31-33 Oliver St 212/233-8728
Lee Aija
  38 W 32nd St Ste 1007 ....212/239-5559
Lum Isis Chen
  341 E 5th St 212/477-4553
McKenzie Kevin
  258 W 22nd St 212/255-1429
Merrell Woodson MD
  44 E 67th St 212/535-1012
Millefleurs Day Spa
  130 Franklin 212/966-3656
Moenich Margaret
  244 E 21st St Ste 1 ....212/228-1187
Perez Olaya
  200 E 16th St Apt 6K 212/722-6242
Peterburgsky Joseph V
  176 W 94th St Apt 12C 212/222-4868
Pettorino Paulette
  231 Thompson St Apt 18 ....212/473-1837
Prensky William OMD DAC
  133 E 73rd St 212/861-9000
Rabin Mitchell J
  653 E 14th St Ste 70 ....212/420-0800
Reilly Richard L
  110 Seaman Ave Apt 7C 212/304-3586
Schoultz Elizabeth Ann
  214 W 16th St Apt 5 ....212/366-4936
Seem Mark
  20 W 86th St................................212/496-7514
Smith Mary Anne
  280 Mott St #5R 212/431-8088
Strickler James M LAC DIPL AC

242 E 72nd St 212/772-2838

Sun Ya Hua
65 E 59th Street 212/935-8409

Temchin Mona H
509 E 81st St Apt 16 ....212/744-7452

Terlitzky Stephen Fenning LAC
484 W 43rd St Ste 29 ....212/564-5324

Trahan Christopher OMD LAC
50 W 34th St #17-A-10 ....212/714-0856

Tsao Roger Wei-Ming
210 E 68th St Suite 1-G 212/517-4040

Two Hon-Jen
36 E Broadway #2F 718/575-3717

Xu Xiao Lan
48-21 44th St Woodside 718/361-8369

Zeller Barbara
243 W 98-5C 212/769-6485

Zhang Fu Qiang
396 Broadway Ste 803 ....212/966-6015

Nyack
Dechar-Wish Lorie E
112 Highmount Ave 914/359-4815

Pelzig Naomi MD
3 S Broadway 914/353-3267

Old Bethpage
Schecter Daniel Jay OMD ACDIP
11 Voorhis Dr 516/752-0274

Peekskill
Amazalorso Roy
12 Valerie Lane Courtlandt Manor .914/739-6387

Port Washington
Rice William J
20 E Vanderventer Ave 516/944-9460

Port Jefferson
Harrington Hubert C
302 E Broadway 904/737-8291

Queens
Lau Chui Yiu
66-51 Saunders St 718/268-5836

Rego Park
Leviton Gary R
63-70 Wood Haven Blvd 718/898-8388

Ridgewood
Clegg Suzanne
348 12th St 1L.............................718/788-5924

Rochester
Lee Thomas Koangho
424 White Spruce Blvd 716/272-0690

Rocky Point
Behr William T
19 Aloma Rd 516/744-3511

Sag Harbor
Aqua Roberta W

Corwin RdRR 3 Box 522 ....516/725-1684

Gohring Mikal P
RR 3 Box 522 ....516/725-1684

Syosset
The New Center for Wholistic Health
6801 Jericho Turnpike 516/364-0808

Valhalla
Kluepfel-Kiris Erika
115 E Stevens Ave 914/238-6142

Valley Stream
Fenton Herbert F
44 S Central Ave 516/561-1151

Voor
Pang Jane O 5750 Hennessey Rd ...518/861-8567

Woodstock
Nielsen Arya A
1923 Glasco Tpk 914/679-8428

North Carolina

Asheville
Kuai Shi Ying
114 Arlington St 704/254-2167

Majebe M Cissy OMD
369 Montford Ave 704/258-9016

Ricker Philip R
518 Hendersonville Rd 704/277-8000

Black Mountain
Garvy Jack
115 Richardson Blvd 704/669-7762

Blowing Rock
Worthington Elizabeth MA LAC
PO Box 554 ....704/295-9630

Burnsville
Solomon Jennifer A LMTC
PO Box 806 ....718/398-2911

Chapel Hill
Dotson Ercel E
307 S Columbia St 919/967-8831

Erickson Cholena LAC DAC
976 Airport Rd Ste 250 ....919/968-1198

Hawes Diana L
307 N Columbia St 919/929-9988

Charlotte
Johnson Douglas H
1911 Park Dr 704/344-8231

Matsuda Michel
1218 East Blvd 704/358-3719

Durham
Fendell Lori 807 Wilkerson Ave 919/682-1590

Goldsboro
House Richard J 1008 E Ash St 919/734-7772

Allyn-Peck Diane

512 Woodlawn Ave 919/370-4399
Peck Tracy
512 Woodlawn Ave 919/370-4399
Sullivan Linda
3100-18D North Elm St 919/282-3207

Oxford
Pfister Joseph James
3184 Tar River Rd 919/528-2842

Pfafftown
Fitzgerald Macleod
3495 Transou Rd 919/924-0192

Pittsboro
Stewart Susanna LAC RN
RR 5 Box 114 ....919/542-4379

Wilmington
Colios Nikos
4701 Wrightsville Ave #2 ....919/272-1129
Paterson Page
3941 Market St #A 919/343-9811

Chesterland
Wang Peter C PO Box 8 ....216/729-9937

Cincinnati
Kim Sung S
9600 Colerain Ave Ste 410 ....513/385-4333

Cleveland
Dreu Mark M
18601 Shawnee Ave 216/692-0853
Grotte Lee B
5399 Mayfield Rd 216/321-1388
Weeks Douglas MD
24700 Center Ridge Rd 216/835-0104

West Chester
Kim Sung Soo
5638 Eagle Nest Ct 513/874-8033

Albion
Turner R Michael
PO Box 116 ....918/567-2343

Norman
Hagglund Howard MD
2227 W Lindsey St Ste 1401 ...... 405/329-4457

Oklahoma City
Farr Charles H MD PHD
10101 S Western Ave 405/691-1112
Gumman Amit BSC BAMS DAC ND PHD
OKC Family Health & Pain Clinic
41 South Walker #102 ....405/631-5450
Manning Clark A
3632 NW 21st St 405/943-8131
Nayeri Bobak
4720 South Western Ave 405/634-5529

Tohgi Fumimoto
5320 N Portland Ave 405/948-1177
Weathers Ray DIPL AC DAC OMD
OKC Family Health & Pain Clinic
8241 S Walker Ste 102 ....405/631-5450

Tahlequah
Nicholson Jeff D
209 N Muskogee Ave 918/456-2292

Tulsa
Weathers Ray DIPL AC DAC OMD
Tulsa Family Health & Pain Clinic
1211 S Harvard Ave #A 918/836-5454

Ashland
Abelle Mark S
611 Siskiyou Blvd Ste E 503/488-5719
Boldon Bruce Edward
670 C St #2 ....503/488-3912
Goldman Jonathan M
7051 Old Siskiyou Hwy 503/482-5381
Stott Benjamin W LAC OMD
64 N 3rd St 503/488-3612
Weiss Shandor ND LAC
238 E Main St Ste E 503/488-1198

Beaverton
Ch'En Joan C
4562 SW 103rd Ave 503/643-2818
Chon Catherine Hamdu
12655 SW 10th Street 503/646-3731
Marinelli Rick ND OM
2445 SW Cedar Hills Blvd............503/644-4446
Stargrove Mitchell B
4720 SW Watson Ave 503/526-0397

Bend
Hauser James S
587 NE Greenwood Ave Ste C...... 503/382-5897
Rosen Ronald D MD
124 Hawthorne 503/388-3804

Cannon Beach
Rice Robert E PO Box 193 ....503/436-1911

Corvallis
Oxenhandler Harry S
3546 NW Thrush Dr 503/757-1481

Elkton
Brooks Sherrie A PO Box 578 ....503/584-2725

Eugene
Ch'En Betty Pei
132 E Broadway 503/686-9424
Eugene Beverly Jaeger
132 E Broadway 503/484-0177
Finkelstein Malvin H
2767 Friendly St 503/683-9230
Hobbs Jerome B

1661 Willamette St 503/344-1162

Jaeger Beverly DAC TC
580 E 40th Ave 503/484-0177

Weinstein Larry
260 E 15th Ave Ste A 503/344-5882

Grants Pass

Doss Gregory K OMD DAC
118 NE Manzanita Ave 503/476-4611

Gresham

Batie Jeffry J PO Box 1404 ....503/666-7195

Bliatout Hollis Yap
133 NE 3rd St 503/760-6855

Gemmato Frank
1685 NW 1st St 503/661-6701

Soloway Nathaniel Alan
655 W Burnside 503/666-2325

Tshinili Yap-Bliatou Holly
200 SW Nancy Cir 503/661-2327

Hood River

Franklin Kelly Kay 1237 State St 503/386-4489

La Grande

March Kevin John
1303 O Ave #1 ....503/288-0578

Lake Oswego

Germain Kathleen MS ND LAC
West River Natural Health Clinic
545 First St....................................503/635-6643

Lamont Sally Ctr for Traditional Medicine
560 1st St Ste 204 ....503/636-2734

Northrup Lynda M
1 Jefferson Pky Apt 169 ....503/655-9536

Peterson Noel
560 1st St Ste 204 ....503/636-2734

Manning

Dodge Jeanette E
PO Box 50 ....503/324-1630

McMinnville

Zeff Jared L
18540 NW Baker Creek Rd 503/255-4860

Medford

Senogles Gerald J
832 E Main St #3 ....503/779-6223

Newport

Edmisten K E ND LAC
344 SW 7th St Ste B 503/265-6378

Portland

Adler Nigel D
2515 SE 67th Ave 503/239-6843

Arndt Natalie K
4351 SE Hawthorne Blvd 503/588-9480

Bae Ildowe
18078 NW Sylvania Ln 503/777-5079

Bayard Robin G DC LAC

10360 NE Wasco St 503/252-8125

Bayard Bernie S
1722 NE Schuyler St 503/288-9793

Binder Gary
921 SW Washington St Ste 880 ..503/239-2321

Blank John S
1917 NE Loth Avenue 503/238-6621

Boyajian Laurel Dawn
2707 NE Jarrett St 503/231-0960

Brewer Marilyn
PO Box 18001 ....503/786-0281

Brust-Thille Evelyn K
3114 NE Irving St 503/252-9166

Burke John L
2614 SE 115th Ave # 1 ....503/760-4382

Chang Jeffry Liang
4226 SE Ash St 503/235-3236

Chiasson Marcelle
4055 SW Garden Home Rd 503/245-3156

Coletto Joseph J
10525 SE Cherry Blossom Dr 503/254-3566

Crosby John
811 NW 20th Ste 101-A 503/221-6232

Desylvia Michael Eugene
3701 SE Milwaukie Ave 503/667-1604

Downs Allen B
729 SE 33rd Ave 503/239-4065

Eisen David C
2230 NE Brazee St 503/289-9666

Fenske Philip Dean
2806 NE 12th Ave 503/287-1307

Freeman James
2835 SE Yamhill St 503/989-8599

Frierman David H
4134 SE 14th Ave 503/233-9827

Hofvendahl Camille L
2322 N Webster St 503/285-9075

Jacobson Rayna Joyce
303 NE 69th Ave 503/257-6334

Kim Hwacha
19840 NW Quail Hollow Dr 503/646-5703

Levine Karen June
2348 NW Lovejoy St 503/224-7224

Li Frances F
4226 SE Ash St 503/235-3236

Liggett Laura Jean
1125 SE Spokane St 503/233-9079

Lin Zheng-Fei
7920 SE Washington St 503/254-5818

Littlefield Kathy Jo
2606 SE Tarbell Rd 503/653-0014

Madison Beverly M
4107 NE Tillamook St 503/288-7661

Manning Eric Edward
2129 SE Ladd 503/233-2854

Marion Daye

10835 SE Powell Blvd #33 ....503/760-3227
Marz Russell B
2002 SE 50th Ave 503/233-0585
Meeker Stephen R
1804 NE 25th Ave 503/284-2627
Moore Roxanna Lee
6625 SE 46th Ave 503/777-9083
Mulrooney Debra Lynn
3065 NW 178th Ave 503/645-9666
Murphy Patricia A ND LAC
4511 SE Hawthorne Blvd Ste 112 ....503/238-1032
Paetzhold Pamela Z
4616 SW Vermont St 503/282-8367
Page Edie Baldwin
7912 SW 35th Ave 503/244-8476
Quinn Dorian D
5927 NE Davis St 503/236-8697
Rollo Peggy M ND LAC
833 SW 11th Ave Ste 612 ....503/223-7067
Sandler Maureen
2625 SE Hawthorne Blvd 503/238-9788
Scott Mary Ellen
1025 SE 27th Ave 503/232-8786
Shefi Ellen L
2041 SW 58th Ave Ste 207 .... 503/297-7656
Sieckman Arlett K
1920 NW Johnson St Ste 110 .....503/222-7174
Smith Julia Ann
1011 E Burnside St 503/232-3857
Soloway Nick DC LMT L
12335 NE Brazee St 503/253-4694
Soprani Joseph Lee
3424 NE 36th Ave 503/223-7458
Soprani Marian T
3424 NE 36th Ave 503/287-8831
Stiastny Elizalbeth Maur
915 SE 70th Ave 503/253-3157
Trumbo Warren D
1218 SE 18th Ave 503/232-0585
Van Geest-Green Lida C
1390 NW 131st Ave 503/626-8108
Vickers Edythe M
2348 NW Lovejoy 503/224-7224
Wang Lihua
14325 SE Stark St 503/761-8145
Weih Jeffrey A
3414 N Kaiser Center Dr 503/249-8555
Weinreb Brandon
2225 SE Brooklyn St 503/233-0339
Wieland Gregory M
5772 SE 117th Ave 503/761-5045
Winter Brooke
316 NE 28th 503/230-0812

Salem
Bruno Gene Clark
1880 Lancaster Dr NE Ste 111 ....503/371-8770

Shedd
Maus Benedict J
29706 Main St 503/232-6583

Silverton
Eng Margaret P
612 N 1st Street 503/873-6705

Tigard
McClellan Marnie Carol
12050 SW Summercrest Dr 503/624-0198

Veneta
Kassel Joseph ND LAC
25632 Jeaus Rd 503/935-3453

West Linn
Rifkin Kenneth Harvey
990 SW Long Farm Rd 503/638-8195

Wilsonville
Dreger Gary C
PO Box 1041 ....503/538-6059

Pennsylvania

Allentown
Wang Ching-Chang
447 E Lexington St 215/797-1365

Ambler
Yu Ruey J OMD DAC
4 Lindenwold Ave 215/628-9088

Bethlehem
Fritz George 1370 Sycamore Ave 215/861-7744
Kuo Rong Chin
321 E Laurel St 215/861-8879

Boyertown
Shay W William DO PHD RAC
407 E Philadelphia Ave 215/367-5505

Brookhaven
Lester Mary Ellen
6113 Hilltop Dr 215/892-9009

Catasauqua
Molony David Edgar RA CA PH
101 Bridge St 215/264-2768
Pan Molony Ming Ming OMO
101 Bridge St 215/964-2755

Cheltenham
Kaplan Ross H PO Box 318 ....215/379-6000

Coudersport
Miller Howard J MD 360 E 2nd St ...814/274-7070

Dallas
Oh Dong-Joon 25 Kingswood Dr 717/675-8117

Darby
Xi Mu-Shi 27 S 14th St 215/734-1127

Doylestown
Goldstein Donald A
47 W Oakland St 215/345-5821

Erie

Tsui Ying-Lin
4437 W Ridge Rd 814/833-4060

Harrisburg

Spivey Nathan J
1510F High Pointe Dr 717/238-3106

Indiana

Reilly James B
257 N 6th St 412/463-7165
Sinha Chandrika MD
1177 S 6th St 412/349-1414

Lancaster

Steinman Sandy MAc
2416 Lititz Pike 717/581-0351

Langhorne

Schwartzman Nicolette DAC
409 Executive Dr 215/968-5550

Lansdale

Green Leland J MD
PO Box 508 ....215/855-9501

Lansdowne

Flanagan Bethleigh
22 Linden Ave 914/434-2000

New Hope

Brown Roland M
5011 Toll Gate Rd 215/297-8808
Mackenzie Janice A DAC
5011 Toll Gate Rd 215/297-8806
Rinkel Bert J
PO Box 14128 S Main St #1 .... 215/862-3686

Norristown

Scola David A
179 Hughes Rd 215/687-8586

Philadelphia

Debevoise Mark Alan
3619 Fisk Ave #1 ....215/844-4488
Diamond Elliot
2429 Brown St 215/236-4088
Dong Gangyi
Med School-Temple University
3420 N Broad St 215/221-3695
Frank Cara
6333 Wayne Ave............................ 215/438-2977
Freedman Randi F
The Town House 301 S 19th St 215/735-5705
Goldstein Cathy L
1700 Sanson St Ste 503 ....215/988-9898
Lariccia Patrick J
51 N 39th St 215/662-8988
Post Nancy RAC
5515 Wissahickon Ave Apt C202 .215/438-2657
Rothman Irwin VO MD VM
6420 City Ave 215/473-8900

Sampathachar K R MD
6366 Sherwood Rd 215/473-4226
Sheng Zufang
2R330 S 43rd St 215/898-8348
Wah Laila LAC CERT
225 S 15th St................................215/731-0177
Walsh Bryn Cathryn
5700 Wissahickon Ave Ste 510B 212/371-5829
Yin Wheeler Hui Luo
7513 Oak Lane Rd 215/782-8063
Zhu Chenghui CMD DAC
1644 Bridge St 215/744-8260

Pipersville

Price Cheryl
6075 Covered Bridge Rd 215/345-0166

Pittsburgh

Jacob W Lindsay
417 S Craig St 412/687-3633
Mortell David DAC
5830 Ellsworth Ave Ste 303 ....412/621-2610

Reading

Lisbin Eric 309 Madison Ave 215/929-8430

Sharpsville

Ham Tong Ho 290 Koehler Dr 412/342-4052

Warren

Sanghi J K MD FRCS
106 Pennsylvania Ave W 814/726-3202

Washington Cross

Cassidy Dick MA DAC
1313 Lord Sterling Rd Ste 5........ 215/493-9077
Hudson Christopher LAC
1082 Taylorsville Road...................215/493-8530

Wayne

Michelland Joan 700 Knox Rd 215/687-8595

Windance

Silva Linda Jean 8805 Patton Rd 215/233-1733

Wyncote

Dishler Michael V
1451 Ashbourne Rd 215/884-9921

Yardley

Khalsa Deva K
1724 Yardley Langhorne Rd 215/493-0621

Rhode Island

Newport

Allwell Carol S 25 Bull St 401/849-9412

North Kingstown

Graham Nancy
1130 Tenrod Road 401/294-1644

Providence

Yan Ying 43 William Ellery Pl 401/946-9750

Warwick

Tsai Nai Che
322 Post Rd 401/461-8304
Woonsocket
Aubuchon Paul L
172 Pond St 401/765-6363

South Carolina

Columbia
Skelton William D
2719 Middleburg Dr Ste 106........803/799-7755
Hilton Head Island
Vos Marguerite J
112 Forest Cove 803/785-7257
Travelers Rest
Demyan Jeanne R
409 Old Buncombe Rd 803/834-7334

South Dakota

North Sioux City
Bronson Allen Wd
338 Streeter Dr Box 440 ....605/232-4383
Webster
Smith William John
511 Main St 605/345-3130

Tennessee

Knoxville
Cobble Stephen R DDS PHD DDS
7301 Middlebrook Pk...................615/691-2910

Texas

Amarillo
Taylor John T DO
4714 S Western St 806/355-8263
Arlington
Chang Nancy Yangying
705 Foxford Trl 817/467-5471
Chemly Sunny OMD LAC
2301 N Collins St Ste 118 ....817/461-6700
Zhang William
308 W Park Rd 817/261-8498
Zhang William Y
4309 Murwick Dr 817/483-1001
Austin
Davidson Marion Robert CAC
3939 Bee Caves Rd #B 512/327-6562
McKenna Brian J
3006 Bee Caves Rd Ste 300.......512/327-2883
Moose Elizabeth S
4105 S 1st St................................512/328-3308
Newbold Dee Ann DAC
1301 W 25th St Ste 401.............512/458-6211
Scott John Arthur OMD DAC
4105 S 1st St 512/444-6744

Sutton-Wyss Danielle W
4032 S Lamar Blvd Ste 500-179 512/282-2344
Tarnower Karen R
PO Box 3563 ....512/482-8496
Tummins Ward L
703 E 45 1/2 St 512/451-8332
Wadlington Truman Caylor
3006 Bee Caves Rd #D-300 ....512/327-2883
Beaumont
Phan Tam T MDH PHD
1995 Broadway 409/833-6097
Big Spring
Ng Po(Paul) Man
706 Edwards Blvd 915/267-7878
Brenham
Thai Tam Khai
1100 E S Market St 409/830-9111
Brownsville
Rogers Charles L MD MDH CDM
Matamoro.......................................512/541-7182
Crawford
Snowden Janet A
RR 1 Box 89D 817/848-4114
Dallas
Bureau Colette
13154 Coit Rd Ste 100 ....214/480-9355
Fortune Richard J DAC
6440 N Central Expy Ste 303 ......214/369-8532
Koryo In Kim
2880 LBJ Freeway 214/484-3147
Lim-Peck Iva RN DAC
17194 Preston Rd Ste 222 .... 214/380-9070
Mauro Stuart S
5626 Bell Ave 214/521-2001
Nabeshima Hideko T
13789 Noel Rd Ste 118 ....214/385-6426
Peck Richard A LAC
17194 Preston Rd Ste 222 .... 214/380-9070
Xing Zhaoxu LAC
13154 Coit Rd Ste 100 ....214/480-9355
El Paso
Arroyo Maximo
4700 N Mesa St Ste S-2 ....915/544-5663
Arroyo Maximo E
237 Ferrari Ct 915/584-9511
Lee Sang Kuen
9861 Dyer St Ste 21 ....915/755-5959
Euless
Fabres Vicki L
1520 El Camino Real 817/354-6421
Fort Worth
Krayem Elhadi M
2901 Montgomery St 817/737-7401
Houston

Chen Shuang MD
8911 Grape St 713/541-0052
Cheng Yin Bong
6910 Bellaire Blvd Ste 5 .... 713/776-3442
Greenfield Zion Ben
606 Marshall St Apt 3 ....713/880-5505
Harmon Robert B
907 El Dorado Blvd Ste 110 ....713/486-5425
Lee Emma Y
One West Loop S Ste 214 .... 713/960-1069
Li Jessie
10703 Sandstone St 713/777-7605
Li Pang Y 1500 Sandy Springs 713/785-3142
Liang Shen P
1200 Post Oak Blvd Ste 516 ....713/622-8881
Liu Chi-Chang
3113 St Charles St 713/521-2356
Liu Jan Shiow LAC RN
9319 Rowan Ln 713/777-9505
Lu Lin 10047 Westpark Dr Apt 3 .....713/952-2626
Lu Chun Hui
13034 Meadowline Dr 713/952-6826
Luk Choi Wai
7502 Eichler Dr 713/981-1385
Ma Shun Mei
1303 Eaton St 713/797-9043
Pang Ya Li 1500 Sandy Springs 713/785-3142
Pao June DAC 713/444-8310
Puddy Phillip A
5720 Parwill St Ste 3 ....713/858-3235
Sun Lan-Ying
1801 S Dairy Ashford St Ste 10 ..713/589-6800
Wang Yuh-Fen Ku
8107 Riptide Dr 713/568-9988
Wang Theresa
9600 Bellaire Blvd Ste 221 ....713/778-0659

Humble

Tomsheck Mary J
2719 Longleaf Pines Dr 713/358-0718

Hurst

Chemly Chung-Hwei MS DAC
124-E Grapevine Hwy 817/498-8449

Katy

Liu Quingchuan Cath
1430 Shillington Dr 713/787-9423

Kerrville

Evans-Stark Adrienne E
245 Guadalupe St 512/257-4811

McAllen

Schramm Kenneth L
2221 Primrose Ave 512/630-3018

Midland

Jon Amy
2109 W Texas Ave Ste F 915/694-2293

Paris

Tang Zhenkai
1017 S Collegiate Dr 214/612-1662

Pasadena

Liu Adam TI CMD TAA
2222-G Southmore Ave 713/473-0001

Pecos

Reeves County Hospital
2323 Texas St 915/447-3551

Richardson

Chan Lomina
817 Canyon Creek Sq 214/669-0186
Chuang Wei
1315 Northlake Dr 214/783-9822
Guo Xiang Ming
110117 E Main St 214/783-6388
Zhou Afu
817 Canyon Creek Sq 214/669-0186

San Angelo

Thurman Ben 107 N Main St 915/655-0601

San Antonio

Ho Hoang X
2900 Mossrock Ste 330 ....512/366-0959
Ho Mobi
10606 Benchmark Way 512/826-4251
Jin Ser-Ling
6625 Sawyer Rd 512/680-8600
Wong Edmund DIPLAC
4411 Walzem Rd 512/590-2861

Spring

Yokoyama Hidenbo
6450 Louetta Rd #120 ....713/251-9566

Utah

Heber City

McNeely Florence J
PO Box 457 ....801/654-2670

Orem

Yu Ming De 698 Heather Rd 801/371-2740

Provo

Yu Shiping
5B-268 Wymount Trail 801/371-2448

Saint George

Zhang Shize 18 N 500 E 801/628-8040

Salt Lake City

Brewton Wendelyn Ann
989 E 900 S 801/359-6538
Clausen Natalie J
667 E 100 S 801/359-2705
Cook Vaughn LAC
1720 Fort Union Blvd #101......... 801/944-4070
Earl Glenn L OMD PHD
644 S 900 E 801/355-8226

Fang Chaohua
874 E South Temple Apt 19 .... 801/596-2765
Justesen Dr Kristelle
545 E 4500 S Ste E 230............. 801/263-9380
Liu Delu
3804 Highland Dr Ste 9 ....801/277-8048
Jewkes L Scott
4568 Highland Dr #300 ....801/261-4260

Sandy
Sterling Leslie
3562 E 9800 S 801/943-2773
Tan Tao
1446 Marbella St 801/568-0630

Vermont

Brattleboro
Sinclair Janet
139 Main St Ste 404 ....802/254-4103
Valentine-Marshall Sean C
4 Walnut St 802/257-2622

Burlington
Ernandez Serge C
323 Pearl St 802/425-2258
Fleming Molly C ND 41 Main St.......802/863-7099
Powell Donna M
41 Main Street 802/863-7099

Marshfield
Degraff Deborah A
RR 1 Box 1540 ....802/454-8687

Montpelier
Brady Pamela A 23 Tracy St 802/223-6360

Ripton
Kiczkowski Francois D
PO Box 141 ....802/864-1417

Rutland
Brown Daniel W
56 1/2 Merchants Row 802/773-3780

Saxtons River
Jonas Julian J PO Box 515 ....802/869-2883

Shrewsbury
Heathcote Marlee A
Upper Cold River Road 802/773-7994

Virginia

Alexandria
Traditional Acupuncture Assoc
8601 Fort Hunt Rd 301/565-2700
Chen Yongs
4600 Duke St Apt 410 ....703/671-4905
Joy M Dee
240 S Reynolds St 703/548-0442
Kim Sun Dong
375 S Reynolds St Apt 214 .... 703/370-6518

Annantale

Park Chan
4512 Old Columbia Pike 708/941-6611

Arlington
Nie Yun Lin
333 S Glebe Rd Apt 429 ....202/625-1603

Burke
Herdrich Floyd M DIPLAC (NCCA)
The Traditional Acupuncture Clinic
10415 Todman Landing Ct 703/978-4956

Fairfax
Park Chan S
5266 O'Faly Rd 708/941-6611

Falls Church
Kim Luke Kap Sok
3536 Carlin Springs Rd #20........ 703/379-4442
Tran Canh Q MD
5621 Columbia Pike 202/659-0515

Mc Lean
Rhee Richard
7028 Benjamin St 703/448-0266

Orange
Taylor Julie Everett
RR 3 Box 222 ....703/672-2065

Richmond
Nguyen Tien Duc MD CA
5500 Monument Ave Ste O 804/285-0176

Springfield
Bulin Edward
PO Box 6002 ....703/569-3742

Stafford
Suh David H
650 Courthouse Rd 301/587-4292

Vienna
Tang Trinh Thi
9825 Faust Dr 703/759-7834

Woodbridge
Rosemblat Aldo MD
1948 Opitz Blvd (DC Metro)...................690-6030

Washington

Bainbridge Is
Eggleston Diane CA DIPLAC NCCA
600 Ericksen Ave NE #320 .... 206/842-0553

Bellevue
Morrissey E Stephen
1370 116th Ave NE Ste 106 ...... 206/454-9727

Bothell
Meshew Christine Alain
23304 35th Ave SE 206/481-0169

Des Moines
Reinhard Mark G
21606 29th Ave S Ste A 206/824-7346

Duvall

Mati Jeff A PO Box 1062 ....206/788-6657

Edmonds
Kruthers PA LAC
   23200 Edmonds Way 206/542-5595

Issaquah
Chin Kenneth C
   85 NW Alder Pl Ste C 206/392-7449

Kent
Imlay Marc A
   24625 148th Ave SE 206/631-0099

Kirkland
Covert Lionnell
   10437 NE 113th Pl.......................206/827-2036
Covert Loretta
   10437 NE 113th Pl.......................206/827-2036
Covert Lionnel
   10437 NE113th Pl 206/828-6751
Dunn-Merit Sheila B
   607 Market St 206/822-3716
Frey Jill Suzanne
   607 Market St 206/365-0164

Langley
Sadow Shoshana CA
   PO Box 660 ....206/221-6010

Lynnwood
Conlon Carol J
   20102 Cedar Valley Rd 206/776-5353

Mill Creek
Sang Wong 15015 16th Ave SE 206/338-3915

Mukilteo
Mukilteo Chiropractice & Acupuncture
   PO Box 218 ....206/355-3433

Olympia
Stiritz Robin Dianne
   4711 Brech St SE 206/781-0352

Port Townsend
Holland Alex 907 Rose St 206/385-4383
O'Connor Linda S
   210 Polk St Ste 3 ....206/385-4383

Richland
Liu Sheung Siu J
   218 Sitka Ct 509/627-2878
Poe Barbara Sue
   2105 Pullen St Apt 15 ....509/946-7412

Seattle
Bastyr University Natural Health Clinic
   1307 N 45th St #200.................. 206/632-0354
Bayer Sara
   1535 11th Ave #204 ....206/322-9363
Blair James R
   525 Minor Ave 206/622-0246
Boehm Jennifer
   144 NE54th St 206/523-9585

Boyd Karen Ann
   2908 9th Ave W 206/285-7656
Chan Hoy Ping Yee
   1021 1/2 NE 125th St 206/367-3242
Chan Jimmy C
   7201 5th Ave NE 206/525-4660
Chen Amy Zhuan
   2611 NE 125th St Ste 240......... 206/364-5000
Chiong Chu-Lan S
   7714 16th Ave NE 206/522-8589
Cohen Stewart L
   2345 NE 95th St 206/527-3152
Conaty Neil P
   3009 3rd Ave W Ste 6 ....206/284-8265
Curcio Dorothea J
   130 Nickerson St 206/286-1802
Hein Dirk P 2201 E Howe St 206/448-1199
Ji Kun Won 1234 SW 150th St 206/241-7800
Karsten Paul 1307 N 45th St 206/633-2419
MacDonald Robert R
   7722 24th Ave NE 206/523-5258
Martinez Steven M
   525 Minor Ave Ste D 206/622-0246
Peterson Lori Diane
   2914 NW 75th St 206/633-2097
Ptacek Gail
   4320 Latona Ave NE 206/634-2061
Reibman Mark Philip
   215 11th Ave E 206/323-5277
Reinstein Julia Shad
   619 N 35th St Ste 317 ....206/547-4583
Roush Gwendolyn Joyce
   5120 25th Ave 206/725-2521
Scott Susan E
   4110 Stone Way N 206/547-1745
Sonia Paul D
   2427 NW 64th St 206/783-2667
St Clair Torri
   933 Lake Washington Blvd S 206/323-7000
Thoreson Michelle
   3019 NW 57th St 206/781-1690
Vosova Julie
   1307 N 45th St Ste 300 ....206/633-2419
Wang Xue-Zhi
   3115 Univ Way NE Ste 111 .... 206/547-2435
Wulsin William F ND MA DI
   753 N 35th St Ste 302 ....206/632-0411
Yun Jong Suk Theres
   4942 SW Forney St 206/937-6822
Zizza Daniel J
   2820 Eroy St 206/329-5466

Spokane
Acu Care...800/974-5664
Krull Kim P
   1422 S Dickinson Dr 509/927-8097
Stephan Robert B DDS

731 W Indiana Ave 509/325-2051

Tacoma

Acupuncture Clinic of Tacoma
3001 6th Ave Ste 6......................206/572-1050
Chinese Acupuncture Center
5900 100th SW #22 .... 206/581-4111
Calpeno Anthony
4111 Bridgeport Way W Ste A...... 206/565-2444
Liu Jei-Shi
5900 100th St SW Ste 22 .... 206/581-4111

Woodinville

Park Wong Ho
17632 140th Ave NE Ste A 206/481-2542

West Virginia

Beckley

Kostenko Michael DO DC
114 E Main St 304/253-0591

Wisconsin

Beloit

Blahnik Jennifer A
2101 Riverside Dr 608/365-6771

Dresser

Leef Linda DAC PO Box 266 ....715/755-3807

Lake Geneva

Alwa Rathna MD
717 Geneva St 414/248-1430

Madison

Behrens Kathleen
2037 Winnebago St 608/244-2446
Carey Donna Marie
533 Ohio Ave 608/251-7879
Chung Jae Bock
PO Box 384 ....608/256-0808
Hassert Susan
6506 Schroeder Rd 608/273-4458
Kohn N Mike D DVM
1014 Williamson St 608/255-1239

Manitowoc

Arndorfer Ellen S
2143 S 17th St 608/233-3600

Milwaukee

Jin Guan-Yuan MD LAC
260 E Highland Ave 414/821-5968
Keuler Helen RN DAC
4701 W National Ave 414/645-1616
Li Yee-Kit MD
155 E Silver Spring Dr Ste 208.... 414/963-0903
Luo Henley
8405 W Burleigh St 414/871-1228
Luo Marie
8405 W Burleigh St 414/871-1228

New Berlin

Tillman Keith D 13815 W Robin Trl .708/295-5436

Plover

Chang James C LAC DAC
PO Box 908 ....715/345-0655
Ensweiler Mark S PO Box 908 ....715/345-0655

Sun Prairie

Chung Jae Bock
918 Camp Fire Dr 608/837-7740

Suring

Cook Douglas L DDS
10971 Clinic Rd 414/842-2083

Washburn

Jensch Kristine M MA DAC
502 E 4th St 715/373-5491

Watertown

Hidde Orval DC 1434 E Main St 414/261-5607

Wyoming

Moose

Mersereau Carol Ann PO Box 331 ...307/733-3863

Canada

Alberta

Bayrock Roman G
9617-111 Ave EDMONTON 403/422-7656
Yawrenko David Murray DAC DCHIR
10216-124 St #300 ....403/482-6071

British Columbia

Bennett Peter W
Box 1343 Ganges WINDSOR 604/537-4419
Kuramoto D ND
#202-55 Victoria Rd NANAIMO.....604/753-0280
Watterson Mary S
5621 Dunbar St VANCOUVER 604/261-8700

Manitoba

Naturopathic Medical Clinic Conyette Paul NMD ND
708 10th St BRANDON 204/727-3524

Nova Scotia

Stick Kermit C
49 Anchor Dr HALIFAX...................902/477-7217

Ontario

Aubry Jean R MD PO Box 223065B
QUEEN STURGION FALLS...............705/753-2300
Campbell Lauri ND
2525 Roseville Gdn Dr #203 ....519/944-6000
Devgan Ravi MD
42 Redpath Ave TORONTO.............416/487-0882
Pei Paul P H
18 Banff Rd TORONTO 416/489-0552
Wine William DD MA PHD DSC DAC FA
32 Gothic Ave TORONTO 416/766-6069

Quebec

Goldman David LAC
Ste 182425 Grand Blvd MONTREAL

....514/481-4028

Paquin Dominique Manue
    210 Main St GATINEAU 819/6630375
    877 W Fremont Ave 408/736-8103

AROMATHERAPY

Aromatherapy is the science of using the essential oils from botanical sources with anti-viral, anti-fungal properties for the treatment of illness. The essential oils can be inhaled, applied topically, and, in some cases, ingested. In France, aromatherapy is recognized as a system of medicine and is used in hospitals. Many aspects of aromatherapy also make it a valuable system of self-care.

Arizona

Chandler
Magyar Teri 750 W Toledo St.............602/963-7644
Flagstaff
New-Jenkins Pat
    12205 N Peaks Pky......................602/526-8515
Parks
Morris Connie PO Box 50425...........602/635-2331
Phoenix
Addesso Anthony DC
    2525 W Greenway.........................602/843-9249
Damian Kate Windrose Aromatics
    12629 N Tatum Blvd......................602/861-3696
Fritsche Anna Marie
    4113 E Alan Ln 602/494-7332
Kane Lou Ann
    4108 W Kaler Dr 602/934-7929
May Kathleen Body Balance
    844 E Bell Rd Apt 3112 ....602/493-3872
Strong Maria
    4341 E Redfield Rd 602/493-3513
Tucson
Morris Lance J WMD
    1001 N Swan Rd 602/323-7133

California

Alameda
Northrop Margaret
    2325 Clement Ave #275 ....510/522-0189
Zdral Claudia
    512 Westline Dr #102 ....510/522-0998
Diamond Bar
Welke Lynne RN HYP Family Wellness Clinic
    1111 Grand Ave Ste J 619/225-2197
Lake Forest
Grossman Michael J MD Wellness Ctr of Lake Forest
    24432 Muirlands Blvd 714/770-7301

Mill Valley
Garnder Nancy 333 Miller Ave 415/383-7224
Sacramento
Luthra Yugal K
    PO Box 1103 ....916/442-4945
San Diego
Kahn Linda Anne
    Beauty Kliniek
    3268 Governor Dr 619/457-0191
Santa Rosa
Thomas Helen DC
    1260 N Putten Ave #160 ....707/527-7313
Sherman Oaks
Steele John Lifetree Aromatix
    3949 Longridge Ave 818/986-0594
South Pasadena
Buhler Annemarie Time Laboratories
    PO Box 694 ....818/300-8096

Florida

Clearwater
D'Costa Harriet M MD D
    1481 Belleair Rd 813/584-7246
Orlando
Carr Arlene FS LMT Bodyworks Healing Center
    1720 S Orange Ave #204 ....407/649-8162
West Palm Beach
Kratz Cynthia J LMT
    2601 N Flagler Dr #212 ....407/835-6821

Idaho

Pocatello
Davis Annette PO Box 638 ....208/232-5250

Illinois

Chicago
Steenvoorden Marianne Chicago Holistic Center
    2400 N Ashland Ave 312/296-6700

Massachusetts

Amherst
Lentz John
    33 Long Plain Rd Rfd 3 ....413/548-9763
Harvard
Beaty Janet K ND PO Box 661 ....508/772-0222

New Jersey

Ramsey
Lindberg Elisabeth MTH
    263 E Main St 201/934-1751

Pennsylvania

Allentown
Cassell Bonita MT Lehigh Valley Healing Arts
5677 Greens Dr 215/398-9642

Washington

Seattle
Contento Elise
2117 Nob Hill Ave N #2 ....206/283-2819

Tacoma
Alexandar School
4032 Pacific Avenue 206/473-1142

AYURVEDIC

Ayurvedic medicine is an ancient system of medicine from India based upon treating patients according to three metabolic types. Ayurveda places a high value on diet, detoxification, exercise, herbal medicine, and meditation, and is effective in treating a wide range of chronic conditions.

Arizona

Phoenix
Addesso Anthony Marharishi Ayurveda
2525 W Greenway 602/843-9249

California

Brea
Zamarra John M Maharishi Ayurveda
603 Valencia Ave #201 ....714/993-5200

Encino
Lichtenfeld Philip Maharishi Ayurveda
16542 Ventura Blvd 818/784-7784

Lake Forest
Grossman Michael MD
24432 Muirlands Blvd 714/770-7301

Oakland
Sternlieb Lisa
230 Grand Ave 510/444-1804

Pasadena
Lichtenfeld philip
960 East Green St L 102 ....818/796-7676

Richmond
Steele Spencer Maharishi Ayurveda
12855 San Pablo Ave 510/233-8650

San Anselmo
Hardy Leonard G DC Maharishi Ayurveda
25 Tamalpais Ave #D 415/485-5768

Santa Barbara
Doner David MD
2410 Fletcher Ave #301 ....805/682-5879

Santa Monica
Martin Lucien DC Maharishi Ayurveda
612 Colorado Ave #10 ....310/392-8184

San Francisco
Aouyago Sho DC
2107 Van Ness #309 ....415/922-3091

Santa Rosa
Thomas Helen DC Maharishi Ayurveda
1260 N Putten Ave #160 ....707/527-7313

Colorado

Boulder
Lyon Peter DC
2299 Pearl St #208 ....303/444-1212

Connecticut

Canaan
Vyas Rajesh P 10 Church St 203/259-2700

Hartford
Ranade Rekha 530 Silas 203/721-7911

Stratford
Gunn Richard F DC
2875 Main St 203/378-3398

Westport
Vishvanath K Pramica ND
299 Greens Farms Rd 203/259-2700

Delaware

New Castle
Rosenthal Melvin J DC Maharishi Ayurveda
208 Delaware St 302/322-3030

District of Columbia

Washington DC
Lonsdorf Nancy MD
4910 Massachusetts Ave NW 202/244-2700

Florida

Alachua
Sylvester Joseph
PO Box 1090 ....904/462-7909

Boca Raton
Hedendal Bruce DC
301 Crawford Blvd 407/391-4600
Willix Jr Robert D MD Maharishi Ayurveda
1515 S Federal Hwy 407/362-0724

Clearwater
D'Costa A Harriet M MD D
1481 Belleair Rd 813/584-7246

Naples
Perlmutter David MD
720 Goodlette Rd N 813/262-8971

Stuart

McKay Kevin DC
971 Central Pky 407/283-0109

Tampa
American Natural Hygiene Society Inc
11816 Race Track Rd 813/855-6607

Georgia

Albany
Woodard Jr Otis J MD Maharishi Ayurveda
533A Pine Ave 912/436-9535

Atlanta
Hurd Philip A DC Maharishi Ayurveda
4633 Buford Hwy 404/455-6767
Sayer William DC
5075 Roswell Rd NE 404/256-1161

Brunswick
Dill J Darcy 4109 Atlanta Ave 912/264-2424

Roswell
Dawson Stan 740 Grimes Bridge Rd 404/993-9820

Hawaii

Kaneohe
Hoffman T MD
Maharishi Ayurveda
47-655 Hui-Kelu #2 ....808/239-5859

Illinois

Chicago
Ganges Herbs
155 N Harbor Dr............................312/565-0486
Bhavnani Lata Herbal Esthetician
2400 N Ashland Ave 312/296-6700

Indiana

Muncie
Peterson John C MD Maharishi Ayur'vedic
Consult Svc 317/286-5087

Maine

Farmington
Fuson Jeffery Maharishi Ayurveda
RR 4 Box 5104 ....207/778-9531

Yarmouth
French Camille N DC
14 Pleasant St................................207/846-3247

Maryland

Bethesda
Beech Douglas DC Maharishi Ayurveda
9213 Seven Locks Rd 301/469-6700

Silver Spring
Ginsberg Robert J MD

Maharishi Ayurveda
9301 Colesville Rd 301/588-1577
Placenta Jr Nicholas J DO
Maharishi Ayurveda
11018 Lockwood Dr 301/681-4277

Massachusetts

Boston
Carballeira Nicolas P ND
95 Berkeley St 617/350-6900

Michigan

Pontiac
Reddy Hema MD
Maharishi Ayurveda Health
Center of Michigan
909 Woodward #117 ....810/855-8030

Minnesota

Saint Paul
Donohoe Joseph
821 Raymond Ave 612/645-1050

Missouri

Kirkwood
Neeb Norman DO
Maharishi Ayurveda
12166 Old Big Bend Rd 314/984-0033

New Jersey

Elizabeth
Locurcio Gennaro
610 3rd Ave 908/351-1333

Toms River
Dichiara Frank DO
2446 Church Rd 908/255-3636

New Mexico

Albuquerque
Pool Thomas DC
1950 Zuan Tabo Ne 505/296-3340
Lad Vasant
1231 Setter Dr NE 505/292-7268

New York

New York
Gerson Scott MD PC
13 W 9th St 212/505-8971

Ohio

Rocky River
Smith D Edwards MD FACP Maharishi Ayur-Veda
Medical Center....................................216/333-6700

Oklahoma

Oklahoma City
Gumman Amit BSC BAMS DAC ND
OKC Family Health & Pain Clinic
8241 South Walker 405/631-5450
Taylor Charles D MD
3715 N Classen Blvd 405/525-7751

Oregon

Lake Oswego
Morris Prafulla 10 Eagle Crest Dr 503/699-2547
Portland
Elder Leslie D MD Maharishi Ayruveda
16575 SE Sager Rd 503/661-3349

Texas

Arlington
Davis Jim DO
1916 Valleywood #153 ....817/795-1513

Washington

Bellevue
Marmorstein Barry L MD Maharishi Ayurveda
1603 116th Ave NE #112 .... 206/455-4929
Sodhi Virender MD ND
10025 NE 4th St 206/453-8022
Bremerton
McGregor Marianne MD Maharishi Ayurveda
1907 Madrona Pt Dr 360/373-0497
Leavenworth
Hamner Lynda S MD Maharishi Ayurveda
911 commercial 509/548-7090
Port Townsend
Rienstra J Douwe Maharishi Ayurveda
242 Monroe St 360/385-5658

West Virginia

Huntington
Sharma Tara C MD Maharishi Ayurveda
1401 6th Ave..................................304/523-8800

Biofeedback

Biofeedback training teaches one how to consciously control the autonomic nervous system through the use of biofeedback devices in order to alleviate stress, migraine headaches, asthma, high blood pressure, and a host of other health conditions.

Alabama

Birmingham
James George C PHD
956 Montclair Rd Ste 112 .... 205/951-5113

Alaska

Anchorage
Kappes Bruno PHD
Psychology Department
University Of Alaska 907/786-1719

Arizona

Tucson
Nicholson Elaine PHD
2330 N Rosemond Blvd 602/881-1977

Arkansas

North Little Rock
Doyle Robert B PHD
2500 McCain Blvd Ste 120 .... 501/771-4442

California

Beverly Hills
Holmes Mark OMD LAC Center for Regeneration
9730 Wilshire Blvd Ste 108 ....310/271-6467
Sandweiss Jack H MA
436 N Bedford Dr Ste 301 .... 310/274-0981
Garden Grove
Balodis Jacquie PHD Amparo Biotherapy Institute
10332 Hill Rd 714/530-4369
Irvine
Bio Health Inc 12 Hughes D101 .....800/500-4246
Los Angeles
Creative Sound Technologies Inc
Elena Renner RN PHD
800 W 1st St Ste 103....................213/746-7900
Los Gatos
Wickowicz Diana M RN MFCC
15619 Los Gatos Blvd 408/356-9989
Newport Beach
Byers Rogee PHD
2525 E 16th St 714/760-3607
Palo Alto
Rosche Christine MPH CHT
4157 El Camino Way #C 415/856-3151
Placentia
Marino Virginia BA CHT
601 E Yorba Linda Blvd Ste C 714/993-7757
Riverside
Tresselle Leo
2900 Adams Bldg A Ste 435 ....909/352-6577
San Diego
Rubio Geronimo MD
American Metabolic Institute
555 Saturn Blvd Bldg B 800/388-1083

San Rafael
The Atma Group
185 N Redwood Dr Ste 220 ....415/499-3319

San Ramon
Halpin Lisa
2819 Crow Canyon Rd #219C..... 510/820-5860

Santa Barbara
McKenna Maureen
319 W Valerio St #2 ....805/682-6363

Colorado

Littleton
Sheehan Kay M
2305 E Arapahoe Rd Ste 214 .....303/795-1761

Connecticut

Westport
Cunningham Paul
1 Turkey Hill Rd S Ste 2H 203/454-4485

Florida

Fort Lauderdale
Montgomery Doil PHD
311 SE 13th St 305/463-5256

Winter Park
Rowe Anna L PHD PO Box 2363 .....305/644-2121

Georgia

Marietta
Michaud Betsy MA
522 North Ave Ste A 404/425-0483

Hawaii

Kahuliu
Davison Kevin J ND LAC
444 Hana Hwy #211.....................808/871-4722

Illinois

Chicago
Carpenter Phyllis R Certified MD Chicago Holistic Ctr
2400 N Ashland Ave 2nd Fl 312/296-6700

Evanston
Good Nancy L LCSW
1740 Ridge Ave Ste 200 ....708/679-0486

Indiana

Indianapolis
Leon-Roth Vanessa MS VOTR
1261 W 86 St #E4 ....317/251-1607

Kansas

Lawrence
Stucky Rita
1012 Massachusetts St Ste 206 .913/841-4114

Topeka
Boeving Hue MS PO Box 829 ....913/273-7500
Fahrion Steven PHD PO Box 829 ....913/273-7500
Kleiger James PHD PO Box 829 ......913/273-7500
Nicholls Jeff MD PO Box 829 ....913/273-7500
Norris Patricia PHD PO Box 829 ......913/273-7500
Parks Peter MS PO Box 829 ....913/273-7500
Snarr Carol RN PO Box 829 ....913/273-7500
Walters Dale PHD PO Box 829 ....913/273-7500
Werder Doris MS PO Box 829 ....913/273-7500

Kentucky

Paducah
Johnson Jack B LCSW
155 Woodcreek Blvd 502

Louisiana

Baton Rouge
Jacques III Charles G LPC
8017 Jefferson Hwy Ste 3A 504/924-4903

Maryland

California
Miller H Joseph PHD
2190 Kingston Village Rd 410/535-5400

Massachusetts

Boston
Lee Susan 15 Kenwood St 617/625-8840

Brookline
Mehler Bruce L
1415 Beacon St 617/738-4817

Quincy
Ding Wenjing MD 59 Mill St 617/472-8428

Michigan

Spring Lake
Moss Donald PHD
109 S Jackson St 616/842-1277

Minnesota

Brainerd
Baltzell James W MD
555 Edgewood Dr N 218/829-1845
Baltzell Karen B MS
555 Edgewood Dr N 218/829-1845

Thompson Andrew MS
  555 Edgewood Dr N 218/829-1845
Edina
Jeffrey Smith Lilli A PHD
  7300 France Ave S Ste 200 ....612/893-9400
Mankato
Anderson Patricia M RN MS
  114 Cedar St 507/389-8568
Minneapolis
Ross Scott M MD
  2545 Chicago Ave S 612/863-4700

Missouri

Chesterfield
Wlitte Hermann PHD
  222 S Woods Mill 314/851-6054
Saint Louis
Russ Kenneth PHD
  200 S Hanley Rd #514 ....314/863-9111
Springfield
Shealy C Norman PHD
  1328 E Evergreen St......................417/865-5940

Mississippi

Jackson
Stanley Charlton PHD
  1050 N Flowood Dr #C1 ....601/932-1178

North Carolina

Pinehurst
Schulte Don R PHD
  PO Box 1388 ....919/295-6851

Nebraska

Lincoln
Rose Connie M ED
  2300 S 16th St 402/473-5629

New Jersey

Boonton Turnpike
Alson Eli PHD
  Powerville Rd St Clares Riverside...201/316-1949

New Mexico

Albuquerque
Waybright III Edgar PHD
  4308 Carlisle Blvd NE Ste 201 ....505/881-2184

New York

Brooklyn
Bindler Paul PHD

  1060 E 26th St 718/377-7187
New York
Biofeedback & Stress Management
  62nd & Broadway..........................212/265-1983

Ohio

Toledo
McGrady Angele V PHD
  PO Box 10008 ....419/381-4141

Oklahoma

Oklahoma City
Plowman Paul E DDS
  4801 Richmond Sq 405/840-5600
Tulsa
Wall Delynda MS
  6585 S Yale Ave #620 ....918/481-4781

Oregon

Eugene
Weintraub Skye
  911 Country Club Rd #290 .... 503/345-0747
Portland
Davis Susan
  10615 SE Cherry Blossom Dr #1 .503/256-1930

Pennsylvania

Allison Park
Rosen Rhonda K LSW
  4284 Route 8 ....412/487-1967
PA Society of Behavioral Medicine
  46 E Sedgwick St 215/848-2297

South Carolina

Charleston
Kaiser Charles F PHD
  Dept Psychology 66 George St 803/792-5590

Tennessee

Jackson
Vickery J David
  460 N Parkway Ste #B 901/668-1818

Texas

Bellaire
Alexander Helen M MA
  104 Calvi Ct 713/447-5536
Houston
Brown George A MA
  6560 Fannin St Ste 1224 ....713/790-1225
Matagorda

Looney Penny CHT RCT
PO Box 202 ....409/863-7445
Wilson Richard DOMD RMT
PO Box 202 ....409/863-7445

Utah

Logan
Striefel Sebastian PHD......................801/797-1985

Washington

Seattle
Bradley Sharon R
10626 3rd Ave SW 206/242-2596
Cahn Timothy S PHD
901 Boren Ave Ste 1010 ....206/624-1856

Spokane
Peptide Inc
828 S Adams.................................509/624-4868
Wells Katherine M RNBSN
1412 W Bellwood Dr 509/326-6900

Wisconson

Madison
Rubow Rick PHD PO Box 470 ....608/251-7702

Chelation

Chelation therapy is a simple, painless medical process involving intravenous drips of EDTA to remove heavy metals and toxins from the blood and to reverse atherosclerosis. Chelation therapy provides an alternative to bypass surgery and angioplasty, reduces high blood pressure, and helps reverse age-related degenerative diseases.

Alabama

Birmingham
Prosch Jr Gus J MD Biomed Associates PC
759 Valley St 205/823-6180

Alaska

Anchorage
Denton Sandra MD
4115 Lake Otis Pky #200 ....907/563-6200
Manuel F Russell MD
4141 B St Ste 209 ....907/562-7070
Rowen Robert MD
615 E 82nd Ave Ste 300 ....907/344-7775

Wasilla
Martin Robert MD
PO Box 870710 ....907/376-5284

Arizona

Glendale
Armold Lloyd D DO
4901 W Bell Rd Ste 2 ....602/939-8916

Mesa
Halcomb William W DO
4323 E Broadway Ste 109 ....602/832-3014

Parker
Meyer S W DO
332 River Front Dr PO Box 1870 ..602/669-8911

Phoenix
Olsztyn Stanley R MD
3610 N 44th St Ste 2 ....602/954-0811

Prescott
Josephs Gordon H DO
315 W Goodwin St 602/778-6169

Scottsdale
Friedmann Terry S MD
10565 N Tatum Blvd Ste B115 ....602/381-0800
Josephs Gordon H DO
7315 E Evans Rd 602/998-9232

Tempe
Gordon Garry MD
5535 S Compass Rd 602/838-2079

Arkansas

Hot Springs
Wright William MD
1 Mercy Lane 211 ....501/624-3312

Little Rock
Becquet Norbert J MD
115 W 6th St 501/375-4419

North Little Rock
Gustavus John L
4721 E Broadway 501/758-9350

California

Albany
Gordon Ross B MD
405 Kains Ave 510/526-3232

Auburn
Kime Zane MD
1212 High St Ste 204 ....916/823-3421

Azusa
Bryce William C MD
400 N San Gabriel Ave 818/334-1407

Bakersfield
Seibly Ralph G MD
1311 Columbus St 805/873-1000

Colton
Shaw Hiten MD

22807 Barton Rd 714/783-2773

Concord
Toth John P MD
2299 Bacon St Ste 10 ....510/682-5660

Covina
Privitera James
105 N Grandview Ave 818/966-1618

Del Mar
Nathan Pamela S LAC
13983 Mango Dr Ste 206 ....619/755-3340

El Cajon
Saccoman William J MD
505 N Mollison Ave Ste 103.........619/440-3838

Encino
Abraham Iona MD
17815 Ventura Blvd 818/345-8721
Klepp A Leonard MD
16311 Ventura Blvd Ste 725 ....818/981-5511

Escalon
Verigin Gary M DDS
1415 Oklahoma Ave 209/838-3522

Escondido
Wilson Jacquelyn J MD
536 Brotherton Rd 619/747-2144

Fresno
Edwards David J MD
360 S Clovis Ave 209/251-5068

Grand Terrace
Smith-Halstead Clinic
22805 Barton Road 909/783-2773

Hemet
Meadowlark Health Center
26126 Fairview Ave 909/927-1343

Hollywood
Julian James J MD
1654 Cahuenga Blvd 213/467-5555

Huntington Beach
Resk Joan M DO
18821 Delaware St Ste 203........ 714/842-5591

Lake Forest
Steenblock David A DO
22706 Aspen Ste 500 ....714/770-9616
Health Restoration Center
22706 Aspen St #501................. 714/770-9616

Laytonville
Finkle Eugene D MD
PO Box 309 ....707/984-6151

Long Beach
Casdorph H Richard MD PHD
1703 Temino Ave Ste 201 ....310/597-8716

Los Altos
Cathcart III Robert F MD
127 2nd St Ste 4 ....415/949-2822

Marquette Claude MD
5050 El Camino Real #110 .... 415/964-6700

Los Angeles
Belenyessy Laszio MD
12732 Washington Blvd #D......... 213/822-4614
Jahangirl M MD
2156 S Santa Fe Ave 213/587-3218
Park Byung S MD
2211 Corinth Ave #204 ....310/477-8151
Sciabbarrasi Joseph MD
2211 Corinth Ave #204 ....310/477-8151
Susser Murray MD
2211 Corinth Ave #204 ....310/477-8151

Los Gatos
Waiton R O
221 Almendra Ave 408/354-2300

Mission Viejo
Kim Duke D MD
27800 Medical Center Rd Ste 11 714/364-6040

Monterey
Work Lon B MD
841 Foam St #D 408/655-0215

Morro Bay
Odell Stephen W
625 Main St 805/772-6006

Newport Beach
Whitaker Julian MD
4321 Birch St Ste 100 ....714/851-1550

North Hollywood
Freeman David C MD
11311 Camarillo St #103 .... 818/985-1103

Pacific Palisades
McBroom F Pearl MD
1515 Palisades Dr Ste P 310/454-7227

Palm Springs
Degnan Sean MD
2825 E Tahquitz McCallum Way.....619/320-4292

Rancho Mirage
Farinella Charles B MD
University Executive Park
69-730 Hwy 111 Ste 106A 619/324-0734

Redding
Tillman Bessie J MD
2054 Market St 916/246-3022

Sacramento
Kwiker Michael DO
3301 Alta Arden Ste 3 ....916/489-4400

San Diego
Taylor Lawrence MD
3330 3rd Ave #402 ....619/296-2952

San Francisco
Kunin Richard A MD
2698 Pacific Ave 415/346-2500

Lemesh Russell A MD
595 Buckingham Way #320 ....415/731-5907
Lynn Paul MD
345 W Portal Ave 415/566-1000
Mark Denise R MD
345 W Portal Ave 415/566-1000

San Jacinto
Shah Hiten MD
229 W 7th St 909/658-7246

San Jose
Gilford T MD
2674 N First St #101 ....408/433-0923

San Leandro
Gee Steven H MD
595 Estudillo Ave 510/483-5881

San Luis Obispo
Dorman Thomas A MD
171 N Santa Rosa St #A 805/781-3388

San Marcos
Kubitschek William C DO
1194 Calle Maria 619/744-6991

San Rafael
Gordon Ross B MD
4144 Redwood Hwy 415/499-9377

Santa Ana
Wempen Ronald MD
3620 S Bristol St Ste 306 ....714/546-4325

Santa Barbara
Hoegerman H J MD
101 W Arrellaga Ste D 805/963-1824
Moharram Mohamed MD
101 W Arrellaga St Ste B 805/965-5229

Santa Maria
Reiner Donald E MD
1414-D S Miller St 805/925-0961

Santa Monica
Rosenbaum Michael MD
2730 Wilshire Blvd #110 ....310/453-4424

Santa Rosa
Su Terri MD
1038 4th St #3 ....707/571-7560

Seal Beach
Green Allen MD
909 Electric Ave Ste 212 .... 714/851-1550

Sherman Oaks
Fraser Clifford MD
4910 Van Nuys Blvd Ste 110 ...... 818/986-2199

Smith River
Vipond JoAnn MD
12559 Hwy 101 N 707/487-3405

Stanton
Goldwag William J MD

7499 Cerritos Ave 714/827-5180

Studio City
Law Jr Charles E MD
3959 Laurel Canyon Blvd Ste 1 ... 818/761-1661

Torrance
Millen Anita
1010 Crenshaw Blvd Ste 170...... 310/320-1132
Skinner Suzanne M PHD ND DSC HHD
2424 Torrance Blvd 310/518-4555

Ventura
Colquitt James W DDS
10883 Telegraph Rd 805/647-1322

Walnut Creek
Charles Alan S MD
1414 Maria Ln 510/937-3331

Colorado

Colorado Springs
Denton Sandra C MD
5080 List Dr 719/548-1600
Fish James R MD
3030 N Hancock Ave 719/471-2273
Juetersonke George DO
5455 N Union Blvd Ste 200 ....719/528-1960

Connecticut

Milford
Cohen Alan R
67 Cherry St 203/877-1936

Orange
Sica Robban MD
325 Post Road 203/799-7733

Torrington
Finnie Jerrold N MD
333 Kennedy Dr #L-204 ....203/489-8977

Delaware

Georgetown
Yossif George MD
546 S Bedford St 302/856-5151

District of Columbia

Washington DC
Mitchell George H MD
2639 Connecticut Ave NW Ste C...202/265-4111

Florida

Boca Raton
Haimes Leonard MD
7300 N Federal Hwy Ste 107 ....407/994-3868

Bradenton
Melnikov Eteri MD DC

116 Manatee Ave E 813/748-7943

Crystal River
Borromeo Azael MD
700 SE 5th Terrace 904/795-7177

Fort Lauderdale
Dooley Bruce MD
1493 SE 17th St 305/527-9355

Fort Myers
Pynckel Gary L DO
3940 Metro Pky Ste 115 ....813/278-3377

Hollywood
Pardell Herbert DO
210 S Federal Hwy Ste 302 ....305/922-0470

Jacksonville
Mauriello John MD
4063 Salisbury Rd Ste 206 ....904/296-0900

Jupiter
Ahner Neil MD
1080 E Indiantown Rd 407/744-0077

Lakeland
Robinson Harold MD
4406 S Florida Ave #30 ....813/646-5088

Longwood
Rogers Robert MD
2170 W State Rd 434 #190.........407/682-5222

Maitland
Schoen Joya L MD
341 N Maitland Ave Ste 200 ....407/644-2729

Miami
Dayton Martin DO
18600 Collins Ave 305/931-8484
Godorov Joseph G DO
9055 SW 87th Ave Ste 307 .... 305/595-0671
Ramirez-Calderon Carlos MD
1800 SW 27th Ave Ste 601 .... 305/441-6669

Milton
Watson William MD PA
600 Stewart St NE 904/623-3836

North Miami Beach
Dayton Martin DO
18600 Collins Ave 305/931-8484

Ocala
Graves George DO
3501 NE 10th St 904/236-2525

Orange City
Herring Travis L MD
106 W Fern Dr 904/775-0525

Ormond Beach
Chaim Hana T DO
595 W Granada Blvd Ste D 904/672-9000

Oviedo
Kupsinel Roy MD
1325 Shangri-La Ln 407/365-6681

Palm Bay
Ahner Neil MD
1200 Malabar Rd SE 407/729-8581

Panama City
Elghany Naima A MD
710 Venetian Way 904/763-7689

Pompano Beach
Lenzi Roehm Medical Center
3400 Park Central Blvd 800/554-6170
Post William MD
3400 Pk Central Bl N Ste 3450 ...305/977-3700

Port Canaveral
Parsons James MD
707 Mullet Dr Ste 110 ....407/784-2102

Port Saint Lucie
Barbaza Ricardo V MD
1541 SE Port Saint Lucie Blvd 407/335-4994

Saint Petersburg
Wunderlich Jr Ray MD
666 6th St S #206 ....813/822-3612

Sarasota
McNaughton Thomas M
1521 Dolphin St 813/365-6273
Ossorio Joseph MD
3900 Clark Rd Ste H-5 ....813/921-6338

Tampa
Carrow Donald J MD
3902 Henderson Blvd Ste 206 ....813/832-3220
Lee Eugene H MD
1804 W Kennedy Blvd #A 813/251-3089

Wauchula
Massam Alfred S MD
528 W Main St 813/773-6668

Winter Park
Parsons James M MD
2699 Lee Rd #303 ....407/628-3399

Georgia

Atlanta
Environmental & Prevention Health Center of Atlanta
Edelson Stephen MD FAAP
3833 Roswell Rd Ste 110............ 404/841-0088
Epstein David DO
427 Moreland Ave #100 ....404/525-7333
Fried Milton MD
4426 Tilly Mill Rd 404/451-4857
Mlaver Bernard MD
4480 N Shallowford Rd 404/395-1600
Richardson William E MD
1718 Peachtree St NW #552 ....404/607-0570

Camilla
Gunter Oliver L MD
24 N Ellis St 912/336-7343

Clayton
Douglas William C MD
PO Box 888 ....404/782-7222
Marietta
Lee Ralph C MD
110 Lewis Dr #B...........................404/423-0064
Warner Robins
Schneider Terril J MD
205 Dental Dr Ste 19 ....912/929-1027

Kealakekua
Arrington Clifton MD PO Box 649 ....808/322-9400

Coeur D'alene
McGee Charles T MD
1717 Lincolnway Ste 108 ....208/664-1478
Nampa
Thornburgh Stephen DO
824 17th Ave S 208/466-3517
Sandpoint
McCallum K Peter MD
2500 Selle Rd 208/263-5456

Arlington Heights
Haws Terrill K DO
121 S Wilke Rd Ste 111 ....708/577-9451
Sukel Phillip P DDS
1640 N Arlington Heights Rd.........708/253-0240
Aurora
Hesselink Thomas MD
888 S Edgelawn Dr Ste 1743......708/844-0011
Chicago
Jenkins Hugh A MD
2148 W 95th St 312/445-6800
Metamora
Elsasser Stephen DO FACAM
205 S Engelwood 309/367-2321
Oak Park
Dunn Paul J MD 715 Lake St 708/383-3800
Ottawa
Love Terry W DO
645 W Main 815/434-1977
Rolling Meadows
Stone Thomas L MD
1811 Hicks Rd 708/934-1100
Tinley Park
Dieska Daniel R DDS
17726A Oak Park Ave 708/429-4700
Woodstock

Tambone John R MD
102 E South St 815/338-2345
Zion
Senatore Peter DO
1911 27th St 708/872-8722

Evansville
Sparks Harold T DO
3001 Washington Ave 812/479-8228
Highland
Strecter Cal DO
9635 Saric Ct 219/924-2410
Indianapolis
Darbro David A MD
2124 E Hanna Ave 317/787-7221
Jeffersonville
Wolverton George MD
647 Eastern Blvd 812/282-4309
Mooresville
Whitney Norman E DO
PO Box 173 ....317/831-3352
Valparaiso
Trowbridge Myrna D DO
850-C Marsh St 219/462-3377

Sioux City
Blume Horst G MD
700 Jennings St 712/252-4386

Andover
Acker Stevens B MD
310 W Central #D 316/733-4494
Garden City
Hunsberger Terry DO
602 N 6th 316/275-7128
Hays
Neil Roy N MD 105 W 13th 913/628-8341

Bowling Green
Tapp John C MD
414 Old Morgantown Rd 502/781-1483
Louisville
Morgan Kirk MD 9105 Us Hwy 42 ..502/228-0156

Newellton
Whitaker Joseph R MD
PO Box 458 ....318/467-5131

Shreveport
Prakasam Felix K MD
PO Box 3153 ....318/226-1304

Maine

Van Buren
Cyr Joseph MD 62 Main St 207/868-5273

Maryland

Annapolis
Brown-Christopher Cheryl MD
1419 Forest Dr Ste 202 ....410/268-5005

Laurel
Beals Paul MD
9101 Cherry Ln Ste 205 ....301/490-9911

Pikesville
Parks Ronald MD 410/486-5656

Rockville
Health Management Institute
11140 Rockville Pike Ste 550 ......301/816-3000

Massachusetts

Barnstable
Janson Michael MD
275 Mill Way PO Box 732 ....508/362-4343

Boston
Commonwealth Chelation Center
Ruben Oganesov
39 Brighton Ave 617/254-2500

Cambridge
Janson Michael MD
2557 Massachusetts Ave 617/661-6225

Hanover
Cohen Richard MD
51 Mill St Ste 1 ....617/829-9281

Michigan

Atlanta
Modzinski Leo DO MD
100 W State St 517/785-4254

Detroit
Farris Lovell L DDS
19207 Schaefer Hwy 313/861-2100

Farmington
Parenta Paul ADO
30275 Thirteen Mile Rd 810/626-7544
Scarchilli Albert JDO
30275 Thirteen Mile Rd 313/626-7544

Flint
Bernard William M DO
1044 Gilbert St 313/733-3140

Grand Haven
Lowe Thomas J DDS

605 Beacon Blvd 616/842-5640

Grand Rapids
Born Grant DO
2687 44th St SE 616/455-3550

Greenville
Nutt James DO
420 S Lafayette 616/754-3679

Linden
Penwell Marvin D DO
319 S Bridge St 313/735-7809

Montague
Coller Gary H DO
9883 US 31 N 616/894-2641

Muskegon
Walkotten Ruth DO
427 Seminole Rd 616/733-1989

Ortonville
Regiani David W DDS
101 South St 810/627-4934

Pontiac
Agbabian Vahagn DO
28 N Saginaw St #1105 ....810/334-2424

Saint Clair Shores
Ziobrn James DO
23550 Harper Ave 313/779-5700

Southfield
Nugent Stephen D
25755 Southfield Rd Ste N201... 810/557-1776

Williamston
Nelson Seldon DO
4386 N Meridian Rd 517/349-2458

Minnesota

Minneapolis
Dole Michael MD
10700 Old Cty Rd 15 #350 ....612/593-9458
Eckerly Jean R MD
10700 Old Cty Rd 15 #350 ....612/593-9458
Klos Steven E MD
2421 W 42nd St 612/929-4568

Tyler
Carlson Keith J MD PO Box 62 ....507/247-5921

Mississippi

Columbus
Sams James H MD
11220 Lehmburg Rd 601/327-8701

Ocean Springs
Waddell James H MD
1520 Government St 601/875-5505

Shelby
Hollingsworth Robert MD
PO Box 87 ....601/398-5106

Missouri

Festus
Schwent John T DO
1400 Truman Blvd 314/937-8688

Florissant
Sultan Tipu MD
11585 W Florissant Rd 314/921-5600

Independence
Dorman Lawrence DO
9120 E 35th St S 816/358-2712

Kansas City
McDonagh Edward W DO
2800-A Kendallwood Pkwy 816/453-5940
Rowland James DO
8133 Wornall Rd 816/361-4077
Rudolph Charles J DO PHD
2800-A Kendallwood Pkwy 816/453-5940

Mountain Grove
Hill Doyle B DO
601 N Bush 417/926-6643

Saint Louis
Walker Jr Harvey MD PHD
Yu Simon M MD
138 N Meramec Ave 314/721-7227

Springfield
Sunderwirth William C DO
2828 N National Ave 417/837-4158

Sullivan
Scott Ronald H DO
131 Meridith Ln 314/468-4932

Union
Hayes Clinton C DO
100 W Main St 314/583-8911

Montana

Hamilton
Binder Timothy A DC ND
173 Blodgett Camp Rd 406/363-4041

Nebraska

Omaha
Oliveto Eugene C MD
8031 W Center Rd #208 ....402/392-0233

Ord
Miller Otis W MD
408 S 14th St 308/728-3251

Nevada

Las Vegas
Pfau Terry DO
2810 W Charleston Blvd Ste 55 ..702/258-7860

Vance Robert DO
801 S Rancho Dr Ste #F2............ 702/385-7771

Reno
Gerber Michael L MD
3670 Grant Dr 702/826-1900
Soli Donald E MD
708 N Center St 702/786-7101

New Jersey

Cherry Hill
Magaziner Allan DO
1907 Greentree Rd 609/424-8222

Edison
Lee C Y MD
952 Amboy Ave 908/738-9220
Lev Ralph MD MS
952 Amboy Ave 908/738-9220
Sy Rodolfo T MD
952 Amboy Ave 908/738-9220

Elizabeth
Locurcio Gennaro MD
610 3rd Ave 908/351-1333

Fort Lee
Klingsberg Gary DO
1355 15th St #200 ....201/585-9368

Princeton
Braverman Eric MD
212 Commons Way Bldg #2 ....609/921-1842

Toms River
Harris Charles MD
1520 Route 37 E 908/506-9200

West Orange
Munito Faina MD
51 Pleasant Valley Wy 201/736-3743

New Mexico

Albuquerque
Taylor John T DO
6208 Montgomery Blvd NE.......... 505/271-4800

Los Alamos
Krohn Jacqueline MD
Los Alamos Med Ctr #136 ....505/662-9620

Roswell
Stoesser Annette MD
112 S Kentucky 505/623-2444

Santa Fe
Shrader W J MD
141 Paseo De Peralta Ste A 505/983-8890

New York

Brooklyn
Yutsis Pavel MD

1309 W 7th St 718/259-2122

East Meadow
Calapai Christopher DO
1900 Hempstead Tpke 516/794-0404

Falconer
Hill Reino MD
230 W Main St 716/665-3505

Huntington
Corsello Serafina MD
175 E Main St 516/271-0222
Kramer Jennie
175 E Main St 516/271-0222
St Germain Joyce
175 E Main St 516/271-0222

Lawrence
Kurk Mitchell MD
310 Broadway 516/239-5540

Massena
Snider Bob MD
HC 61 Box 43D 315/764-7328

New Hyde Park
Pei Sun F 1 Fairfield Ln 516/775-5285

New York City
Ash Richard N MD
860 Fifth Ave 212/628-3133
Atkins Robert C MD
152 E 55th St 212/758-2110
Corsello Serafina MD
200 W 57th St #1202 ....212/399-0222
Hoffman Ronald MD
40 E 30th St 212/779-1744

Niagara Falls
Cutler Paul MD
652 Elmwood Ave 716/284-5140

Rhinebeck
Bock Kenneth A MD
108 Montgomery St 914/876-7082

Staten Island
Lopez Del Castillo Alfredo N MD
126 Wieland Ave 718/966-8120

Suffern
Schachter Michael B MD
2 Executive Blvd #202 ....914/368-4700

Westbury
Yurkovsky Savely MD
309 Madison St 516/334-5926

North Carolina

Asheville
Wilson John L Jr MD
1312 Patton Ave 704/252-9833

Leicester
Laird John L MD RR 1 Box 7.............704/252-9833

Roanoke Rapids
Power Bhaskar D MD FRCS
PO Box 1132 ....919/535-1411

North Dakota

Grand Forks
Leigh Richard H MD
2314 Library Ln 701/775-5527

Minot
Briggs Brian MD
718 6th St SW 701/838-6011

Ohio

Akron
Aronica Josephine MD
1867 W Market St 216/867-7361

Bluffton
Chappell L Terry MD
122 Thurman St Box 248 ....419/358-4627

Canton
Slingluff Jack DO
5850 Fulton Dr NW 216/494-8641

Cincinnati
Cole Ted DO
9678 Cincinnati-Columbus Rd 513/779-0300
Westerdorf William S DDS
2818 Blue Rock Rd 513/923-3839

Cleveland
Baron John DO
4807 Rockside Rd #100 ....216/642-0082
Frackelton James P MD
24700 Center Ridge Rd 216/835-0104
Weeks Douglas MD
24700 Center Ridge Rd 216/835-0104

Columbus
Mitchell William D DO
3520 Snouffer Rd 614/761-0555
Shearer Ernest F DO
4191 N High St 614/262-1308

Dayton
Fricke Donald E DDS
513 E Stroop Rd 513/293-1012
Goldberg David D DO
100 Forest Park Dr 513/277-1722

Dublin
Cates William J
6065 Memorial Dr 614/764-4600

Lancaster
Sielski Richard MD PO Box 1010 ....614/653-0017

Madison
Krabill Richard DO
6231 N Ridge Rd 216/428-2141

Paulding

Snyder Don K MD
  11573 State Rt 111 ....419/399-2045
  West Chester
Pitman Gregory M DC
  7908 Cincinnati Dayton Rd 513/777-0024
  Westlake
Lonsdale Derrick MD
  24700 Center Ridge Rd 216/835-0104

Oklahoma

  Jenks
Anderson Leon DO
  121 2nd St 918/299-5039
  Norman
Hagglund Howard MD
  2227 W Lindsey St Ste 1401 ......405/329-4457
  Oklahoma City
Farr Charles H MD PHD
  10101 S Western Ave 405/691-1112
Taylor Charles D MD
  3715 N Classen Blvd 405/525-7751
  Tulsa
Snitker Gaylord D
  5531 S Lewis Ave 918/749-8349

Oregon

  Ashland
Peters Ronald L MD
  1607 Siskiyou Blvd 503/482-7007
  Eugene
Gambee John E MD
  66 Club Rd #140 ....503/686-2536
  Murphy
Fitzsimmons James WM
  PO Box 130 ....503/474-2166
  Portland
Sklovsky Robert ND
  6910 SE Lake Rd 503/654-3938
  Salem
Young Terence H MD
  1205 Wallace Rd NW 503/371-1558

Pennsylvania

  Allentown
Schmidt Robert H DO
  1227 W Liberty St Ste 303 ....215/437-1959
Von Kiel D Erik DO
  501 N 17th St #200 ....215/776-7639
  Bangor
Cinelli Francis J DO
  153 N 11th St 215/588-4502
  Bedford

Illingworth Bill DO
  120 W John St 814/623-8414
  Bethlehem
Rex Sally Ann DO
  1343 Easton Ave 215/866-0900
  Chaddsford
Maulfair Conrad G JR DO
  6 Wilminton W Chester Pike #2.... 800/733-4065
  Coudersport
Miller Howard J MD
  360 E 2nd St 814/274-7070
  Cranberry Township
Donald Mantell DO
  6505 Mars Rd 412/776-5610
  Fountainville
Byer Harold H MD
  5045 Swamp Rd #A-101 ....215/348-0443
  Greensburg
Miranda Ralph A MD
  RR 12 Box 108 ....412/838-7632
  Indiana
Sinha Chandrika MD
  1177 S 6th St 412/349-1414
  Langhorne
Luxembourg Medical Dental Center
  303 Corporate Dr E 215/968-4781
  Mertztonn
Maulfair Conrad G Jr DO
  1413 State Street..........................800/733-4065
  Morrisville
Kosmorsky PAUL M DO
  303 Floral Vale 215/860-1500
  Mount Pleasant
El-Attrache Mumduh F
  20 E Main St..................................412/547-3576
  Newtown
Peterson Robert J DO
  64 Magnolia Dr 215/579-0330
  Philadelphia
Burton Frederick MD
  69 W School House Ln 215/844-4660
Galperin Mura MD
  824 Hendrix St 215/677-2337
Sampathachar K R MD
  6366 Sherwood Rd 215/473-4226
  Pittsburgh
Stewart Roger DC
  2022A Mt Troy Rd 412/322-1945
  Quakertown
Buttram Harold E MD
  5724 Clymer Rd 215/536-1890
  Quarryville

Royal Dan DO
937 Little Britain Rd N 717/786-1314
Somerset
Peirsel Paul MD
RR 4 Box 267-1A 814/443-2521

South Carolina
Columbia
Rozema Theodore C MD
2228 Airport Rd 803/796-1702
Landrum
Rozema Theodore C MD
1000 E Rutherford St 803/457-4141
Rock Hill
Rozema Theodore C MD
2915 N Cherry Rd 800/992-8350

South Dakota
Chamberlain
Matheny Theodore MD
300 S Byron Blvd 605/734-6958

Tennessee
Knoxville
Carlson James DO
509 N Cedar Bluff Rd 615/691-2961
Nashville
Reisman Stephen L MD D/C
28 White Bridge Rd #400 ....615/356-4244

Texas
Abilene
Fox William I MD
1227 N Mockingbird Ln 915/672-7863
Alamo
Carr Herbert DO
PO Box 1179 ....210/787-6668
Amarillo
Parker Gerald DO
4714 S Western St 806/355-8263
Taylor John T DO
4714 S Western St 806/355-8263
Austin
Rizov Vladimir MD
8235 Shoal Creek Blvd 512/451-8149
Dallas
Myer Brij MD DC
4222 Trinity Mills Rd Ste 222 ....214/248-2488
Samuels Michael G DO D/C
7616 LBJ Fwy #230 ....214/991-3977
El Paso
International Medical Center
1420 Jeronimo Ste D2 ....800/621-8924

Hall Gerald DC
10904 Lakewood Ave 915/598-0601
Soto Francisco MD
1420 Geronimo D-2 ....915/534-0272
Houston
Battle Robert MD
9910 Long Point 713/932-0552
Borochoff Jerome L MD
8830 Long Point Ste 504 ....713/461-7517
Humble
Trowbridge John P MD
9816 Memorial Blvd Ste #205.... 713/540-2329
Kirbyville
Sessions John L DO
1609 S Margaret Ave 409/423-2166
Madison
Winslow J Robert DO
5025 Arapaho Ste 500 ....214/702-9977
Pecos
Reeves County Hospital MD
2323 Texas St 915/447-3551
Plano
Martin Linda DO
1524 Independence Pky Ste C 214/985-1377
Port Arthur
Taylor Jack K DO
3749 39th St 409/982-1391
San Antonio
Archer Jim P DO
8434 Fredericksburg Rd 210/697-8445
Jennings James F MD
7300 Blanco Rd #103 ....210/340-1717

Utah
Murray
Harper Dennis DO DC
5263 S 300 W #203 ....801/288-8881
Provo
Remington D MD DC
1675 N Freedom Blvd Ste 11E.... 801/373-8500
West Jordan
Logan Cordell E PHD ND
9265 S 1700 W #A 801/562-2211

Vermont
Saint Albans
Lee Alan T MD
PO Box 306 ....802/524-1062

Virginia
Chantilly
Levin Norman
4510 Daly Dr Ste 200 ....703/802-8900

Falls Church
Rosemblat Aldo MD
6316 Castle Place Ste 2E 703/241-8989
Hinton
Huffman Harold MD D/C
PO Box 197 ....703/867-5242
Midlothian
Gent Peter C DO
11900 Hull Street Rd 804/744-3551

Washington
Kent
Wright Jonathan MD
24030 132nd Ave SE 206/631-8920
Kirkland
Collin Jonathan MD
12911 120th Ave NE 206/820-0547
Port Townsend
Collin Jonathan MD
911 Tyler St 360/385-4555
Spokane
Hart Burton B DO
12104 E Main Ave 509/927-9922
Vancouver
Bickle Paula MD
406 SE 131st Ave Bldg C-303......360/253-4445
Yakima
Black Murray L DO
609 S 48th Ave 509/966-1780

West Virginia
Beckley
Corro Prudencio MD
251 Stanaford Rd 304/252-0775
Kostenko Michael DO DC
114 E Main St 304/253-0591
Charleston
Zekan Steve M MD
1208 Kanawha Blvd E 304/343-7559
Wheeling
Jellen Albert V MD
2097 National Rd 304/242-5151

Wisconsin
Green Bay
Leutner Thomas J DC
1792 E Mason St 414/465-1431
Vander Heyden Richard L DDS
2313 S Webster Ave 414/435-5915
Lake Geneva
Alwa Rathna MD
717 Geneva St 414/248-1430

Madison
Galvez Timoteo L MD
2705 Marshall Ct 608/238-3831
Milwaukee
Spaeth Alan W DDS
8200 W Appleton Ave 414/463-1956
Yee Jerry N DO D/C
2505 N Mayfair Rd 414/258-6282
Suring
Cook Douglas L DDS
10971 Clinic Rd 414/842-2083
Wisconsin Dells
Waters Robert S MD
PO Box 357 ....800/200-7178

Canada
Alberta
Oklo G OMD
9535 135th Ave EDMONTON........403/472-7900
British Columbia
Chan Jim MD 101-3380 Maquinna Dr.
VANCOUVER 605/435/3786
Strauts Zigurts MD 16088-84th Ave #304
SURREY..604/543-5000

Chinese Medicine

Traditional Chinese Medicine is the worlds' oldest continuously practiced medicine. One quarter of the world's population makes use of one or another of TCM's therapies. These therapies include acupuncture, herbal remedies, massage, meditation, and internal energy.

Alabama
Fairhope
Stump John L DC OMD PHD
401 N Section St 334/928-5058

Arizona
Lake Havasu City
Kuhns Bradley OMD PHD
1641-25 McCulloch Blvd 602/453-6245

California
Albany
Magin Sandra RN OMD
1172 San Pablo Ave #201 .... 510/525-3016
Aptos
Beilin Daniel OMD
9057 Soquel Dr #3 ....408/685-1125
Berkeley
Kalfus Frances OMD LAC

2615 Ashby Ave 510/841-1753
Marcus Alon LAC DOM
  1650 Alcatraz Ave 510/652-5834
Sordean John R OMD LAC
  3021 Telegraph Ave #C 510/849-1176

Burbank

Ebert Patricia DC
  3808 Riverside Dr Ste 406 ....818/558-5613
Jensen Muffitt DC
  3808 Riverside Dr Ste 406 ....818/558-5613

Calabasas

Mann Laura OMD CA
  24009 Ventura Blvd #250 .... 818/702-0717

Carmel

Lerner Melanie G OMD
  PO Box 221144 ....408/625-6161

Chula Vista

Hung Marguerite M LAC OMD
  353 H St Ste E 619/422-1200

Del Mar

Roland Melinda
  1349 Camino Del Mar Ste A 619/259-1553

Eureka

McCarty Patrick
  1122 M St 707/445-2290
Zhao William MD
  1122 M St 707/445-2290

Fair Oaks

Gantt Roc H
  9915 Fair Oaks Blvd Ste D 916/961-4268

Huntington Park

Archer Gary OMD HMD
  2670 E Gage Ave Ste #1 ....213/584-4230

Kensington

Dreyfuss Robert N CA OMD
  267 Arlington Ave 415/528-0132

La Mesa

Riley David R OMD LAC
  4711 4th St 619/462-7890

La Puente

Chen Alex Y OMD PHD
  1124 N Hacienda Blvd 818/917-2121

Los Angeles

Bienenfeld Linda PHD OMD
  2211 Corinth Ave Ste 204 .... 310/477-8151

Malibu

Zand Janet ND OMD
  PO Box 4144 ....310/457-7749

Mill Valley

Reich Gatya LAC
  642 Northern Ave 415/927-0776

North Hollywood

Katz David OMD LAC

10628 Riverside Dr #5 ....818/508-6188
Penner Joel OMD LAC
  5223 Corteen Pl Apt 8 ....818/344-1983

Oakland

Fong Byron B LAC DOM
  220 Grand Ave 510/451-8244

Pacific Palisades

Gregory Scott OMD
  PO Box 1445 ....310/394-2693

Palo Alto

Dittmer Sharon DC
  605 Cowper St 415/325-9200
Neustaedter Randall OMD LAC
  360 Bryant St 415/324-8420
Wood Diandra DC
  605 Cowper St 415/325-9200

Petaluma

Prange William LAC OMD
  245 Kentucky St #A 707/778-3171

Reseda

McSweyn Joe DOM
  19231 Victory Blvd #151 .... 818/344-9973

San Anselmo

Kutchins Stuart OMD DAC
  32 City Hall Ave 415/459-1868

San Clemente

China Healthways Institute
  117 Avendia Granada Ave 800/743-5608

San Diego

Fusco Henry LAC OMD
  2611 Denver St 619/276-4188
Ivey Martha OMD LAC
  4254 5th Ave 619/543-9904

San Francisco

Koon-Hung Lau MD
  1333 Pacific Ave Ste E 415/697-8989
Korngold Efrem LAC OMD
  1201 Noe St 415/285-0931

San Jose

Chen Daren LAC OMD
  167 N Bascom Ave 408/998-1838

San Luis Obispo

Kavanagh Kimberly OMD DAC
  2103 Broad St 805/541-6242

Santa Barbara

Jahnke Rober OMD LAC
  Health Action
  19 E Mission St #102 ....805/682-3230
Merryweather Bambi OMD PHD
  PO Box 5573 ....805/684-7099
Wu M Lonnie RN LAC OMD
  4046 Foothill Rd 805/682-2153

Santa Clarita

Morris-Devine Leitia OMD LAC
18285 Soledad Canyon Rd 805/250-9010

Santa Cruz
Tierra Michael LAC OMD
912 Center St 408/429-8066

Santa Monica
Birch Patricia OMD LAC
1150 Yale St Ste 7 ....310/828-5588
Chilkov Nalini OMD LAC
530 Wilshire Blvd Ste 206 ....310/395-4133
Forbes Linda LAC DC OMD
1514 Franklin St Apt 5 ....310/453-1918
Lehrer Danise LAC OMD HMD
1411 5th St Ste 405 ....310/395-9525
Ni Daoshing LAC OMD
1314 2nd St Ste 101 ....310/917-2200
Ni Maoshing DOM
1314 2nd St #101 ....310/917-2200
Paris Laura
1514 17th St Ste 203 ....310/453-0286

Thousand Oaks
Nielsen Erik OMD LAC
1864 Orinda Ct 805/492-1811

Torrance
Sakamoto Jenny OMD LAC
23441 Madison St Ste 215 .... 310/373-0368
Skinner Suzanne M PHD ND DSC HHD
2204 W Torrance Blvd....................310/518-4555

Van Nuys
Martin Randy W PHD OMD
15165 Ventura Blvd Ste 335 ....818/905-5755

Colorado

Denver
Colorado School of Traditional Chinese Medicine
1441 York St #202........................303/329-6355
Kitchie George H OMD LAC
2525 S Madison 303/584-9714
Le Victoria DC
3611 Cherry Creek N Dr 303/322-8977

District of Columbia

Washington DC
Wu Jing-Nuan LAC OMD
5524 Macarthur Blvd NW 202/363-3236

Florida

Aventura
Grossbard Harvey J OMD DH DAC
19022 NE 29th Ave 305/937-2281

Miami
Canali Charlene DC
6350 Sunset Dr 305/667-8174

Canali Paul DC
6350 Sunset Dr 305/667-8174
Karman Robert R OMD
253 SW 8th St 800/753-9792

Sarasota
Center for Traditional Chinese Medicine
RJ Zhoa OMD PHD Clinic Dir
1299 S Tamiami Tr #1209.............813/365-8008
Kaltsas Harvey J DAC
The Healing Center
505 S Orange Ave 813/955-4456

Illinois

Chicago
Marino Mary Ellen
2400 N Ashland Ave 2nd Fl 312/296-6700
Plovanich Dan
2400 N Ashland Ave 2nd Fl 312/296-6700
Qi Rebecca
2400 N Ashland Ave 2nd Fl 312/296-6700
Wallach Pamela
2400 N Ashland Ave 2nd Fl 312/296-6700
Yurasek Frank
2400 N Ashland Ave 2nd Fl 312/296-6700

Dekalb
Faivre Patricia DIPLAC
6776 Fairview 815/758-4494

Oak Park
Akiyama Teena OMT 708/848-3526

Kansas

Wichita
Gao Qizhi DOM
550 N Hillside Ste 203 ....316/688-7154

Kentucky

Louisville
Odell James P OMD
305 N Lyndon Ln 502/429-8835

Louisiana

Breaux Bridge
Churchill Hether M OMD CA
513 Grant Ave 318/269-0444

Maine

Kingfield
Allen Janet R OBT
PO Box 235 ....207/628-2582

Maryland

Bethesda
Brenner Zoe Dee

4733 Bethesda Ave Ste 804.........301/718-0953

Massachusetts

Arlington
Cox Donald 9 Lakehill Ave 617/641-0807

Kensington
Wong Grace OMD 9709 Hill St 652/2828

Wellfleet
McCarthy Maryann PO Box 744 ......508/349-7592

Michigan

Paw Paw
Bayha Carl DS DIPLAC
   27231 38th Ave 616/668-4730

New Jersey

Middletown
Gallagher Dean DC 4 RT 36 ....908/291-5656

Nutley
Shiuey Su-Jung OMD CA
   331 Bloomfield Ave 201/667-2394

New Mexico

Albuquerque
Polasky Diane H OMD
   540 Chama St NE Ste 9 ....505/262-0555
Pool Thomas DC
   1950 Zuan Tabo NE 505/296-3340

Placitas
Monda Lorena C OMD DAC
   3 Calle Taraddei #B 505/867-1879

Santa Fe
Caissie Judith S OMD.......................505/988-7117
Frawley David OMD
   PO Box 8357 ....505/983-9385
Gardner-Abbate Skya LAC OMD
   712 W San Mateo Rd 505/988-3538
McRostie Govindha OMD ND
   1468 S St Francis Dr 505/988-4210
Skardis Jonas R OMD DRAC
   411 St Michael's Dr 505/988-5551
Zeng Michael D MD
   10 Calle Zanate 505/471-5258

New York

Elmhurst
Guo-Guang Chen MD MS
   81-18 Broadway............................718/478-8828

Forest Hills
Kirsch Lisa DC
   70-20 Austin St 718/544-8282

Hastings-on-Hudson
Ehrich Cindy DC

615 Broadway 914/478-1300

Monsey
Friedman Carolyn H DC
   190 Grandview Ave 914/362-1680

New York
Behr Alice S DC
   530 E 20th St #MB 212/995-5379
Musso Deborah DC
   530 E 20th St #MB 212/995-5379
Strickler James M LAC DIPLAC
   242 E 72nd St 212/772-2838
Trahan Christopher OMD LAC
   50 W 34th St #17-A-10 ....212/714-0856
Prensky William OMD DAC
   133 E 73rd St 212/861-9000

Rochester
Graber Robyn DC
   3300 Monroe Ave 301 ....716/381-8130

Syosset
Byrd Julia LMT AMMA
   6801 Jericho Tpke 516/496-7766
Picone Karen RN LMT A
   6801 Jericho Tpke 516/496-7766

Oklahoma

Oklahoma City
Weathers Ray DIPLAC DAC OMD
   OKC Family Health & Pain Clinic
   8241 S Walker Ste 102 ....405/631-5450

Tulsa
Weathers Ray DIPLAC DAC OMD
   Tulsa Family Health & Pain Clinic
   1211 S Harvard Ave #A 918/836-5454

Oregon

Ashland
Stott Benjamin W LAC OMD
   64 N 3rd St 503/488-3612

Veneta
Kassel Joseph ND LAC
   25632 Jeaus Rd 503/935-3453

Pennsylvania

Ambler
Yu Ruey J OMD DAC
   4 Lindenwold Ave 215/628-9088

Catasauqua
Molony Ming Ming P OMO
   101 Bridge St 215/964-2755

Texas

Arlington
Chernly Sunny OMD LAC
   2301 N Collins St Ste 118............817/461-6700

Austin
Scott John A OMD
4105 S 1st St 512/444-6744

Utah

Salt Lake City
Earl Glenn L OMD PHD
644 S 900 E 801/355-8226

Biological Dentistry

Biological dentistry is a rapidly growing field of alternative medicine. It stresses the use of nontoxic restoration materials for dental work and focuses on the unrecognized impact that dental toxins and hidden dental infections can have on overall health.

Nationwide

Alternative Dental Consultants..........800/756-7431
DAMS, INC 6025 Osuna Blvd NE Ste B
Albuquerque NM.............................800/311-6265
Manna Marketing
PO Box 22911 Carmel CA.............800/692-8743

Alaska

Anchorage
Connell Charles T DDS
4200 Lake Otis Pky #301 ....907/562-7909
Miller Burton A DDS
2600 Denali St Ste 500 ....907/277-2600
Walsh John D DDS PC
550 W 7th Ave Ste 1390 ....907/258-1390

Arkansas

Harrison
Sinclair John H DDS
702 N Main 501/741-2254

Arizona

Scottsdale
Barton Cecil C DDS
7500 E Angus Dr 602/990-9544

Tucson
Ayers A J DDS
1505 N Swan Rd #A 602/881-8585
Farnum Stan DDS
6119 E Grant Rd 602/721-7874

California

Burney
Kersten Timothy A DDS
PO Box 1460 ....916/335-5491

Carmel Valley

Arana Edward M DDS
PO Box 856 ....408/659-5385

Carmichael
Howe Frederick W DDS
5615 Manzanita Ave 916/334-1730

Chico
Colbie Carl K DDS
1601 Oleander Ave 916/343-5571
Schuchard George DDS
5389 Riverside Dr 714/628-4783

Del Mar
Olmsted Michael J DDS
2640 Del Mar Heights Rd #253 ...619/551-0252

Escalon
Verigin Gary M DDS
1415 Oklahoma Ave 209/838-3522

Fresno
Garabedian Robert L DDS
1616 W Shaw Ave Ste C2 ....209/229-6553

Fullerton
Olson Robert L DDS
1966 E Chapman Ave 714/526-2860

Healdsburg
Lipelt Michael J DDS ND D
8201 W Drycreek Rd 510/466-5680

Los Angeles
Alpan Jack DDS
2440 W 3rd St 213/383-3833
Prescott Marvin DDS
833 Moraga Dr Apt 15 ....310/476-8302
Stan Joseph DDS
2440 W 3rd St 213/383-3833

Los Gatos
Adams Jim DDS
14513 S Beacom Ave 408/356-8146

San Diego
Rubio Geronimo MD American Metabolic Institute
555 Saturn Blvd Bldg B................800/388-1083
Hall James DDS
2115 Bacon St 619/224-2986

San Leandro
Eccles S Ward DDS
299 Juana Ave Ste B 510/352-5017

Santa Monica
Sheily Aaron H
1260 15th St Ste 802 ....310/394-0247

Sherman Oaks
Bleicher Howard H DDS
4910 Van Nuys Blvd Ste 208 ......818/981-3130

Torrance
Skinner Suzanne M PHD ND DSC HHD
2204 W Torrence Blvd 310/518-4555

West Los Angeles
Ravins Harold DDS
  12381 Wilshire Blvd #103 ....213/207-4617

Colorado
Boulder
Koral Stephen M DMD
  2006 Broadway St 303/443-4984
Denver
McAdoo Scott DDS
  201 University Blvd #203 ....303/393-0039
Lakewood
McFerrann Robert E DDS
  2290 Kipling St 303/237-3306

Connecticut
Bridgeport
Sunshine Morris DMD
  4695 Main St 203/374-5777
Westport
Baer Stephen S DDS
  225 Main St 203/227-6338

District of Columbia
Washington DC
National Integrated Health Assoc
  5225 Wisconsin Ave NW Ste 401
  ....202/237-7000

Florida
Hialeah
Brody Martin DDS MD
  7100 W 20th Ave 305/822-9035
Keystone Heights
Parsons Phillip K DDS
  PO Box 266 ....904/473-4595
Lake Worth
Harrison James A DDS
  3015 Congress Ave 407/965-9300
Miami
Green Steven N DDS PA
  8740 N Kendall Dr #214 ....305/271-8321
Orlando
McIlwain Milton L DDS
  5400 Hernandes Dr 407/293-3185
Ziff Michael DDS
  5400 Hernandes Dr 407/293-3185
West Palm Beach
Medlock James W DDS PA
  2326 Congress Ave Ste 1-D 407/439-4620
Winter Park
Hardy James E DMD PA
  7221 Aloma Ave 407/678-3399

Georgia
Atlanta
Dressler Ronald M DDS
  3071 Campbellton Rd SW 404/349-2088

Idaho
Boise
Pfost James E DDS
  9502 Fairview Ave 208/375-7786

Illinois
Arlington Heights
Sukel Phillip P DDS
  1640 N Arlington Heights Rd 708/253-0240
Hoffman Estates
Rothchild John A DDS
  1585 Barrington Rd Ste 106 ....708/884-1220
Northbrook
Gottlieb Seymour DDS
  821 Sunset Ridge Rd 708/272-7874
Tinley Park
Dieska Daniel R DDS
  17726A Oak Park Ave 708/429-4700

Kansas
McPherson
Payne William M DDS
  306 S Main St 316/241-0266

Kentucky
Louisville
Lavely Robert W DMD MBA
  7300 La Grange Rd 502/426-4110

Maryland
Ellicott City
Sombataro Eugene A DDS
  5012 Dorsey Hall Dr Ste 205 ......410/964-3118

Michigan
Bloomfield Hills
Rousseau Robert D DDS
  6405 Telegraph Rd #J-3 ....313/642-5460
Bloomfield Township
Lielais John DDS
  6405 Telegraph Rd #J-3 ....810/642-5460
Detroit
Farris Lovell DDS
  19207 Schaefer Hwy 313/861-2100
Ortonville
Regiani David W DDS
  101 South St 810/627-4934

Minnesota

Maplewood
Olin Gary J DDS
1701 Cope Ave E 612/770-8982

Minneapolis
King Ronald L DDS
1201 Lagoon Ave 612/824-0777

Montana

Carson City
Christian Duane E DDS
810 N Nevada St 702/882-4122

New Jersey

South Amboy
Tortora John J DDS
210 Augusta St 908/721-0210

New Mexico

Albuquerque
Wolfe Bill DDS NMD
8501 Candelaria NE Ste A-2 ....505/292-8533

Santa Fe
Norton Chris DDS
1533 St Francis #F 505/988-1616

New York

Buffalo
Barber Donald R DDS
5782 Main St 716/632-7310

Cold Spring
Lerner David L DDS
55 Chestnut St 914/265-9643

Flushing
Friedman Drelsa M DDS MS
142-22 37th Ave 718/353-3303

Kingston
Sorrin Bruce M DDS
76 Maiden Ln 914/338-7200

New York
Winick Reid DDS
275 Madison Ave #2118 ....212/867-4223

North Bellmore
Bressack Norman DDS
1692 Newbridge Rd 516/221-7447

Roslyn
Wolski Krystyna DMD DDS
38 Mineola Ave.............................516/484-5871

Southampton
Cantor Mitchell J DMD
97 N Main St 516/283-6362

Ohio

Cincinnati
Chanin Richard J DMD
800 Compton Rd Apt 9256 ....513/729-2800
Westendorf William A DDS
2818 Blue Rock Rd 513/923-3839

Dayton
Quinttos Richard C DDS
30 W Rahn Rd ....

Oklahoma

Oklahoma City
Plowman Paul E DDS
4801 Richmond Sq 405/840-5600

Oregon

Beaverton
Thom Dick W
4720 SW Watson Ave 503/526-0397

Lake Oswego
Williamson Jeffrey A DDS
5 Centerpointe Dr Ste 260 ....503/684-4174

Pennsylvania

Bala-Cynwyd
Krausz Alan D DMD
111 Bala Ave 215/668-2330

Butler
Pawk Michael L DDS
210 N Washington St 412/285-3305

Camp Hill
Niklaus Ronald DMD
3456 Trindle Rd 717/737-3353

Langhorne
Luxembourg Medical Dental Center
303 Corporate Dr E 215/968-4781
Smith Gerald H DDS
303 Corporate Dr E 215/968-4781

Paoli
Roeder Anthony G DDS
45 Darby Rd 215/647-7272
Smith Stephen D DMD
Rt 252 & Waynesborough Rds 215/647-2755

Philadelphia
Rogal Owen Dds
260 S Broad St Ste 1310 ....215/545-2104

Verona
Gupta Som N DDS
550 Jones St 412/828-1920

South Dakota

Rapid City
Lytle Larry 3312 Jackson Blvd 605/342-0989

Texas

Arlington
Snowden Jack B
801 E Border Ste A 817/275-2633

Brazoria
McCann Michael DDS NMD
PO Box 66 ....409/798-9103

Utah

Logan
Hansen Joseph DDS
195 N 200 E 801/753-2322

Virginia

Annandale
Fischer Richard D DDS
4222 Evergreen Ln 703/256-4441

Fredericksburg
Whitley Wayne L DDS
443 Bridgewater St 703/371-9090

Washington

Anacortes
Borneman Ruos
1004 7th St 206/293-8451

Bainbridge Island
Kitamoto Frank Y
Grow Ave NW & High School Rd ..206/842-4772

Lake Stevens
Lamarche Michael G DDS
515 Hwy 9 Ste 101 ....206/334-4087

Seattle
Marder Mitchell L
822-A NE Northgate Way 206/367-6453

Spokane
De Felice Armand V DDS BS
4703 N Maple St 509/327-7719
Stephan Robert B DDS
731 W Indiana Ave 509/325-2051

Tacoma
Grobins George J DDS
7810 27th St W 206/564-2722

Wisconsin

Greendale
Owen Allen C DDS
5310 W Loomis Rd 414/421-1700

Suring

Cook Douglas L DDS
10971 Clinic Rd 414/842-2083

Canada

Alberta
Komlodi Michael J DDS
472-115 9th Ave SE CALGARY......403/262-1775

British Columbia
Paulos Kostadino DMD VANCOUVER
805 W Broadway Ste 701 ....604/224-2601
Paulos Dino DMD VANCOUVER
701-805 W Broadway 604/876-9228

Detoxification

Detoxification therapy helps to rid the body of chemicals and pollutants and can facilitate a return to health. Forms of detoxification therapy include Colon Therapy, Hydrotherapy, Hyperthermia, Fasting, Juice Therapy, and Massage. For more information, look under each alphabetical listing for specific therapies.

Alaska

Anchorage
Rowen Robert MD
615 E 82nd Ave Ste 300 ....907/344-7775
Walsh John D DDS
550 W 7th Ave Ste 1390 ....907/258-1390

Arizona

Tucson
Deloe Paul NMD
6161 E Speedway Blvd 602/886-9988

Arkansas

Leslie
Taliaferro Melissa 101 Cherry St. 501/447-2599

California

Beverly Hills
Campanelli Eve PHD
8530 Wilshire Blvd Ste #209........310/855-1111
Holmes Mark OMD LAC
9730 Wilshire Blvd Ste 108.........310/271-6467

Carmel Valley
Arana Edward M PO Box 85610 .....408/659-5385

Cottonwood
Colema Boards of California
PO Box 1879 ....916/347-5868

Fountain Valley
Broadwell Robert J ND DMD
18837 Brookhurst St Ste 205 ......714/965-9266

Huntington Beach

Cactu-Life
209 Frankfort Ave............................800/500-1713
Lake Forest
Steenblock David A DO
22706 Aspen Ste 500......................714/770-96
Los Angeles
Gardener Nancy
333 Miller Ave................................415/383-7224
Monterey
Work L B MD
841 Foam St Ste D 408/655-0215
San Diego
Rubio Geronimo MD American Metabolic Institute
555 Saturn Blvd Bldg B MS #432 800/388-1083
San Francisco
Kunin Richard A MD
2698 Pacific Ave 415/346-2500
San Rafael
Preventive Medical Center of Marin
25 Mitchell Blvd Ste 8 ....415/472-2343
Santa Barbara
Jahnke Roger OMD Health Action
243 Pebble Beach 805/682-3230
Santa Monica
Herbal Magic
2821 3rd St 310/396-6648
Saratoga
Loscalzo Ritamarie
1848 Saratoga Ave Ste 5 ....408/374-6161
Torrance
Skinner Suzanne M PHD ND DSC HHD
2424 W Torrance Blvd 310/518-4555

Colorado
Colorado Springs
Adele Ruth
1625 W Uintah St Ste I 719/636-0098

Connecticut
Middletown
Reneson Joseph PHD
148 College St 203/347-8894

Florida
Boca Raton
Haimes Leonard MD
7300 N Federal Hwy Ste 107 ......407/994-3868
Cooper City
Johnson Jim W DC Cooper City Chiropractic
9532 Griffin Rd 305/434-1800
Miami
Dayton Martin DO

18600 Collins Ave 305/931-8484
Holder Jay M DC PHD DAAPM
5990 Bird Rd..................................305/661-3474
Miami Beach
Holder Jay M DC PHD DAAPM
975 Arthur Godfrey (41st St).........305/534-3635

Georgia
Atlanta
Environmental & Prevention Health Ctr of Atlanta
Edelson Stephen MD FAAP
3833 Roswell Rd Ste 110 ....404/841-0088

Hawaii
Honolulu
Kenyon Paul ND
1314 S King St Ste 664 ....808/591-2872

Illinois
Chicago
Jenkins Hugh
2400 N Ashland Ave 2nd Fl 312/296-6700
Oak Park
Yurosek Frank MA ACT OMD
816 S Oak Park Ave 708/319-0192

Indiana
Indianapolis
Darbro David A MD
2124 E Hanna Ave 317/787-7221

Kansas
Leavenworth
Emery Dorothy MS DC
PO Box 504 ....913/682-4848

Kentucky
Louisville
Lavely Robert W DMD MBA
7300 La Grange Rd 502/426-4110
Murray
Broeringmeyer Mary DC
RR 3 Box 121 ....800/626-3386

Louisana
Saint Martinville
Dupois Sidney RPH PHD
PO Box 125 ....318/394-3350

Maryland
Rockville
Health Management Institute
11140 Rockville Pike Ste 550 .....301/816-3000

Massachusetts

Harvard
Beaty Janet K
  PO Box 661 ....508/772-0222

Michigan

Ortonville
Regiani David W DDS
  101 South St 810/627-4934

Minnesota

Saint Paul
Stowell Thomas W ND
  1365 Englewood Ave 612/644-4436

Missouri

Saint Louis
Walker Jr Harvey MD PHD
Yu Simon M MD
  138 Meramec Ave 314/721-7227

Montana

Billings
Strong Gary A DDS
  503 Wicks Ln 406/252-1221

Bozeman
Moore Willow T DC ND
  214 S Black Ave 406/586-9413

Kalispell
Lang Michael
  124 3 Mile Dr 406/752-0727

New Hampshire

Nashua
Larmer Jack M
  Northbridge Business Ctr 603/595-7755

New Jersey

West Orange
Munito Faina MD
  51 Pleasant Valley Way 201/736-3743

New Mexico

Santa Fe
Dean Willard H MD 912 Baca St 505/983-1120

New York

Huntington
Corsello Serafina MD
  175 E Main St 516/271-0222
Kramer Jennie 175 E Main St 516/271-0222
St Germain Joyce
  175 E Main St 516/271-0222

New York
Ash Richard N MD
  860 Fifth Ave 212/628-3133
Gerson Scott MD PC
  13 W 9th St 212/505-8971
Margolin Shoshana MA DH ND 212/961-1378

Rhinebeck
Bock Kenneth A MD
  108 Montgomery St 914/876-7082

Suffern
Schachter Michael B MD
  2 Executive Blvd #202 ....914/368-4700

Syosset
Borzone Sharon DC AMMA
  6801 Jericho Tpke 516/496-7766
Picone Karen RN LMT A
  6801 Jericho Tpke 516/496-7766
Schenkman Faye MA LMT A
  6801 Jericho Tpke 516/496-7766
Wittink Marian RN LMT A
  6801 Jericho Tpke 516/257-6070
Young Anneke RN LMT A
  6801 Jericho Tpke 516/496-7766

North Dakota

Minot
Briggs Brian MD
  718 6th St SW 701/838-6011

Ohio

Bluffton
Chappell L Terry MD
  122 Thurman St 419/358-4627

Centerville
Morgan Heather MD
  138 N Main St 513/439-1797

Oregon

Beaverton
Marinelli Rick ND OMD
  2445 SW Cedar Hills Blvd 503/644-4446
Shefrin David
  12525 SW 3rd St 503/644-7800

Eugene
Weintraub Skye
  911 Country Club Rd Ste 290 .....503/345-0747

Lake Oswego
Lamont Sally
  560 1st St Ste 204 ....503/636-2734
Peterson Noel
  560 1st St Ste 204 ....503/636-2734
Prafulla Morris
  10 Eagle Crest Dr 503/699-2547

Medford

Kadish A NMD
1012 E Jackson St 503/773-3191

Portland
Bettenburg Rita
10360 NE Wasco St 503/252-8125
Collins John G
800 SE 181st Ave 503/667-1961
Gillaspie Elaine B ND
2606 NW Vaughn St 503/224-8083
Jeanne Pamela S RN ND
800 SE 181st Ave 503/667-1961
Kruzel Thomas A
11231 SE Market St 503/255-4860
Massey James B ND
3285 SW 78th Ave 503/292-1895
McClure Steven ND
1507-B SE 122nd Ave 503/254-1522
Melead Leia ND
1405 NE Broadway St 503/282-1224

Salem
Serkalow Alex ND
665 12th St SE 503/588-2333

Pennsylvania

Philadelphia
Jayalashmi P MD
6366 Sherwood Rd 215/473-4226

Pittsburgh
Stewart Roger DC
2022A Mt Troy Rd 412/322-1945

Rapid City
Just Lili CMT PO Box 3394 ....605/341-5696

South Dakota

Rapid City
Lytle Larry 3312 Jackson Blvd 605/342-0989

Tennessee

Johnson City
Neely William
512 E Unaka Ave 615/928-9355

Washington

Anacortes
Borneman Ruos
1004 7th St 206/293-8451

Concrete
Mincin Karl MS PO Box 126.............206/853-7610

Edmonds
Wood Cheryl L
7614 195th St SW 206/778-5673
Wood David B
7614 195th St SW 206/778-5673

Everett
Prentice John R
12619 Waltham Dr 206/338-2702

Lake Stevens
Lamarche Michael G DDS
515 Hwy 9 Ste 101 ....206/334-4087

Leavenworth
Hamner Lynda S MD
911 Commercial 509/548-7090

Olga
Mische Magda PO Box 22 ....206/376-5454

Seattle
Faith Hope ND
8315 5th Ave NE Ste A 206/527-1366
Lind Amy
4141 California Ave SW 206/938-1393
Roberts Nancy
14546 Greenwood Ave N 206/362-3250

Spokane
Miller Alan L ND
3154 E 29th Ave M 509/535-913

Energy Medicine

Energy Medicine is a rapidly emerging field encompassing traditional systems such as acupuncture and homeopathy as well as electro-magnetic frequency devices and electro-acupuncture biofeedback devices which can diagnose and, in some cases, restore imbalances in the individual's energy field.

Arizona

Phoenix
Ber Abram MD
20635 N Cave Creek Rd Ste B 602/279-3795

Tucson
Flagler Lila NMD DHANP
6737 E Camino Principal Ste C.....602/721-8821
Flagler Samuel NMD DHANP
6737 E Camino Principal Ste C.....602/721-8821

California

Fountain Valley
Broadwell Robert J ND DMD
18837 Brookhurst St Ste 205 ..... 714/965-9266

Long Beach
Casdorph H Richard MD PHD
1703 Temino Ave Ste 201 ....310/597-8716

Los Angeles
Alpan Wendy
2440 W 3rd St 213/383-3833
Creative Sound Technologies Inc

Elena Renner RN PHD
800 W 1st St Ste 103................. 213/746-7900

Newport Beach
Whitaker Julian MD
4321 Birch St Ste 100 ....714/851-1550

Pacific Palisades
Estes Don
Aha Spa
1515 Palisades Dr 310/459-6880

San Clemente
Luck Nicole
117 Avendia Granada Ave 800/743-5608

San Diego
Keller Loisanne OMD LAC
3737 Moraga Ave Ste A5 ....619/272-8215

Torrance
Skinner Suzanne M PHD RNC ND DSC HH
2204 W Torrance Blvd 310/518-4555

Truckee
Sarrat Nancy ND
PO Box 3390 ....916/587-7746

Colorado

Aspen
Krakovitz Rob 430 W Main St...........303/927-4394

Boulder
Lange Andrew ND
3011 Broadway Ste #14 ....303/443-8678

Carbondale
Goddard Sally
1680 Sunset Ln 303/963-9165

Snowmass
Krakovitz Rob
94 Elk Range Dr 303/927-4394

Florida

Sarasota
Center for Traditional Chinese Medicine
R J Zhao OMD PHD Clinical Director
1299 S Trail #1209 ....813/365-8008

Hawaii

Hilo
Carson Jacqueline ND
324 Kauila St 808/934-3233

Honolulu
Kenyon Paul ND
1314 S King St Ste 664 ....808/591-2872

Illinois

Chicago
Pelovska Eugenia BD
Chicago Holistic Center

2400 N Ashland Ave 2nd Fl 312/296-6700

Indiana

Evansville
Sparks Harold T DO
3001 Washington Ave 812/479-8228

Maryland

Annapolis
Teiterbaumm Jacob E
139 Old Solomons Island Rd....... 410/224-2222

Massachusetts

Newton Highlands
Fagan Trudy S BC
30 Lincoln St 617/964-2551

Missouri

Peculiar
Kanion Dorothy
15706 E 245th St 816/779-4844

Nevada

Reno
Edwards David A MD
6490 S McCarran Blvd #C24........702/827-1444

New Mexico

Roswell
Stoesser Annette MD
112 S Kentucky 505/623-2444

Santa Fe
Dean Willard H MD 912 Baca St 505/983-1120

New York

Hicksville
Schaeffer Cheryl A LMT OBT
17 Peachtree Ln 516/433-4536

Huntington
Corsello Serafina MD
175 E Main St 516/271-0222
Kramer Jennie
175 E Main St 516/271-0222
St Germain Joyce
175 E Main St 516/271-0222

New York
Gerson Scott MD
13 W 9th St 212/505-8971
Margolin Shoshona MA DHM ND
Futuristic Approach Free Info 212/961-1378

New York City
Chin Richard M OMD
121 E 37th St #4B 212/686-9227

North Dakota

Grand Forks
Leigh Richard H MD
2314 Library Ln 701/775-5527

Oregon

Ashland
Craddick Joy MD
1206 Linda St 503/488-0478

Beaverton
Stargrove Mitchell B ND LAC
4720 SW Watson Ave 503/526-0397

Eugene
Gambee John E MD
66 Club Rd 503/686-2536

Medford
Donohoe Patrick K BS ND
1603 E Barnett Rd 503/770-5563

Portland
Bettenburg Rita ND
10360 NE Wasco St 503/252-8125
Garcia Gregory ND
1405 SW 17th 503/228-6959
Melead Leia ND Woodrose National Health Clinic
1405 NE Broadway St 503/282-1224

Pennsylvania

Chadds Ford
Maulfair Jr Conrad DO
Box 71 Main St 215/682-2104

Philadelphia
Jayalashmi P MD
6366 Sherwood Rd 215/473-4226

Texas

Mineral Wells
Electromedical Products
2201 Garrett Morris Pkwy 817/328-0788

Virginia

Vienna
Van landingham ruth
Terra Christa
431-B Maple Ave W.......................703/281-9140

Washington

Freeland
Jongaard Robert ND
PO Box 130 ....206/331-6470

Mount Vernon
Shupe Jack R ND CA
3267-B N Shore Dr 206/422-6004

Olga
Mische Magda ND RPHARM
PO Box 22 ....206/376-5454

Roy
Post International
PO Box 788 ....206/843-1321

Seattle
International SHEN Therapy Association
3213 W Wheeler St #202 ....206/542-6199
Page Sarah ACSW Lake City Professional Center
2611 NE 125th #203...................206/361-7306
Roberts Nancy ND Sequoia Naturopathic
14546 Greenwood Ave N 206/362-3250

Wisconsin

Madison
Meyer Emily
2152 Linden Ave 608/249-1206

Canada

British Columbia
King Christoph ND
S-652 C-19 RR #6 COURTENAY....604/336-8349
Pontius D Eugene ND
393 Kinchant St QUESNEL............604/992-5712
Herington Heather ND
212-2760 W Broadway
VANCOUVER...................................604/732-4325

Herbal Medicine

*Herbal Medicine involves the use of plant sub-
stances as medicine and has been practiced successfully for thousands of years throughout the world.
Today research into herbal medicine has shown it
to be effective in a wide range of conditions.*

Alabama

Birmingham
The Healthy Way
3161 Cahaba Heights Rd..............205/967-4372

Arizona

Phoenix
Ber Abram MD
20635 N Cave Creek Rd Ste B 602/279-3795

Sedona
Heron Silena ND
2081 W US Hwy 89A #1-C.......... 520/282-6909

Tucson
Deloe Paul NMD
6161 E Speedway Blvd 602/886-9988
Flagler Lila NMD DHANP

6737 E Camino Principal Ste C.....602/721-8821
Flagler Samuel NMD DHANP
6737 E Camino Principal Ste C ...602/721-8821

Arkansas

Leslie
Taliaferro Melissa Leslie Medical Center
PO Box 400 ....501/447-2599

California

Agoura Hills
Gentile Teresa PHD ND Agoura Healing Arts
28247 Agoura Rd 818/707-3126

Albany
Canavan Don
555 Pierce St Apt 724 ....510/524-8652

Auburn
Dry Creek Herb Farm & Learning Center
13935 Dry Creek Rd 916/878-2441
Kime Zane MD
1212 High St Ste 204 ....916/823-3421

Colton
Chavez Mitch BS CN
Nutrapham Consulting
1220 E Washington St Ste #2 .....909/824-2203

Cotati
De Monterice Anu MD
680 E Cotati Ave 707/795-2141

Eureka
Zhao William MD
1122 M St 707/445-2290

Lake Forest
Grossman Michael MD
24432 Muirlands Blvd...................714/770-7301

Mill Valley
Alexander Gregory ND
333 Miller Ave...............................415/383-7224

San Diego
Broadwell Robert J
PO Box 15210...............................714/965-9266
Rubio Geronimo MD American Metabolic Institute
555 Saturn Blvd Bldg B MS#432
....800/388-1803
Head Kathi ND
2496 E St Ste 300 ....619/236-8285
Rosenberg Z'ev DOM LAC
6667 Fisk Ave 619/546-8309

San Dimas
Bauer Matthew D
451 W Bonita Ave #1 ....909/599-2347

San Rafael
The Atma Group
185 N Redwood Dr Ste 220 .... 415/499-3319
Preventative Medical Center Of Marin

25 Mitchell Blvd Ste 8...................415/472-2343

Santa Ana
Wempen Ronald MD
3620 S Bristol St Ste 306 .... 714/546-4325

Santa Barbara
Davis Deborah LAC 805/969-1992
Jahnke Roger OMD LAC
Healing Action
243 Pebble Beach..........................805/682-3230

Santa Monica
Hirsh Roger OMD LAC
1247 7th St Ste #201 ....310/319-9478
Lehrer Danise LAC OMD HMD
1411 5th St Ste 405.....................310/395-9525
Sandler Elisabeth LAC
Herbal Medicine & Homeopathy
3301 Ocean Park Blvd 310/339-1362
Shoden Skip ND
429 Santa Monica Blvd Ste 350 .310/451-4419

Soquel
McIlwaine Sharon MA LAC
3121 Park Ave #H 408/475-1749

Thousand Oaks
Nielsen Erik OMD LAC
1864 Orinda Ct 805/492-1811

Torrance
Skinner Suzanne M PHD ND DSC HHD
2204 W Torrance Blvd 310/518-4555

Vacaville
Nelson Linda S
607 Elmira Rd Ste 113................ 707/447-2556

Colorado

Aspen
Goodrich Mary C PO Box 2245........303/927-9617

Boulder
Lange Andrew ND
3011 Broadway Ste #14 ....303/443-8678

Colorado Springs
Adele Ruth
1625 W Uintah St Ste I 719/636-0098

Connecticut

Branford
Klass Jeffrey J
625 E Main St 203/481-5219

Greenwich
Kallenborn Gabriele
54 Lafayette Pl 203/454-5989
Meade Babs DIPLAC
523 E Putnam Ave 203/661-2933

Middletown
Germain Jacqueline

87 Bernie O'Rourke Dr 203/347-8600
Liva Ehrico
87 Bernie O'Rourke Dr 203/347-8600
Samuelson Keli
87 Bernie O'Rourke Dr 203/347-8600

Norwalk
Schweitzer Marvin P
71 E Ave Ste F 203/853-6285

Westport
Schmid Ronald ND
39 Richmondville Ave....................201/227-0887

Florida

Altamonte Springs
Lam Nghiem K PT..............................904/357-8351

Boca Raton
Willix Robert D Jr MD
1515 S Federal Hwy Ste 306 ...... 407/362-0724

Clearwater
D'Costa Harriet M MD DAC
1481 Belleair Rd 813/584-7246

Maitland
Schoen Joya L MD
341 N Maitland Ave Ste 200 .... 407/644-2729

Miami
Holder Jay M DC PHD DAAPM
5990 Bird Rd..................................305/661-3474
Pagani Luis
1720 79th St Causeway Ste 1......305/868-6801

Miami Beach
Holder Jay M DC PHD DAAPM
975 Athur Godfrey Rd (41st St) 305/534-3635

Sarasota
Ctr for Traditional Chinese Medicine
RJ Zhao OMD PHD Director
1299 S Tamiami Trail #1209.........813/365-8008
Kaltsas Harvey J DAC
The Healing Center
505 S Orange Ave...........................813/955-4456

West Palm Beach
Carianna Ember AP
2601 N Flagler Dr Ste #212 ....407/835-6821

Illinois

Arlington Heights
Mauer William J DO Atkins Center
3401 N Kennicott Ave 708/255-8988

Chicago
Bhavnani Lata Herbal Est
2400 N Ashland Ave 2nd Fl 312/296-6700
Marino Mary Ellen
2400 N Ashland Ave 2nd Fl 312/296-6700
Qi Rebecca

2400 N Ashland Ave 2nd Fl 312/296-6700
Naperville

Indiana

Evansville
Martin Joy L
600 E Walnut St #11 ....812/425-5811

Indianapolis
Jacques Frank
3725 Kentucky Ave 317/856-5211

Lousiana

Saint Martinville
Dupois Sidney RPH PHD
PO Box 125 ....318/394-3350
Maine
Richmond
Fingerman Eileen MD
24 Gardiner St 207/737-4359

Maryland

Bethesda
Beech Douglas DC
9213 Seven Locks Rd 301/469-6700
Brenner Zoe Dee
4733 Bethesda Ave Ste 804 ....301/718-0953

Pikesville
Porks Ronald MD
3655 B Old Court Rd....................410/486-5656

Massachusetts

Boston
Barton Shivanatha
1152 Beacon St 617/277-4150

Concord
Umphress Catherine M
42 Thoreau St 508/371-1228

Newburyport
Silbert Barbara S 4 Federal St 508/465-0929

Michigan

Paw Paw
Bayha Carl DS DIPLAC
27231 38th Ave 616/668-4730

Minnesota

Minneapolis
Gallagher Robert Present Moment
3546 Grand Ave S.........................612/824-3157
Lucking Andrew J ND
3546 Grand Ave 612/924-8112

Saint Paul

Stowell Thomas W ND Wellspring Naturopathic Clinic
1365 Englewood Ave 612/644-4436

Missouri

Peculiar
Kanion Dorothy
15706 E 245th St..........................816/779-4844

Montana

Arlee
Lane Sarah B ND
PO Box 540 ....406/726-3000

Nevada

Las Vegas
Schwartzman Lynn ND MH
3023 Peridot St 702/435-7501

New Jersey

Millville
Mintz Charles H MD
10 E Broad St 609/825-7372

Morristown
Kadar Peter CA OMD
40 Franklin St 201/984-2800

New York

Levittown
Alyn Barbara LMTH ND
650 Wantagh Ave 516/421-4807

New York City
Chin Richard M OMD
121 E 37th St #4B 212/686-9227
Fuller Karen ND MSW
601 W 110th St 212/932-8442
Gerson Scott MD Ayurvedic Medicine Of NY
13 W 9th St 212/505-8971
Hancock Nancy
152 E 55th St 212/758-2110
Strickler James M LAC DIPLAC
242 E 72nd St...............................212/772-2838

Syosset
Chow Chi OMD Wholistic Health Center
6801 Jericho Tpke 516/496-7766

North Dakota

Minot
Briggs Brian E MD
718 6th St SW 701/838-6011

Oklahoma

Tulsa
Frye Bruce A DC
6349 S Memorial 918/250-1072

Oregon

Beaverton
Stargrove Mitchell B
4720 SW Watson Ave 503/526-0397

Canby
Dev Prem S ND
101 N Grant St Ste 212 ....503/266-3888

Lake Oswego
Australasian College Of Herbal Medicine
PO Box 57......................................800/48-STUDY
German Kathleen MS ND LA
Westriver's Natural Health Clinic
545 1st St 503/635-6643

Medford
Petherbridge Carol ND
1603 E Barnett Rd 503/770-5563

Newport
Edmisten K E ND LAC
344 SW 7th St Ste B 503/265-6378

Portland
Collins John G
800 SE 181st Ave 503/667-1961
Dev Prem S ND
15925 SE Stark St 503/254-3051
Jeanne Pamela S RN ND
800 SE 181st Ave 503/667-1961
Sklovsky Robert ND
6910 SE Lake Rd 503/654-3938
Wood Ray ND
3126 NE 11th Ave 503/249-2957

Pennsylvania

Cranberry Township
Mantell Donald MD
6505 Mars Rd 412/776-5610

Philadelphia
Frank Cara
6333 Wayne Av 215/438-2977

Pittsburgh
Stewart Roger DC
2022 A Mt Troy Rd 412/322-1945

Quakertown
Buttram Harold E MD
5724 Clymer Rd 215/536-1890

Texas

Dallas
Stroup Glenda DHT ND The Health Institute
13154 Coit Rd Ste 100 ....214/480-9355

Houston
Manso Gilbert MD
5177 Richmond Ave #125 ....713/840-9355

Utah

Salt Lake City
Jamison K Brent
   65 W Louise Ave 801/467-3007
Nunn William A ND Salt Lake Naturopathic Clinic PC
   345 E 4500 S Ste H 801/265-0077

Springville
School of Natural Healing
   25 West 200 S 800/372-8255

Washington

Anacortes
Clapp Debra 1213 14th St 206/299-9038

Battle Ground
Stansbury Jill L ND
   506 E Main St 206/687-2799

Concrete
Mincin Karl MS PO Box 126 ....206/853-7610

Freeland
Jongaard Robert PO Box 130 ....206/331-6470

Kirkland
Collin Jonathan MD PO Box 8099 ...206/820-0547

Mukilteo
Mukilteo Chiropractic & Acupuncture
   PO Box 218 ....206/355-3433

Port Townsend
Rienstra J Douwe Monroe Street Medical Clinic
   242 Monroe St 206/385-5658

Redmond
Siegler Larry DVM
   8015 165th Ave NE.......................206/885-5400

Roy
Post International PO Box 788 ....206/843-1321

Seattle
Brown Donald
   600 1st Ave Ste #205 ....206/623-2520
Faith Hope ND The Hope Clinic
   8315 5th Ave NE Ste A 206/527-1366
Lin Chun-Ming RPH ND
   815 S Weller St Ste 107A 206/624-4663

Spokane
Hole Linda Chiu MD
   S 2814 Grand 509/747-2902

Suquamish
School of Herbal Medicine
   PO Box 168 ....206/697-1287

Tacoma
Hall Ursula Family Health
   8303 97th St SW 206/581-0408

West Virginia

Wheeling
Jellen Albert V MD
   2097 National Rd 304/242-5151

Canada

British Columbia
Kuramoto D ND
   #202-55 Victoria Rd NANAIMO.....604/753-0280
Kuprowsky Stefan MA ND
   105-2786 W 16 VANCOUVER.......604/738-2111

Ontario
Macneil J R
   RR 4 PERTH...................................613/267-7470
Devgan Ravi MD
   42 Redpath Ave TORONTO.............416/487-0882
Campbell Lauri ND
   2525 Roseville Gdn Dr WINDSOR.519/944-6000

Saskatchewan
Schafer Leo Box 251 UNITY..............306/228-2512

High Blood Pressure

Also called hypertension, it often occurs due to a strain on the heart, which can arise from a variety of factors including diet, atherosclerosis, diabetes, environment, and lifestyle.

California

Los Gatos
Waiton R O DO MD
   221 Almendra 408/354-2300

San Diego
Rubio Geronimo MD American Metabolic Institution
   555 Saturn Blvd Bldg B MS#43 .. 800/388-1083

Santa Barbara
Jahnke Roger DOM Health Action
   243 Pebble Beach.........................805/682-3230

Torrance
Skinner Suzanne M PHD ND DSC HHD
   2204 W Torrance Blvd 310/518-4555

New York

New York City
Margolin Shoshana MA DHM ND 212/961-1378

Homeopathy

Homeopathy is the use of minute amounts of medicinal substances to stimulate the healing response of the body in order to restore health and normal body functions. Though not as well-

known in the U.S., it is widely used in England (including by the Royal Family), Europe, Mexico, and India.

Alaska

Anchorage
Minor Mary A ND
4050 Lake Otis Pky Ste 206B.......907/563-8180
Smith Torrey DR ND
1407 West 31st 4th Fl 907/277-0932

Juneau
Jamison Scott L ND
369 S Franklin St #300 ....907/586-6810

Arizona

Flagstaff
James Mark ND
809 N Humphreys St 602/774-1770

Phoenix
Ber Abram
20635 N Cave Creek Rd Ste B 602/279-3795
Davidson Stephen M DO
1303 W Bethany Home Rd 602/246-8977
Reed John MD.................................602/956-4444

Scottsdale
Bigelson Harvey MD
9755 N 90th St Ste A-200 .... 602/451-4488
Feingold Jeffrey H NMD
5743 E Thomas Rd Ste 1 ....602/945-8773
Gutowski Louise D ND
8300 N Hayden Rd Ste 112 ....602/443-1600

Tucson
Spector Ilene M DO
540 W Prince Rd Ste #F.............. 602/293-2218

Arkansas

Bradley Pat DVM
65 Sunny Gap Road.....................501/329-7727

Harrison
Sinclair John H DDS
702 N Main 501/741-2254

California

Albany
Civerella Christine PA-C
828 San Pablo Ave 510/524-3117
Herrick Nancy MA PA
828 San Pablo Ave 510/524-3117
Morrison Roger N MD
828 San Pablo Ave 510/524-3117
Vuksinich Matthew J MD
828 San Pablo Ave 510/524-3117

Alhambra
Neiswander Allen C MD DHT

1508 S Garfield Ave 818/284-6565

Berkeley
Helms Joseph M MD
2520 Milvia St 510/841-7600
Kalfus Frances OMD LAC
2615 Ashby Ave 510/841-1753
Lourie Carol MD ND LAC
1442 A Walnut St #410 ....510/526-2028
Powelson Joan MSW
570 The Alameda 510/525-6193

Burney
Kersten Timothy A DDS
PO Box 1460 ....916/335-5491

Colton
Shaw Hiten MD
22807 Barton Rd 714/783-2773

Colton
Ladyzhensky Eliza MD
760 Washburn Ave Ste 11 ....909/736-8185

Concord
Boyle Sue RN 2342 Almond Ave......510/602-0582

Costa Mesa
Nature's Resources
2708 Orion Ste #4 ....714/641-9146

Davis
Gray Bill MD DHT 413 F St 916/756-0567

Del Mar
Nathan Pamela S LAC
13983 Mango Dr Ste 206 ....619/755-3340

Escondido
Wilson Jacquelyn J MD
536 Brotherton Rd 619/747-2144

Eureka
Laporta Kevin R LAC
350 E St Ste 507 ....707/445-0586

Fair Oaks
Shanks Pamela E DC
11618 Fair Oaks Blvd Ste 100 ....916/965-4312

Fairfax
Warkentin David K PA-C
PO Box 39 ....415/457-0678

Greenbrae
Shore Jonathan MD DHT M
322 1/2 Miller Ave 415/389-1837

Hayward
Subotnick Steven I DPM MS
19682 Hesperian Blvd 510/783-3255

Healdsburg
Jackson Jessica LAC
513 Center St 310/433-7714

Huntington Park
Archer Gary OMD HMD
2670 E Gage Ave Ste #1................213/584-4230

La Jolla

King Hollis DO 619/587-1822

La Mesa

Riley David R OMD LAC
   4711 4th St 619/462-7890

Larkspur

Ikenze Ifeoma MD
   5 Bon Air Rd Ste 220 ....415/258-9600

Livermore

Hawley Clyde MD
   1038 Murrieta Blvd 510/447-8294

Los Angeles

Alpan Wendy 2440 W 3rd St 213/383-3833
Bienenfeld Linda PHD OMD
   2211 Corinth Ave Ste 204 ....310/477-8151
Family Health and Nutrition Clinic
   PO Box 70247 ....213/969-4970
Galitzer Michael
   12381 Wilshire Blvd 213/820-6042
Jay Dr Olympians International
   Sports Medicine & Therapy............800/579-5787
Sciabbarrasi Joseph MD
   2211 Corinth Ave #204 ....310/477-8151
Uy R MD
   6317 Wilshire Blvd Ste 202 ....213/655-5628

Los Gatos

Rapp Cathleen M ND
   451 Los Gatos Blvd #204 .... 408/358-7797
Waiton RO DO MD
   221 Almendra Ave 408/354-2300

Mill Valley

De Shore Ana PA-C
   322 1/2 Miller Ave 415/389-6205

Morro Bay

Brajkovich Wendy R LAC
   665 Main St Ste C 805/772-5807

North Hollywood

Limehouse John B DVM
   10742 Riverside Dr 818/761-0787
Swope Harry F ND
   12522 Moorpark St 818/786-9627

Ojai

Hiltner Richard MD DHT
   169 E El Roblar Dr 805/646-1495

Palo Alto

Neustaedter Randall OMD LAC
   360 Bryant St 415/324-8420

San Anselmo

Beeley Brenda J LAC
   165 Tunstead Ave 415/459-5430

San Diego

Rubio Geronimo MD American Metabolic Institute
   555 Saturn Blvd Bldg B MS#432 800/388-1083

Dooley Timothy R Nd MD
   4095 Jackdaw St 619/491-0878
Head Kathi ND
   2496 E St Ste 300 ....619/236-8285

San Francisco

Cohen Misha R
   30 Albion St 415/861-1101
Levine Alan S MD DHT
   20 Eagle St 415/861-0168

San Rafael

The Atma Group
   185 N Redwood Dr Ste 220 ....415/499-3319
Gibney Christopher LAC HMD
   185 N Redwood Dr Ste 220 ....415/499-3319
Schreibman Judy 1108 Irwin St 415/455-9766

San Ramon

Stratford Betty MD
   1501 Bollinger Canyon Rd 510/837-6432

Santa Barbara

Health in Balance Chiropractic & Wholistic Center
   330 Park Ave Ste 3........................714/497-2553
Newell Philip G CA
   1642 Calle Canon 805/682-6872
Jahnke Roger OMD Health Action
   243 Pebble Beach.........................805/682-3230

Santa Cruz

Rich Donald S MD
   706 Western Dr 408/423-2078

Santa Monica

Deorio Keith MD DHOM
   2901 Wilshire Blvd Ste 435 ....310/828-4480
Dolgin Eric DO
   2210 Wilshire Blvd #281 ....310/453-9591
Krems Steven M MD
   1437 7th St Ste 301 ....310/458-8020
Lehrer Danise LAC OMD HMD
   1411 5th St Ste 405 ....310/395-9525
Paris Laura OMD LAC
   1514 17th St Ste 203 ....310/453-0286
Sandler Elisabeth LAC
   3301 Ocean Park Blvd 310/339-1362

Santa Rosa

Carlston Michael G MD DHT
   1154 Montgomery Dr Ste 5 ....707/545-1554
Field David ND LAC
   46 Doctors Park Dr 707/576-7388
Green J Claire ND
   1154 Montgomery Dr #5 ....707/527-7525
Su Terri MD
   1038 4th St #3 ....707/571-7560

Saratoga

Kamiak Sandra N MD
   14567 Big Basin Way 408/741-1332

Sebastopol

Vossen Dennis L MD
460 Pitt Ave 707/829-0951

Torrance
Skinner Suzanne M PHD ND DSC HHD
2424 Torrance Blvd 310/518-4555

Van Nuys
Johnston Linda C MD
7549 Louise Ave 818/776-8040
Martin Randy W PHD OMD
15165 Ventura Blvd Ste 335....... 818/905-5755

Walnut Creek
Schneider Howard B DC
1874 Bonanza St Ste A 510/945-1441

Colorado

Aspen
Aspen Chiro & Holistic Health Inc
Teresa Salvadore DC & Andrea Rubel DC
730 E Cooper St 303/920-1247
Krakovitz Rob
430 West Main St.........................303/927-4394

Boulder
Lange Andrew ND DHANP
3011 Broadway Ste #14...............303/443-8678
Rao Nancy A ND RAC
2880 Folsom St #210A 303/449-8581
Shevins Jody K
3985 Wonderland Ave 303/449-8581

Denver
Nossaman Nicholas J MD DHT
1750 High St 303/388-7730
Schor Jacob J
161 Madison St 303/355-4547

Englewood
Kay Dennis H MD
6053 S Quebec St Ste 202 .... 303/290-9401

Connecticut

Avon
Mazur Nancy A
34 E Main St 203/676-2240

Branford
Klass Jeffrey J
625 E Main St 203/481-5219

Canaan
Livingstone Thomas Jr DMD
3 Railroad St PO Box 1078.......... 203/824-0751

Colchester
Mullen Jose M MD
108 Norwich Ave Ste 3 ....203/537-3699

Danbury
Ofgang Harold M
57 North St Ste 323 ....203/798-0533

Enfield
Herscu Paul
115 Elm St Ste 210 ....203/763-1225
Mittman Paul ND
115 Elm St Ste 210 ....203/763-1225
Rothenberg Amy B
115 Elm St Ste 210 ....203/763-1225

Greenwich
Kallenborn Gabriele
54 Lafayette Pl 203/454-5989

Hartford
Byron James A
15 Oakwood Ave 203/523-0741

Meriden
Tobin Stephen DVM
26 Pleasant St 203/238-9863

Norwalk
Schweitzer Marvin P
71 E Ave Ste F...............................203/853-6285

Torrington
Murphy Robert M ND
118 Migeon Ave 203/482-4730

Weston
Grant Ronald A MD
PO Box 1174 ....203/227-2402

Westport
Fine Howard
468 N Main St 203/221-0216
Goodman-Herrick Pearlyn
21 Trails End Rd 203/227-5534

Woodstock
Shevin William E MD DHT
50 Applewood Dr 203/928-4040

District of Columbia

Washington DC
Razi Ioana A MD
3537 R St NW 202/333-1774
Sullivan Andrea D
4601 Connecticut Ave NW 202/244-4545

Deleware

Wilmington
Ehrenfeld David DDS
710 Greenbank Rd 302/994-2582

Florida

Boca Raton
Haimes Leonard MD
7300 N Federal Way Ste 104 ...... 407/994-3868

Clearwater
D'Costa Harriet M MD DAC
1481 Belleair Rd 813/584-7246

Daytona Beach

Fuqua Gayle H AP OD
1635 S Ridgewood Ave Ste 107 ..904/760-7799

Fort Lauderdale

Swift Russell
3511 W Commercial Blvd #227 ..305/739-4416
Tupling Mary Lee
1012 E Broward Blvd 305/566-6203

Jacksonville

Merritt Henry N MD ND PHD
6037 Longchamp Dr 904/771-8934
Wood Cyrus A DC DNBHE
5627 Atlantic Blvd Ste 2 .... 904/725-8800

Miami

Karman Robert R OMD
253 SW 8th St 800/753-9792

Naples

Hobon 3427 Exchange Ave 800/521-7722

Orange City

Herring Travis L MD 106 W Fern Dr ..904/775-0525

Pompano Beach

Fishman Peter DC
2301 W Sample Rd Ste 10-A 305/975-7246

Port Saint Lucie

Blecha William C DC
692 SE Port Saint Lucie Blvd 407/878-1790

Ruskin

Schafer Robert L DC
PO Box 262 ....813/645-6400

St Petersburg

Keane Martin CCH
1432 9th St N 813/821-7771

Tallahassee

Elkjaer Jensen Jan DC
1211 Miccosukee Rd 904/222-2952

Tampa

Heigh Gregory AP MD PHD DNBHE
13014 N Dale Mabry Ste 352 .....813/968-6260

West Palm Beach

Carianna Ember AP
2601 N Flagler Dr Ste #212 ....407/835-6821
Medlock James W DDS PA
2326 Congress Ave Ste 1-D 407/439-4620

Zephyr Hills

Frank Mark B DC
4900 Allen Rd 813/788-0496

Georgia

Atlanta

Miller Rosalyn DC
2531 Briarcliff Rd NE Ste 203 ......404/636-7222

Conyers

Newton Laboratories
612 Upland Trail..............................800/448-7256

Snellville

Mayo Virginia S DC
2840 Main St W 404/297-0022

Stone Mountain

Saadeh Jane DC
4458 Rockbridge Rd 404/297-0022
Tilghman Michelle DVM
1975 Blend Ave 404/498-5956

Hawaii

Hilo

Carson Jacqueline
324 Kauila St 808/934-3233

Honolulu

Ogawa-Lerman Hazel K
1150 S King St #404 ....808/537-2763

Makawao

Baker Jeff ND DHANP PO Box 217 ..808/878-6660

Iowa

Fairfield

Dixon Daniel J ND PO Box 442 ....515/472-0332

Idaho

Boise

Mathieu Brent ND 515 W Hays St ...208/338-5590

Coeur D'alene

Schlapfer Todd ND
1000 W Hubbard Ste 120 ....208/664-1644

Nampa

Thornburgh Stephen DO
824 17th Ave S 208/466-3517

Illinois

Chicago

Kaufman Gregory MD
3029 N Pulaski Rd 312/725-6666
Labeau Mark H DO
46 E Oak St Ste 200 ....312/266-8620
Luban Michael DDS Advanced Center for Chiropractic
55 E Washington #1641 ....312/553-2020
Maes Luc
2400 N Ashland Ave 2nd Fl 312/296-6700

Elgin

Kearns Clifford DC
843 Esmeralda Pl 708/307-8585

Flossmoor

Lin Ming-Te MD FACA
3235 Vollmer Rd Ste 142 ....708/957-7937

Rolling Meadows

Stone Thomas L MD
1811 Hicks Rd 708/934-1100
Tinley Park
Dieska Daniel R DDS
17726A Oak Park Ave 708/429-4700
Wheaton
Martens Ruth C MD DHT
1913 Gladstone Dr 708/668-5595

Kentucky
Louisville
Snelling Victoria DC
7505 LaGrange Rd Ste #100 ......502/426-4325

Maine
Portland
Garner Mary L 4 Milk St 207/772-9812

Massachusetts
Belmont
Raffel Larry L RN
101 Douglas Rd 617/484-2544
Boston
Barton Shivanatha
1152 Beacon St 617/277-4150
Levatin Janet L MD
127 Harvard St 617/265-5277
Spark Elizabeth C MD
1505 Commonwealth Ave 617/254-7700
Taylor Barry
1505 Commonwealth Ave 617/254-7700
Cambridge
Asis Guillermo R MD
2277 Massachusettes Ave 617/661-6225
Clarke Savitri
2166 Massachusettes Ave 617/492-8300
Greenfield
Skinner Sidney Elizabeth RNC
103 Country Club Rd 413/773-0888
Jamaica Plain
Luthra Christine MD
54 Rockview St 617/524-3892
Marblehead
Horowitz Leonard M MD
119 Rockaway Ave 508/631-3486
Newbury
Manson-Webb Marie A RN
53 Old Rowley Rd 508/465-8168
Ward Alan B MD
65 Newburyport Tpke 508/465-9770
Newburyport
Silbert Barbara S
4 Federal St 508/465-0929

North Hampton
Harvey Lisa A MD
16 Center St Ste 523 ....413/586-4551
Shelburne Falls
Miller Jonathan D DC
Mowhawk Trail.................................413/625-8277
Sidorsky Robert G DVM
3 Mohawk Trail 413/625-9517
Stow
Howard Stephen H LAC
150 Harvard Rd 508/897-5979
Watertown
Moskowitz Richard MD DHT
173 Mount Auburn St 617/923-4604
Williamsburg
Levy Jeffrey DVM 71 Ashfield Rd 413/268-3000
Yarmouth Port
Orenstein Robert I DMD
Sunflower Marketplace RR 6A 508/362-8188

Maryland
Baltimore
Scavullo Romi 2612 Talbot Rd 410/367-3429
Bel Air
Tiekert Carvel G DVM
2214 Old Emmorton Rd 410/569-7777
Reisterstown
Lupo Denise A RPH
11813-1/2 Reisterstown Rd 410/833-3930
Rockville
Health Management Institute
11140 Rockville Pk Ste 550 ....301/816-3000
Wember David G MD
26 Guy Ct 301/578-3825
Silver Spring
Aurigemma Anthony M MD
1400 Spring St Ste 200 ....301/495-3060
Sparks
Chambreau Christina B DVM
908 Cold Bottom Rd 410/771-4968
Takoma Park
Maniet Monique DVM
7330 Carroll Ave 301/270-4700

Michigan
Ann Arbor
Chernin Dennis K MD MPH
2345 S Huron Pky 313/973-3030
Linkner Edward J MD
2345 S Huron 313/973-1010
Neuenschwander James R MD
Bio Energy Medical Center
412 Longshore 313/995-3200

Traxler Marsha RN RPP
544 3rd St 313/747-7020

Brighton

Paris Margaret RN FNP
8018 Grand River Ave #1 .... 810/229-2312

Edwardsburg

Dylewski Jerome L DC PO Box 23 ...616/663-8422

Jackson

Israel Robert N MD 2029 4th St 517/782-5700

Lakeland

Eos Nancy Md PO Box 417 ....810/231-2193

Romeo

Kruszewski Gregory RN DHMS
391 S Main St 313/752-7241

Warren

Epstein David A DDS
22741 Van Dyke Ave 810/757-0010

Minnesota

Anoka

Jones G William MD
19644 Cleary Rd NW 612/753-1377

Maplewood

Olin Gary J DDS
1701 Cope Ave E 612/770-8982

Minneapolis

Boraas A Bruce ND
2830 Cedar Ave S 612/721-5882
Gallagher Robert
3546 Grand Ave S 612/824-3157
King Ronald L DDS
1201 Lagoon Ave 612/824-0777
Lucking Andrew J ND
3546 Grand Ave 612/924-8112
O'Hanian Valerie
10700 Old City Rd 15 #350 ....612/593-9458
Sommermann Eric PHD
10700 Old Cty Rd 15 #350 ....612/593-9458

Missouri

Florissant

ICBR Information Office
PO Box 509 ....314/921-3997

Independence

Dutton Carmain F DC
903 W White Oak St 816/252-5147

Montana

Arlee

Lane Sarah B ND PO Box 540 ....406/726-3000

Bigfork

Beans Donald R RN LAC D

245 Commerce St 406/837-5757

Kalispell

Lang Michael ND 124 3 Mile Dr 406/752-0727

Missoula

Haynes Amy G
521 S 2nd St W 406/728-2415
Nagel Glenn D
715 Kensington Ste 24A 406/728-8544

Nebraska

Omaha

Bradley Randall S ND DHANP
7447 Farnam St 402/391-6714

Nevada

Carson City

Christian Duane E DDS
810 N Nevada St 702/882-4122

Las Vegas

Royal Daniel F DO
3720 Howard Hughes Pky 702/732-1400
Royal Fuller MD 3720 Howard Hughes Pky
Ste 270 ....702/732-1400
Stefanatos Joanne
1325 Vegas Valley Dr 702/735-7184

Reno

Gerber Michael L MD
3670 Grant Dr 702/826-1900

New Hampshire

Concord

Naturopathic Clinic of Concord
Pamela Herring ND & Deborah Sellars ND
46 S Main St 603/228-0407

Nashua

Larmer Jack M
Northbridge Business.....................603/595-7755

Portsmouth

Hecht III Leon M ND
500 Marlett St. 603/427-6800

New Jersey

Belleville

Singhal Pratap C MD DHT
431 Washington Ave 201/759-2241

East Brunswick

Gilbert Paul DDS
123 Dunhams Corner Rd 908/254-7946

Elizabeth

Locurcio Gennaro MD FAAFP
610 3rd Ave 908/351-1333

Mountain Lakes

Five Elements Center
115 Rte 46 W Bldg D Ste 29 ....201/402-8510
Cicchetti Jane
115 Rte 46 W Bldg D Ste 29 ....201/402-8510

Skillman
Bahder Paul P MD DHT
149 Bedens Brook Rd 609/924-3132

Voorhees
Claire James F DO
1600 S Burnt Mill Rd 609/627-5600

New Mexico

Albuquerque
Cooper Mary Alice
204 Carlisle Blvd NE 505/266-6522
Marrich Larry DC
3401 Carlisle Blvd NE 505/889-3333

Santa Fe
Riley David MD
539 Harkle Rd Ste A 505/989-9018

New York

Altamont
Malerba Larry DO
PO Box 588 A 518/861-5856

Ausable Forks
Najim George P DDS N Main St 518/647-5150

Candor
Ramirez-Prestas Iris DVM PO Box 5 .607/659-4220

Congers
Schwarz Edwin DC
196 S Conger Ave 914/268-7887

Lagrangeville
Kacherski Stanley E DDS
Box 129 Rte 82 ....914/223-3050

Liverpool
Hsu Wu Mei 4069 Elaine Cir 315/652-6168

New York
Bergman William L MD
50 Park Ave 212/684-2290
Colin Nancy J DC
43 W 12th St-Basement 212/741-2739
Elmaleh Rebecca MD
103 5th Ave 4th Fl.........................212/229-9718
Fuller Karen ND MSW
601 W 110th St 212/932-8442
Kreisberg Joel H DC
333 W 56th St Apt 1E 212/265-4933
Margollin Shoshana MA DHM ND.....212/961-1378
Ofgang Harold M ND
50 Park Ave 212/684-2290

Old Westbury
Gumberich Gregory R DC...................516/294-9494

Sayville
Toner Nancy J BS MT
22-30 Railroad Ave 516/567-1706

Smithtown
Reiter Lloyd C DC DNBHE
192 Maple Ave 516/979-9019

Spencer
Glass Michael
285 Van Etten Rd...........................607/589-7220

Spring Valley
Scharff Paul MD
219 Hungry Hollow Rd 914/356-8494

Suffern
Schachter Michael B MD
2 Executive Blvd #202 ....914/368-4700

Troy
Osborne Therese A DC
406 Fulton St #220 ....518/274-2276

North Carolina

Carrboro
Delaney Susan R ND RN
103 Weaver St 919/929-1132

Durham
Koontz John H DVM CVA
4306 N Roxboro Rd 919/471-1579

Winston Salem
Smith Todd A DC
3410 Healy Dr PO Box 24506 .....910/760-9355

Ohio

Cincinnati
Fabrey David C MD
800 Compton Rd #24 ....513/521-5333
Westendorf William A DDS
2818 Blue Rock Rd 513/923-3839

Columbus
Granger Kevin K DC
1349 McNaughten Rd 614/864-3888

Cuyahoga Falls
Garn Michael C MD
275 Graham Rd Ste 1 ....216/920-8009

Dublin
Griffith Donn DVM
3859 W Dublin Granville Rd 614/889-2556

Newark
Plikerd William DDS
974 N 21st St 614/366-3309

Tipp City
Somerson Michael DO
5850 South County Rd 513/667-2222

Oregon

Ashland
Weiss Shandor ND LAC
238 E Main St Ste E 503/488-1198

Bend
Immel William M ND DHANP
537 NW Wall St Ste E 503/385-8174

Coos Bay
Morgan Joseph T MD
1750 Thompson Rd 503/269-0333

Eugene
Elliott Andrew W ND
260 E 15th Ave Ste F 503/343-0571
Messer Stephen A
400 E 2nd Ave Ste 105 ....503/343-2384
Schaffer Rodney MD
400 E 2nd Ave Ste 105 ....503/484-9229

Lake Oswego
Prafulla Morris
10 Eagle Crest Dr 503/699-2547

McMinnville
Dickson Bruce A ND DHANP
1900 N Hwy 99 W Ste A 503/434-6515
Herdener Larry ND
415 E 3rd St 503/434-6170

Medford
Petherbridge Carol ND
1603 E Barnett Rd 503/770-5563

Portland
Alexander Jonna R ND
635 NE 78th Ave 503/256-0931
Caselli Mary F
2348 NW Lovejoy St 503/224-7224
Collins John G ND DHANP
800 SE 181st Ave 503/667-1961
Hudson Tori
11231 Se Market St 503/255-7355
Jeanne Pamela S RN ND
800 SE 181st Ave 503/667-1961
Kruzel Thomas A ND
11231 SE Market St 503/255-4860
Ladd Adam ND
320 NE 120th Ave 503/252-8125
Lowry Meredith L DO
5909 SE Division St 503/230-2501
Massey James B ND
3285 SW 78th Ave 503/292-1895
Timberlake Patricia L
2625 SE Hawthorne Blvd 503/236-1366
Wood Ray ND
3126 NE 11th Ave 503/249-2957

Salem
Albin Stephen ND
1880 Lancaster Dr NE Ste 109 ...503/399-1255

Pennsylvania

Albion
Shick Clyde D DC
18 W State St 814/756-3648

Allison Park
Wisniewski Nicholas E DC
4084 Mt Royal Blvd Ste 107 ....412/487-6007

Bensalem
Gupta Nand Kishore MD
105B Bensalem Atrium 215/639-7363

Cranberry Township
Mantell Donald MD
6505 Mars Rd 412/776-5610

Devon
Hopkins George H DC
227 Church Rd 215/688-8808

Langhorne
Luxembourg Medical Dental Center
303 Corporate Dr E 215/968-4781

Mechanicsburg
Sheaffer C Edgar DVM
11 Flowers Dr 717/838-4879

Media
Shapiro Mitchel E PAC
6 Roylencroft Ln 215/566-7691

Philadelphia
Nitskansky Lucy MD
9369 Hoff St 215/698-1042

Washington Crossing
Bonnet Philip L MD
1086 Taylorsville Rd 215/321-8321

Yardley
Khalsa Deva K VMD
1724 Yardley Langhorne Rd 215/493-0621

South Carolina

Greenville
Jaynes Roger S DC DNBHE
1521 Augusta St 803/232-0082

Travelers Rest
Demyan Jeanne R DVM CVA
409 Old Buncombe Rd 803/834-7334

South Dakota

Huron
Zike Gregg MD
85 6th Street SW #5 ....605/245-2383

Tennessee

Memphis

Snelling Victoria DC
3206 Scenic Hwy 901/357-9696

Sevierville
Rovetti Corinne S RN-C FNP
2708 Happy Creek Rd 615/428-2186

Texas

Austin
Hazelwood Robert E MD
1610 Northwood Rd 512/479-0101

Dallas
Diabetics Anonymous Inc
2636 Walnut Hill Ln Ste 268.........214/358-3670
Samuels Michael G DO D/C
7616 LBJ Fwy #230 ....214/991-3977
Stroup Glenda DHT ND
13154 Coit Rd Ste 100 ....214/480-9355

Garland
Brooks Donald W DC DNBHE
2045 Forest Ln Ste 140 ....214/272-0682

Houston
Robinson Karl MD
4200 Westheimer Ste 100............713/526-1625

Irving
Okundaye Osa J OD MS
2618 N Belt Line Rd 214/255-1114

San Antonio
Cohen Lawrence M MD
2515 McCullough Ave #103 .... 210/733-0990

Utah

Salt Lake City
Cook Vaughn LAC
1770 E Fort Union Blvd Ste 101 . 801/944-4070

West Jordan
Logan Cordell E PHD ND
9265 S 1700 W #A 801/562-2211

Vermont

Burlington
Roos John R MD
PO Box 172 Church St Ste 2B 802/864-7967

Saxtons River
Jonas Julian J PO Box 515 ....802/869-2883

Virginia

Annandale
Fischer Richard D DDS
4222 Evergreen Ln 703/256-4441

Arrington
Fleisher Mitchell A MD FAAFP
Rr 1 Box 340 ....804/263-4752

Charlottesville

Guess George A MD DHT
617 W Main St Ste 5B 804/295-0362

Chesapeake
Gruber Frank W Md
4323-D Indian River Rd 804/498-8700

Front Royal
Zunka Craig A DDS
107 W 4th St 703/635-3610

Springfield
Evans Richard M RN
5923 Augusta Dr 703/569-2963

Washington

Bellevue
Baruffi Paula
13401 Bel Red Rd Ste A4 ....206/747-9200
Marmorstein Barry L MD
1603 116th Ave NE Ste 112 ....206/455-4929

Eastsound
Sandberg-Lewis Steven
PO Box 493 ....206/376-5689

Edmonds
Jacobs Jennifer MD
23200 Edmonds Way 206/542-5595
Kruthers PA LAC
23200 Edmonds Way 206/542-5595
Maguire Anne L
23405 84th Ave W 206/776-6085
Reichenberg-Ullman Judyth L ND DHANP
131 3rd Ave N 206/547-9665

Everett
Whittaker Melanie
713 SE Everett Mall Way Ste 206/290-5309

Federal Way
Krueger Ray H MD
301 S 320th St 206/874-7042

Kirkland
Collin Jonathan MD
PO Box 8099 ....206/820-0547
Dunn-Merit Sheila B
607 Market St 206/822-3716

Mount Vernon
Bachman Gary A
1910 Riverside Dr #5 ....206/424-3460

Olympia
Adams Suzanne ND
3627 Ensign Rd NE #B 206/459-9082
Dunn Jon
2617 B 12th Ct SW #6 ....206/352-7880

Port Angeles
Marshall Richard
162 S Barr Rd 206/457-1515

Seattle

Donovan Patrick M RN ND
5312 Roosevelt Way NE 206/525-8015
George John W MD
10212 5th Ave NE #230 ....206/525-2425
Goldman Ellen
2024 S Dearborn St 206/322-3046
Gross Barbara E ND
6020 34th Ave NE 206/524-8122
Heron Krista
5502 34th Ave NE 206/522-0488
King Stephen J
5502 34th Ave NE 206/522-0488
Kipnis Sheryl R
5502 34th Ave NE 206/522-0488
Loeb Francine
7201 5th Ave NE 206/525-4660
Lutack Bobbi ND MS
Evergreen Natural Health Clinic
3110 NE 125th St 206/367-3400
Milliman Bruce
5312 Roosevelt Way NE 206/525-8015
Richter Mary MD
901 Boren Ave Ste 1530 ....206/682-0882

Spokane
Hole Linda Chiu MD
S 2814 Grand 509/747-2902

Tacoma
Hall Ursula 8303 97th St SW 206/581-0408

Yakima
Rivers Kaiten A ND
811 W Yakima Ave #105 ....509/576-0811
Wilkinson Richard S MD
302 S 12th Ave 509/453-5506

Wisconsin

Fredonia
Lewis Blair L PAC
N5821 Fairway Dr 414/351-2340
Lipscomb Alice RM MS
N5821 Fairway Dr 414/351-2340

Greendale
Owen Allen C DDS
5310 W Loomis Rd 414/421-1700

Madison
Herbage Sandra A MD
3602 Atwood Ave 608/246-9070
Kohn Mike D DVM
1014 Williamson St.......................608/255-1239

Soldiers Grove
Engel Marta W DVM
RR 1 PO Box 1198 ....608/734-3711

Canada
British Columbia

Water Marijke V RNC
6530 Dumont Rd NANIMO 604/390-2300
Coleman Phyllis RN
1020 Sunset Dr
SALT SPRING ISLAND 604/537-2378
Taylor A A DDS RR 12 PO Box 16 Ste 27
CALGARY 403/686-2808

Ontario
Meissner Julek ND DHANP 174 Victoria St South
KITCHENER.....................................519/570-1942
Hardy Gary J DC ND FC 5762 Hwy #7 Ste 212A
MARKHAM 905/472-2186
Zimmerman Anke 431 Timothy St
NEWMARKET...................................905/895-8285
Kellerstein Joseph DC ND FC 111 Simcoe St N
OSHAWA..905/433-8666
Macneil J R RR 4 PERTH...................613/267-7470
Aubry Jean R MD Sturgeion Falls
PO Box 223065B Queen 705/753-2300
Bakir Nadia ND Ste 20423080 Yonge St
TORONTO 416/489-1236
Jaconello Paul MD 751 Pape Ave #201
TORONTO 416/463-2911
Saine Andre ND DHANP Ste 20423080 Yonge St
TORONTO 416/489-1236
Saunders Paul Richard Nd 3080 Yonge St
TORONTO 416/489-1236
Sowton Christopher G ND FCAH
Ste 20423080 Yonge St
TORONTO 416/489-1236
Chindemi Wayne J DC ND DH 3435 Main St W
VINELAND..416/562-3636
Bender John W ND 22 McDougall Rd
WATERLOO 519/885-3720
Bell Alan J DC ND 3798 Howard
WINDSOR 519/966-3074
Campbell Lauri ND 2525 Roseville Gdn Dr #203
WINDSOR..519/944-6000

Magnetic Therapy

Magnetic field therapy uses magnets and electro-magnetic fields for the medical treatment of numerous conditions, including fractures and pain, rheumatoid disease, circulatory problems, and environmental stress.

Alaska
Anchorage
Connell Charles T DDS
4200 Lake Otis Pky #301 ....907/562-7909

Arizona
Glendale
Arnold Lloyd D DO

4901 W Bell Rd Ste 2 ....602/939-8916

California

Corte Madera
Rosenbaum Michael MD
45 San Clemente Dr Ste B-130 ...415/927-9450

La Jolla
Moss Charles A MD
8950 Villa La Jolla Dr Ste 216 .....619/457-1314

San Diego
Rubio Geronimo MD American Metabolic Institute
555 Saturn Blvd Bldg B MS#432 800/388-1083

Torrance
Skinner Suzanne M PHD ND DSC HHD
2204 W Torrance Blvd 310/518-4555

Colorado

Littleton
Bodyscrapes Therapy
5944 S Kippling St Ste #301 ....303/932-2023

Florida

Oviedo
Kupsinel Roy MD
1325 Shangri-La Ln 407/365-6681

Kentucky

Murray
Broeringmeyer Mary DC
RR 3 Box 121 ....502/753-2962

Missouri

Sedalia
Bryden DC
520 W Broadway Blvd 314/826-7421

Ohio

Cincinnati
Westendorf William A DDS
2818 Blue Rock Rd 513/923-3839

Pennsylvania

Mount Pleasant
El-Attrache Mamduh MD
20 E Main St 412/547-3576

Pittsburgh
Stewart Roger DC
2022A Mt Troy Rd 412/322-1945

Washington

Pullman
Fountain Don 125 SE South St 509/332-1435

Roy

Post International
PO Box 788 ....206/843-1321

Vancouver
Bickle Paula MD
406 SE 131st Ave Bldg C-303 ....360/253-4445

Nutritional Medicine

Nutritional medicine is an emerging science of maintaining a proper balance of nutrients—vitamins, minerals, and amino acids—in the body. Extensive research in recent years has shown the far-reaching impact of various nutrients, including Vitamin C, Vitamin B6, Vitamin B12, Magnesium, Calcium, and others.

Alaska

Anchorage
Denton Sandra MD
4115 Lake Otis Pky # 200 ....907/563-6200

Arizona

Glendale
Armold Lloyd D DO
4901 W Bell Rd Ste 2 ....602/939-8916

Mesa
Halcomb William W DO
4323 E Broadway Ste 109 ....602/832-3014

Parker
Meyer S W DO
332 River Front Dr 602/669-8911

Phoenix
Olsztyn Stanley R MD
Whiton Pl 3610 N 44th St Ste 2 .602/954-0811

Prescott
Josephs Gordon H DO
315 W Goodwin St 602/778-6169

Scottsdale
Josephs Gordon H DO
7315 E Evans Rd 602/998-9232

Tucson
Dommisse John
1840 E River Road Ste 210 ....520/577-1940

Arkansas

Little Rock
Becquet Norbert J MD
115 W 6th St 501/375-4419

North Little Rock
Gustavus John L
4721 E Broadway 501/758-9350

Pine Bluff
Worrell Aubrey M Jr MD

3900 Hickory St 501/535-8200

California

Albany
Gordon Ross B MD
405 Kains Ave 510/526-3232

Azusa
Bryce William C MD
400 N San Gabriel Ave 818/334-1407

Bakersfield
Seibly Ralph G MD
1311 Columbus St 805/873-1000

Bonita
Alsleben Rudolph Md
4364 Bonita Rd #200 ....619/479-4403

Camarillo
Frank Bridget CN
134 Anacapa Dr...........................805/389-0749

Campbell
Shamlin Carol A MD
621 E Campbell Suite 11A 408/378-7970

Colton
Shaw Hiten MD
22807 Barton Rd 714/783-2773

Concord
Toth John P
2299 Bacon St Ste 10 ....510/682-5660

Corte Madera
Anderson Jeffry L Md
45 San Clemete Dr #100B 415/927-7140

Costa Mesa
Stavish Philip C MD
136 Broadway................................714/722-0175

Culver City
Levin Cecile
La East West Center
11215 Hannum Ave 310/398-2228

El Cajon
Saccoman William J MD
505 N Mollison Ave Ste 103........ 619/440-3838

Encino
Klepp A Leonard MD
16311 Ventura Blvd Ste 725 .... 818/981-5511

Fresno
Edwards David J MD
360 S Clovis Ave 209/251-5068

Huntington Beach
Resk Joan M DO
18821 Delaware St #203 ....714/842-5591

La Jolla
Dr Hanna Institute
7742 Caminito Rialto 619/454-0811

Lake Forest
Grossman Michael MD
24432 Muirlands Blvd...................714/770-7301

Laytonville
Finkle Eugene D MD
PO Box 309 ....707/984-6151

Los Altos
Cathcart Robert III MD
127 2nd St #4 ....415/949-2822

Los Angeles
Alpan Jack DDS
2440 W 3rd St 213/383-3833
Bicher James MD Valley Cancer Institute
12099 W Washington Blvd #304..310/398-0013
Lynner Doug
205 1/2 N Larchmont Blvd 213/462-4578
Park Byung S MD
2211 Corinth Ave #204 ....310/477-8151
Sciabbarrasi Joseph MD
2211 Corinth Ave #204 ....310/477-8151
Susser Murray MD
2211 Corinth Ave #204 ....310/477-8151

Los Gatos
Waiton RO DO MD
221 Almendra Ave 408/354-2300

Malibu
Hanley Jesse MD Malibu Health & Rehabilitation Ctr
22917 Pacific Coast Hwy 310/456-7721

Montebello
Molinari Victor....................................213/723-1994

Oakland
Sharps Elisa 401 29th St 510/287-5439

Palm Springs
Degnan Sean MD
2825 E Tahquitz McCallum Way ... 619/320-4292

Rancho Mirage
Farinella Charles B MD
69-730 Hwy 111 Ste 106A 619/324-0734

Redding
Tillman Bessie J MD
2054 Market St 916/246-3022

Sacramento
Kwiker Michael DO
3301 Alta Arden Ste 3 ....916/489-4400
Pace Suzel
3450 Hacienda Rd 916/676-4405

San Diego
Rubio Geronimo MD American Metabolic Institute
555 Saturn Blvd Bldg B.................800/388-1083
Taylor Lawrence MD
3330 3rd Ave #402 ....619/296-2952
Turk Lauren K
17927 Cassia Pl............................619/451-6413

San Francisco
Cohen Misha R
30 Albion St....................................415/861-1101
San Jacinto
Shah Hiten MD
229 W 7th St 909/658-7246
San Luis Obispo
Dorman Thomas A MD
171 N Santa Rosa St #A 805/781-3388
San Marcos
Kubitschek William C DO
1194 Calle Maria 619/744-6991
San Rafael
The Atma Group
185 N Redwood Dr Ste 220 ....415/499-3319
Gordon Ross B MD
4144 Redwood Hwy 415/499-9377
Santa Barbara
Jahnke Roger OMD Health Action
243 Pebble Beach.........................805/682-3230
Santa Maria
Reiner Donald E MD
1414-D S Miller St 805/925-0961
Preventive Medical Center of Marin
25 Mitchell Blvd Ste 8...................415/472-2343
Santa Monica
Deorio Keith MD
2901 Wilshire Blvd Ste 435......... 310/828-4480
Hirsh Roger OMD LAC
1247 7th St Ste #201 ....310/319-9478
Lehrer Danise LAC OMD HMD
1411 5th St Ste 405 ....310/395-9525
Martin Lucien DC
612 Colorado Ave #110 ....310/392-8184
Shoden Skip ND
429 Santa Monica Blvd Ste 350 .310/451-4419
Saratoga
Loscalzo Ritamarie
1848 Saratoga Ave Ste 5 ....408/374-6161
Seal Beach
Green Allen Md
909 Electric Ave Ste 212 .... 714/851-1550
Stanton
Goldwag William J MD
7499 Cerritos Ave 714/827-5180
Studio City
Law Charles E Jr MD
3959 Laurel Canyon Blvd Ste 1 ... 818/761-1661
Thousand Oaks
Nielsen Erik OMD LAC
1864 Orinda Ct 805/492-1811
Torrance
Millen Anita K MD MPH CCN

1010 Crensshaw Blvd 310/320-1132
Skinner Suzanne M PHD ND DSC HHD
2204 W Torrance Blvd....................310/518-4555
Van Nuys
Mosler Frank MD
14428 Gilmore St 818/785-7425
Woodacre
Sullivan Krispin PO Box 961 ....415/488-9636

Colorado
Aspen
Bronson Phyllis J 100 E Main St.......303/920-2523
Krakovitz Rob 430 W Main St...........303/927-4394
Boulder
Koral Stephen M DMD
2006 Broadway St 303/443-4984
Wright Linda C MD
3980 Broadway St #202 ....303/440-5588
Colorado Springs
Adele Ruth
1625 W Uintah St Ste I 719/636-0098
Denver
Malmgren Michael DCPA
6740 E Hampden Ste 311 ....303/782-9277
Englewood
Altshuler John H MD Greenwood Executive Park
7485 E Peakview...........................303/740-7771
Grand Junction
Van Hardenbroek Mechteld C MD
205 Country Club Park 303/241-8554

Connecticut
Branford
Klass Jeffrey J 625 E Main St 203/481-5219
Norwalk
Schweitzer Marvin P
71 E Ave Ste F 203/853-6285
Milford
Cohen Alan R MD
67 Cherry St 203/877-1936
Sica Robban MD
325 Post Road 203/799-7733
Torrington
Finnie Jerrold N MD
333 Kennedy Dr #L-204 ....203/489-8977
Murphy Robert M ND
118 Migeon Ave 203/482-4730

Delaware
Georgetown
Yossif George MD
546 S Bedford St 302/856-5151

District of Columbia

Washington
Nasseri Shahin
  2141 Wisconsin Ave NW 202/363-5664
National Integrated Health Associates
  5225 Wisconsin Ave NW Ste 401 202/237-7000

Florida

Boca Raton
Willix Robert D Jr MD
  1515 S Federal Hwy Ste 306 ...... 407/362-0724

Cooper City
Johnson Jim DC
  9532 Griffin Rd 305/434-1800

Crystal River
Borromeo Azael MD ACAM
  700 SE 5th Ter 904/795-7177

Delray Beach
Rohack Elizabeth E LMT
  1611 NE 2nd Ave 407/278-8358

Fort Lauderdale
Dooley Bruce MD
  1493 SE 17th St 305/527-9355
Swift Russell DVM
  3511 W Commercial Blvd 305/739-4416

Fort Myers
Pynckel Gary L DO
  3940 Metro Pky Ste 115 ....813/278-3377

Hollywood
Pardell Herbert DO
  210 S Federal Hwy Ste 302 ....305/922-0470

Jupiter
Ahner Neil MD
  1080 E Indiantown Rd 407/744-0077

Lakeland
Robinson Harold MD
  4406 S Florida Ave #30 ....813/646-5088

Largo
Russell Marla
  12800 Indian Rocks Rd...............813/593-5933

Lauder Hills
Slavin Herbert R
  7200 W Commercial #210 ....305/748-4991

Longwood
Rogers Robert MD
  2170 W State Rd 434 #190 ...... 407/682-5222

Miami
Green Steven N DDS PA
  8740 N Kendall Dr #214 ....305/271-8321
Holder Jay M DC PHD DAAPM
  5990 Bird Rd.................................305/661-3474

Miami Beach
Holder Jay M DC PHD DAAPM
  975 Arthur Godfrey Rd (41st St) 305/534-3635
Ramirez-Calderon Carlos MD
  1800 SW 27th Ave Ste 601 ....305/441-6669

Milton
Watson William MD
  600 Stewart St NE 904/623-3836

Ocala
Graves George DO
  3501 NE 10th St 904/236-2525

Orange City
Herring Travis L MD 106 W Fern Dr ..904/775-0525

Palm Bay
Ahner Neil MD
  1200 Malabar Rd SE 407/729-8581

Plantation
Krischer Kenneth N MD PHD
  910 SW 40th Ave 305/584-6655

Pompano Beach
Post William MD
  3400 Pk Central Bl N Ste 3450... 305/977-3700

Port Canaveral
Parsons James MD
  707 Mullet Dr Ste 110 ....407/784-2102

Port Saint Lucie
Barbaza Ricardo V MD
  1541 SE Port Saint Lucie Blvd..... 407/335-4994

Wauchula
Massam Alfred S MD
  528 W Main St 813/773-6668

Winter Park
Parsons James M MD
  Great Western Bank Bldg 303 ......407/628-3399

Georgia

Atlanta
Epstein David DO
  427 Moreland Ave #100 ....404/525-7333
Mlaver Bernard MD
  4480 N Shallowford Rd 404/395-1600
Richardson William E Md
  1718 Peachtree St NW #552 ......404/607-0570

Atlanta/Norcross
Shin Young S MD
  3850 Holcomb Bridge Rd #438 .. 404/242-0000

Camilla
Gunter Oliver L MD 24 N Ellis St 912/336-7343

Warner Robins
Schneider Terril J MD
  205 Dental Dr Ste 19 ....912/929-1027

Hawaii

Honolulu
Clark-Wismer VG
   1441 Kapiolani Blvd #1113 ....808/941-0522
Joseph Helen PHD DC
   4614 Kilauea Ave 808/737-3077

Kealakekua
Arrington Clifton MD
   PO Box 649 ....808/322-9400

Idaho

Boise
Mathieu Brent ND
   515 W Hays St 208/338-5590

Coeur D'Alene
McGee Charles T MD
   1717 Lincolnway Ste 108 ....208/664-1478
Schlapfer Todd ND Coeur D'Alene Healing Arts
   W1000 Hubbard Ste 120 ....208/664-1644

Sandpoint
McCallum K Peter MD
   2500 Selle Rd 208/263-5456

Illinois

Arlington Heights
Haws Terrill K DO
   121 S Wilke Rd Ste 111 ....708/577-9451

Aurora
Hesselink Thomas MD
   888 S Edgelawn Dr Ste 1743 ......708/844-0011

Chicago
Jenkins Hugh
   2400 N Ashland Ave 2nd Fl 312/296-6700
Limberg Leslie Chicago Holistic Center
   2400 N Ashland Ave 2nd Fl 312/296-6700
Maes Luc
   2400 N Ashland Ave 2nd Fl 312/296-6700
Rentea Razvan MD
   3525 W Peterson Ste 611 ....312/583-7793
Wiker Judith Chicago Holistic Center
   2400 N Ashland Ave 2nd Fl......... 312/296-6700

Geneva
Hrdlicka Richard E MD
   302 Randall Rd #206 ....708/232-1900

Glendale Heights
Reninger Judith MS
   159 E North Ave Box 330 ....708/653-2272

Gurnee
Stoll Walt MD
   267 Yorkshire Ct 708/233-4273

Oak Park
Dunn Paul J MD
   715 Lake St 708/383-3800

Ottawa
Love Terry W DO 645 W Main 815/434-1977

Urbana
Foster Jim MS
   PO Box 3008 902 E Main St 217/344-1188

Zion
Senatore Peter DO
   1911 27th St 708/872-8722

Indiana

Evansville
Sikes Barbaa F DC
   718 Senate Ave 812/422-7972

Jeffersonville
Wolverton George MD
   647 Eastern Blvd 812/282-4309

Iowa

Sioux City
Blume Horst G MD
   700 Jennings St 712/252-4386

Kansas

Andover
Acker Stevens B MD
   310 W Central #D 316/733-4494

Garden City
Hunsberger Terry DO
   602 N 6th 316/275-7128

Hays
Neil Roy N MD
   105 W 13th 913/628-8341

Kansas City
Gamble John Jr DO
   1509 Quindaro Blvd 913/321-1140

Kentucky

Somerset
Kiteck Stephen S MD
   600 Bogle St 606/677-0459

Louisiana

Chalmette
Tampira Saroj T MD
   800 W Virtue #207 ....504/277-8991

Mandeville
CMS Clinic
   800 Hwy 3228 ....504/626-1985

Natchitoches
Mitchell Phillip MD
   407 Bienville St 318/357-1571

New Iberia
Domingue Adonis J MD

602 N Lewis #600 ....318/365-2196
New Orleans
Carter James P MD
1501 Canal St Ste 810 ....504/588-5136
Newellton
Whitaker Joseph R MD
PO Box 458 ....318/467-5131
Slidell
Graves Christy MD
1850 Gause Blvd #205 ....504/646-4415

Maine

Van Buren
Cyr Joseph MD
62 Main St 207/868-5273

Maryland

Annapolis
Brown-Christopher Cheryl MD
1419 Forest Dr #202 ....410/268-5005
Ellicott City
Sombatoro Eugene A DDS
5012 Dorsey Hall Dr Ste 205 ......410/964-3118
Laurel
Beals Paul MD
9101 Cherry Ln Ste 205 ....301/490-9911
Pikesville
Parks Ronald MD 410/486-5656
Rockville
Health Management Institute
1140 Rockville Pike Ste 550 ....301/816-3000
Silver Spring
Goodman Harold DO
8609 2nd Ave Ste 405B 301/565-2494

Massachusetts

Barnstable
Janson Michael MD
275 Mill Way..................................508/362-4343
Hanover
Cohen Richard MD
51 Mill St Ste 1 ....617/829-9281
Newbury
Kinderlehrer Daniel A MD
65 Newburyport Tpk 508/465-6077
Newburyport
Silbert Barbara S 4 Federal St 508/465-0929
Newton
Englender Carol MD
1126 Beacon St 617/965-7770
West Boylston

La Cava Thomas N MD
360 W Boylston St Rm 508/854-1380
Williamstown
Lux MD 732 Main St 413/663-3701

Michigan

Atlanta
Modzinski Leo DO MD
100 W State St 517/785-4254
Farmington
Parenta Paul A DO
30275 Thirteen Mile Rd 810/626-7544
Flint
Ganapini Kenneth DO
1044 Gilbert Rd 313/733-3140
Novi
Padden Thomas A DO
39555 W Ten Mile Rd #303 ....810/473-2922
Saint Clair Shores
Ziobrn James DO
23550 Harper Ave 313/779-5700
Williamston
Nelson Seldon DO
4386 N Meridian Rd 517/349-2458

Minnesota

Minneapolis
Dole Michael MD DC
10700 Old Cty Rd 15 Ste 350 ....612/593-9458
Eckerly Jean R MD
10700 Old Cty Rd 15 Ste 350 ....612/593-9458
Klos Steven E MD Health Recovery Center
2421 W 42nd St 612/929-4568

Mississippi

Coldwater
Patel Pravinchandra MD
PO Box D 301/622-7011
Columbus
Sams James H MD
11220 Lehmburg Rd 601/327-8701
Ocean Springs
Waddell James H MD
1520 Government St 601/875-5505
Shelby
Hollingsworth Robert MD
PO Box 87 ....601/398-5106

Missouri

Independence
Dorman Lawrence DO
9120 E 35th St S 816/358-2712

Festus
Schwent John T DO
1400 N Truman Blvd......................314/937-8688
Florissant
Sultan Tipu MD
11585 W Florissant 314/921-7100
Joplin
Cooper Ralph D DO
1608 E 20th St 417/624-4323
Kansas City
McDonagh Edward W DO
2800-A Kendallwood Pkwy 816/453-5940
Rudolph Charles J DO PHD
2800-A Kendallwood Pkwy 816/453-5940
Peculiar
Kanion Dorothy
15706 E 245th St.........................816/779-4844
Richmond
Ireland Emerson W DO
703 Wollard Blvd 816/776-6933
Springfield
Sunderwirth William C DO
2828 N National Ave 417/837-4158
Sullivan
Scott Ronald H DO
131 Meridith Ln 314/468-4932
Union
Hayes Clinton C DO
100 W Main St 314/583-8911

Montana
Arlee
Lane Sarah B ND
PO Box 540 ....406/726-3000
Missoula
Nagel Glen ND
715 Kensington Ste 24A 406/728-8544

Nebraska
Ord
Miller Otis W MD
408 S 14th St 308/728-3251

Nevada
Las Vegas
Holper Steven MD
3233 W Charleston Blvd #202 ...702/878-3510
Vance Robert DO
801 S Rancho Dr Ste #F2 ....702/385-7771
Reno
Soli Donald E MD
708 N Center St 702/786-7101

New Jersey
Cherry Hill
Magaziner Allan DO
1907 Greentree Rd 609/424-8222
Denville
All Majld
95 E Main St 201/586-4111
Edison
Lev Ralph MD MS
952 Amboy Ave 908/738-9220
Elizabeth
Locurcio Gennaro
610 3rd Ave...................................908/351-1333
Sy Rodolfo T MD
952 Amboy Ave 908/738-9220
Fort Lee
Klingsberg Gary DO
1355 15th St #200 ....201/585-9368
Millville
Mintz Charles H MD
10 E Broad St 609/825-7372
Mountain Lakes
Five Elements Center
115 Rt 46 W Bldg D #29 ....201/402-8510
Ridgewood
Alfano Constance G MD
Ridgewood Center For Preventative Medicine
104 Chestnut St 201/444-4622
Somerset
Condren Marc J MD
7 Cedar Grove Lane #20 ....908/469-2133

New Mexico
Albuquerque
Parker Gerald DO
9577 Osuna NE Ste M 505/271-4800
Las Vegas
Parcell's System of Scientific Living
805 7th St.....................................505/425-0901
Santa Fe
Scott Shirley B MD
PO Box 2670 ....505/966-9960
Taos
Kirk Joan ND Power Mountain Health
PO Box 1661 ....505/758-9704

New York
Bronx
Izquierdo Richard MD
1070 Southern Blvd Lwr Lvl 718/589-4541
Brooklyn
Sorina Tsilia MD

2026 Ocean Ave 718/375-2600
Teplitsky Michael MD
   415 Oceanview Ave 718/769-0997
Yutsis Pavel MD
   1309 W 7th St 718/259-2122

East Meadow
Calapai Christopher DO
   1900 Hempstead Tpke 516/794-0404

East Northport
Newman Robert
   1 Meadow Rue Ln 516/368-6320

Falconer
Hill Reino MD 230 W Main St 716/665-3505

Lawrence
Kurk Mitchell MD 310 Broadway 516/239-5540

Massena
Snider Bob MD.................................315/764-7328

New Hyde Park
Warshowsky Allan MD
   2001 Marcus Ave 516/488-2877

New York
Ash Richard N MD
   860 Fifth Ave..................................212/628-3133
Corsello Serafina MD
   200 W 57th St #1202 ....212/399-0222
Galland Leo MD
   41 E 60 St 212/698-9668
Lieberman Shari PHD CNS
   103 5th Ave 4th Fl........................212/929-3152
Margolin Shoshana MA DHM ND
   ....212/961-1378
Owusu Maxwell
   220 Church St #1534 ....718/842-0828

Niagara Falls
Cutler Paul MD
   652 Elmwood Ave 716/284-5140

Old Westbury
Gumberich Gregory R DC
   208 Guinea Woods Rd 516/294-9494

Oneonta
Ucci Richard J MD
   521 Main St 607/432-8752

Orangeburg
Block Neil L MD
   60 Dutch Hild Rd 914/359-3300

Plattsburgh
Hassam Driss MD
   50 Court St 518/561-2023

Syosset
Byrd Julia LMT AMMA
   6801 Jericho Tpke 516/496-7766
Picone Karen RN LMT A

6801 Jericho Tpke 516/496-7766
Wittink Marian RN LMT AMMA
   6801 Jericho Tpke 516/257-6070

White Plains
Boczko Miklos L MD
   280 Mamaroneck Ave 914/949-8817

North Carolina

Aberdeen
Johnson Keith E MD
   1111 Quewhiffle Rd 919/281-5122

Asheville
Wilson John L Jr MD
   1312 Patton Ave 704/252-9833

Leicester
Laird John L MD RR 1 Box 7 ....704/252-9833

North Dakota

Minot
Briggs Brian E MD
   718 6th St SW 701/838-6011

Ohio

Akron
Waickman Francis J MD
   544 White Pond Dr Ste B............. 216/867-3767

Bluffton
Chappell L Terry MD
   122 Thurman St 419/358-4827

Cincinnati
Cole Ted DO
   9678 Cincinnati-Columbus Rd 513/779-0300

Cleveland
Frackelton James P MD
   24700 Center Ridge Rd 216/835-0104
Weeks Douglas MD
   24700 Center Ridge Rd 216/835-0104

Columbus
Mitchell William D DO
   3520 Snouffer Rd 614/761-0555

Lancaster
Sielski Richard MD
   PO Box 1010 ....614/653-0017

Lowellville
Ruscitti Ronald DC
   146 S Stateline Rd 216/536-2123

Paulding
Snyder Don K MD
   11573 State Rt 111 ....419/399-2045

Westlake
Lonsdale Derrick MD
   24700 Center Ridge Rd 216/835-0104

Oklahoma

Edmond
Conrad V J MD
1616 S Boulevard St 405/341-5691

Jenks
Anderson Leon DO
121 2nd St 918/299-5039

Norman
Hagglund Howard MD
2227 W Lindsey St Ste 1401 ......405/329-4457

Oklahoma City
Farr Charles H MD PHD
10101 S Western Ave 405/691-1112
Taylor Charles D MD
3715 N Classen Blvd 405/525-7751

Tulsa
Frye Bruce A DC
6349 S Memorial 918/250-1072

Oregon

Hood River
Fisk Bev 108 Oak Street 541/386-3780

McMinnville
Dickson Bruce A ND DHANP
1900 N Hwy 99 W Ste A 503/434-6515

Salem
Young Terence H MD
1205 Wallace Rd NW 503/371-1558

Pennsylvania

Allentown
Schmidt Robert H DO
1227 W Liberty St Ste 303 ....215/437-1959
Von Kiel D Erik DO
501 N 17th St #200 ....215/776-7639

Bala-Cynwyd
Slogoff Harriet....................800/927-2527 Ext 1554

Bangor
Cinelli Francis J DO
153 N 11th St 215/588-4502

Bedford
Illingworth Bill DO
120 W John St 814/623-8414

Bethlehem
Rex Sally Ann DO
1343 Easton Ave 215/866-0900

Boyertown
Shay W William DO PHD RAC
407 E Philadelphia Ave 215/367-5505

Fountainville
Byer Harold H MD
5045 Swamp Rd #A-101 ....215/348-0443

Greensburg
Miranda Ralph A MD
RR 12 Box 108 ....412/838-7632

Greenville
Kerry Roy E MD
17 6th Ave 412/588-2600

Indiana
Sinha Chandrika MD
1177 S 6th St 412/349-1414

Jeannette
Gallagher Martin DC
91 Lincoln Way E 412/523-5505

Lewisburg
Miller George C II MD
3 Hospital Dr 717/524-4405

Morrisville
Kosmorsky Paul M DO
303 Floral Vale 215/860-1500

Philadelphia
Burton Frederick MD
69 W School House Ln 215/844-4660
Galperin Mura MD
824 Hendrix St 215/677-2337
Jayalakshmi P MD
New Life Center
6366 Sherwood Rd 215/473-4226
Sampathachar KR MD
New Life Center
6366 Sherwood Rd 215/473-4226

Pittsburgh
Stewart Roger DC
2022 A Mt Troy Rd 412/322-1945

Somerset
Peirsel Paul MD
RR 4 Box 267-1A 814/443-2521

Southampton
Ferrari June M ND
601 Maple Ave 215-322-6707

State College
Ziegler Monica
510 Fairway Road 814/234-0785

Wyncote
Halbert Steven C MD
1442 Ashbourne Rd 215/886-7842

South Carolina

Columbia
Rozema Theodore C MD
2228 Airport Rd 803/796-1702

Landrum
Rozema Theodore C MD
1000 E Rutherford St 803/457-4141

Texas

Alamo
Carr Herbert DO PO Box 1179 ....210/787-6668
Austin
Rizov Vladimir MD
8235 Shoal Creek Blvd 512/451-8149
Dallas
Myer Brij MD DC
4222 Trinity Mills Rd Ste 222 ....214/248-2488
Samuels Michael G DO DC
7616 LBJ Fwy #230 ....214/991-3977
Winslow J Robert DO
2745 Valwood Pky 214/702-9977
El Paso
Soto Francisco MD
1420 Geronimo D-2 ....915/534-0272
Houston
Borochoff Jerome L MD
8830 Long Point Ste 504 ....713/461-7517
Campbell Andrew MD
14441 Memorial Dr #6 ....713/497-7904
Reeves Thomas E DC
9099 Westheimer Rd Ste 301 .....713/977-0005
SpectraCell Laboratories
515 Post Oak Blvd #830 ....713/621-3101
Humble
Trowbridge John P MD
9816 Memorial Blvd Ste #205 ....713/540-2329
Kirbyville
Sessions John L DO
1609 S Margaret Ave 409/423-2166
Madison
Winslow J Robert DO
5025 Arapaho Ste 500 ....214/702-9977
Plano
Martin Linda DO
1524 Independence Pky..............214/985-1377
San Antonio
Archer Jim P DO
8434 Fredericksburg Rd 210/697-8445
Sweeny
Cole Elisabeth-Anne MD
1002 Brockman 409/548-8610
Tyler
Ram Lakheeshswar DC CCRD
4411 Old Bullard Rd #500 ....903/581-4393
Wichita Falls
Humphrey Thomas R MD
2400 Rushing 817/766-4329

Utah

Murray
Harper Dennis DO D/C
5263 S 300 W #203 ....801/288-8881
Provo
Remington D MD D/C
1675 N Freedom Blvd Ste 11E 801/373-8500
Salt Lake City
Western States Training Associates
346 S 500 East #200...................801/534-1022

Vermont

Essex Junction
Anderson Charles E MD
175 Pearl St 802/879-6544
Saint Albans
Lee Alan T Md PO Box 306 ....802/524-1062

Virginia

Annandale
Annadale Medical Services MD
Anderson Scott V MD
7023 Little River Tpk Ste 207 ......703/941-3606
Patel Sohini MD
7023 Little River Tpk Ste 207 ......703/941-3606
Chantilly
Levin Norman
4510 Daly Dr Ste 200 ....703/802-8900
Hinton
Huffman Harold MD DC
PO Box 197 ....703/867-5242
Marshall
Zimmer Susan RN DC
8430 Main St............................... 703/364-2045
Midlothian
Gent Peter C DO
11900 Hull Street Rd 804/744-3551
Norfolk
Speckhart Vincent MD
902 Graydon Av 804/622-0014

Washington

Auburn
Imkamp A W
30620 Pacific Hwy #103 ....206/839-1433
Bellevue
Buscher David MD
1603 116th Ave NE #112 ....206/453-0288
Concrete
Mincin Karl MS Nutrition Resource Center
PO Box 126 ....206/853-7610

Eatonville

Agell Gun Inc PO Box 1090..............206/233-8880

Eastsound

Sandberg-Lewis Steven
PO Box 493 ....206/376-5689

Federal Way

Payne Tamara 2124 SW 336th St ...206/838-2620

Kent

Lamson Davis ND
515 W Harrison..............................206/854-4900
Wright Jonathan MD
515 W Harrison 206/854-4900

Port Angeles

Marshall Richard ND Natural Healing Clinic
162 S Barr Rd 206/457-1515

Seattle

Bastyr Univ Natural Health Clinic
1307 N 45th St #200...................206/632-0354
Donovan Colleen Capitol Hill Naturopathic Clinic
706 1/2 E Denny Way 206/328-2703
Donovan Patrick M RN ND University Health Clinic
5312 Roosevelt Way NE 206/525-8015
The Hope Clinic
8315 5th Ave NE Ste A 206/527-1366

Spokane

Hart Burton B DO
12104 E Main Ave 509/927-9922
Hole Linda Chiu MD
S 2814 Grand 509/747-2902

Tacoma

Grobins George J DDS
7810 27th St W 206/564-2722

West Virginia

Beckley

Corro Prudencio MD
251 Stanaford Rd 304/252-0775

Charleston

Zekan Steve M MD
1208 Kanawha Blvd E 304/343-7559

Huntington

Sharma Tara C MD
1401 6th Ave 304/523-8800

Wisconsin

Madison

Herbage Sandra MD
3602 Atwood Ave 608/246-9070

Marshfield

Dragt DC
1110 N Central Ave Ste A 715/384-3100

Milwaukee

Faber William J DO

6529 W Fond Du LAC Ave 414/464-7680
Yee Jerry N DO DC
2505 N Mayfair Rd 414/258-6282

Wisconsin Dells

Waters Robert S MD PO Box 357 ...800/200-7178

Bahamas

Freeport

Immunology Researching Center
PO Box F-42689 ....809/352-7455

Canada

British Columbia

Water Marijke V RNC
6530 Dumont Rd NANAIMO 604/390-2300

STROKE

Stroke is a sudden and severe blockage to the brain which results in localized damage where the blockage occured.

California

Los Angeles

Creative Sound Technologies Inc Elena Renner RN PHD
800 West 1st St Ste 103 ....213/746-7900

Torrance

Skinner Suzanne M PHD ND DSC HHD
2204 W Torrance Blvd...................310/518-4555

Florida

Miami

Holder Jay M DC PHD DAAPM
5990 Bird Rd................................305/661-3474

Miami Beach

Holder Jay M DC PHD DAAPM
975 Arthur Godrey (41st St)..........305/534-3635

New York

Albuquerque

Parker Gerald M DO Doctor's Clinic
9577 Osuna NE Ste M 505/271-4800

Oklahoma

Oklahoma City

Gumman Amit BSC BAMS DAC ND PHD
OKC Family Health & Pain
8241 S Walker #102 ....405/631-5450

Washington

Yelm

Cranton Elmer M MD
PO Box 7510 ....360/458-1061